Contents

✔ KU-224-549

Contents

THE TOP 100 DRUGS

CLINICAL PHARMACOLOGY AND PRACTICAL PRESCRIBING

Second Edition

Andrew Hitchings BSc(Hons) MBBS PhD MRCP FHEA FFICM
Senior Lecturer in Clinical Pharmacology, St George's, University of London;
Honorary Consultant in Neurointensive Care, St George's University Hospitals NHS
Foundation Trust, London, UK

Dagan Lonsdale BSc(Hons) MBBS PhD MRCP FHEA FFICM
Honorary Senior Lecturer, St George's, University of London;
Specialty Registrar in Clinical Pharmacology, General Medicine and Intensive Care
Medicine, St George's University Hospitals NHS Foundation Trust, London, UK

Daniel Burrage BSc(Hons) MBBS MSc (Med Ed) MRCP FHEA
NIHR Doctoral Research Fellow, St George's, University of London;
Specialty Registrar in Clinical Pharmacology, General Medicine and Stroke
Medicine, St George's University Hospitals NHS Foundation Trust, London, UK

Emma Baker MBChB PhD FRCP FBPhS
Professor of Clinical Pharmacology, St George's, University of London;
Honorary Consultant Physician, St George's University Hospitals NHS Foundation
Trust, London, UK

ELSEVIER Edinburgh London New York Oxford Philadelphia St Louis Sydney 2019

ELSEVIER

First edition 2015
Second edition 2019

The right of Andrew Hitchings, Dagan Lonsdale, Daniel Burrage and Emma Baker to be identified as authors of this work has been asserted by them in accordance with the Copyright, Designs and Patents Act 1988.

Notices

Practitioners and researchers must always rely on their own experience and knowledge in evaluating and using any information, methods, compounds or experiments described herein. Because of rapid advances in the medical sciences, in particular, independent verification of diagnoses and drug dosages should be made. To the fullest extent of the law, no responsibility is assumed by Elsevier, authors, editors or contributors for any injury and/or damage to persons or property as a matter of products liability, negligence or otherwise, or from any use or operation of any methods, products, instructions, or ideas contained in the material herein.

ISBN: 978-0-7020-7442-4

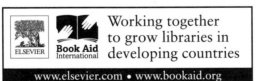

Working together
to grow libraries in
developing countries

www.elsevier.com • www.bookaid.org

Printed in Scotland
Last digit is the print number: 9   8   7

Content Strategist: Pauline Graham
Content Development Specialist: Fiona Conn
Project Manager: Andrew Riley
Design: Miles Hitchen
Marketing Manager: Deborah Watkins

List of abbreviations

5-ASA	5-aminosalicylic acid	COC	Combined oral contraceptive
5-HT	5-hydroxytryptamine (serotonin)	COPD	Chronic obstructive pulmonary disease
ACE	Angiotensin-converting enzyme	COX	Cyclooxygenase
ACS	Acute coronary syndrome	CPR	Cardiopulmonary resuscitation
ACTH	Adrenocorticotropic hormone	CQC	Care Quality Commission
ADH	Antidiuretic hormone	CRH	Corticotropin-releasing hormone
ADP	Adenosine diphosphate	CRP	C-reactive protein
AE	Adverse effect	CT	Computerised tomography
AF	Atrial fibrillation	CTZ	Chemoreceptor trigger zone
ALS	Advanced Life Support		
ALT	Alanine aminotransferase/ transaminase	CYP	Cytochrome P450
AMP	Adenosine monophosphate	CV	Cardiovascular
AMPA	α-amino-3-hydroxy-5-methyl-4-isoxazoleproprionic acid	CVS	Cardiovascular system
		CysLT1	Cysteinyl leukotriene receptor 1
APTR	Activated partial thromboplastin ratio	DEXA	Dual-energy X-ray absorptiometry
APTT	Activated partial thromboplastin time	DOAC	Direct oral anticoagulant
		DMARD	Disease-modifying antirheumatic drug
ARB	Angiotensin receptor blocker	DNA	Deoxyribonucleic acid
AT_1	Angiotensin type 1 (receptor)	DPP-4	Dipeptidylpeptidase-4
		DVT	Deep vein thrombosis
ATP	Adenosine triphosphate	ECF	Extracellular fluid
ATPase	Adenosine triphosphatase	ECG	Electrocardiogram
AV	Atrioventricular	eGFR	Estimated glomerular filtration rate
BCG	Bacillus Calmette–Guérin		
BMI	Body mass index	ENaC	Epithelial sodium channels
BNF	British National Formulary	ER	Estrogen (oestrogen) receptor
BP	Blood pressure		
Ca^{2+}	Calcium ion	FBC	Full blood count
cGMP	Cyclic guanosine monophosphate	FDC	Fixed-dose combination
		FH4	Tetrahydrofolate
CHC	Combined hormonal contraception	FSH	Follicle-stimulating hormone
		FSRH	Faculty of Sexual and Reproductive Healthcare
CKD	Chronic kidney disease		
Cl^-	Chloride ion	G	Gauge
CNS	Central nervous system	g	Gram
CO	Carbon monoxide	G6PD	Glucose-6-phosphate dehydrogenase
CO_2	Carbon dioxide		

GABA	γ-aminobutyric acid
G-CSF	Granulocyte colony stimulating factor
GCS	Glasgow Coma Scale
GFR	Glomerular filtration rate
GI	Gastrointestinal
GIP	Glucose-dependent insulinotropic peptide
GLP-1	Glucagon-like peptide-1
GMP	Guanosine monophosphate
GORD	Gastro-oesophageal reflux disease
GP	General practitioner
GTN	Glyceryl trinitrate
GU	Genitourinary
H^+	Hydrogen ion
HAS	Human albumin solution
HbA_{1c}	Haemoglobin A_{1c} (glycated haemoglobin)
HER2	Human epidermal growth factor receptor 2
HIT	Heparin induced thrombocytopenia
HIV	Human immunodeficiency virus
HMG CoA	3-hydroxy-3-methyl-glutaryl coenzyme A
hr	Hour
hrly	Hourly
HRT	Hormone replacement therapy
HUS	Haemolytic–uraemic syndrome
IBS	Irritable bowel syndrome
Ig	Immunoglobulin
IL	Interleukin
IM	Intramuscular
INR	International normalised ratio
ISMN	Isosorbide mononitrate
IV	Intravenous
K^+	Potassium ion
kg	Kilogram
L	Litre
LABA	Long-acting β_2-agonist
LAMA	Long-acting antimuscarinic
LDL	Low-density lipoprotein
L-dopa	Levodopa
LH	Luteinising hormone
LMWH	Low molecular weight heparin
LRTI	Lower respiratory tract infection
m	Metre
MDI	Metered dose inhaler
mg	Milligram
MHRA	Medicines and Healthcare Products Regulatory Agency
min	Minute
mL	Millilitre
mmHg	Millimetres of mercury
mmol	Millimole
MR	Modified release
MRSA	Meticillin-resistant Staphylococcus aureus
MSK	Musculoskeletal
Na^+	Sodium ion
NAPQI	N-acetyl-p-benzoquinone imine
NHS	National Health Service
NICE	National Institute for Health and Care Excellence
NMS	Neuroleptic malignant syndrome
NO	Nitric oxide
NOAC	Novel oral anticoagulant
NPH	Neutral protamine Hagedorn
NRT	Nicotine replacement therapy
NSAID	Non-steroidal antiinflammatory drug
OPAT	Outpatient parenteral antimicrobial therapy
p	Pence
PaO_2	Partial pressure of oxygen in arterial blood
P_AO_2	Partial pressure of oxygen in alveolar gas
PCR	Polymerase chain reaction
PD	Pharmacodynamic
PDE	Phosphodiesterase

PE	Pulmonary embolism	SSRI	Selective serotonin reuptake inhibitor
PGE_2	Prostaglandin E_2	SV2A	Synaptic vesicle protein 2A
PO_2	Partial pressure of oxygen	SVT	Supraventricular tachycardia
POP	Progesterone-only pill		
PK	Pharmacokinetic	T_3	Triiodothyronine
PPARγ	Peroxisome proliferator-activated receptor γ	T_4	Thyroxine
		TIA	Transient ischaemic attack
PPI	Proton pump inhibitor	TNF	Tumour necrosis factor
Q fever	Query fever	TPMT	Thiopurine methyltransferase
RNA	Ribonucleic acid		
SA	Sinoatrial	TSH	Thyroid stimulating hormone
SC	Subcutaneous		
sec	Second	UC	Ulcerative colitis
SERM	Selective estrogen (oestrogen) receptor modulator	UFH	Unfractionated heparin
		UK	United Kingdom
SGLT-2	Sodium–glucose co-transporter 2	UTI	Urinary tract infection
		VF	Ventricular fibrillation
SIADH	Syndrome of inappropriate antidiuretic hormone	VRE	Vancomycin-resistant enterococcus
SL	Sublingual	VT	Ventricular tachycardia
SNRI	Serotonin and noradrenaline reuptake inhibitor	VTE	Venous thromboembolism
		WCC	White cell count
		WHO	World Health Organization
SpO_2	Saturation of oxygen by pulse oximetry		

Introduction

Why should you use this book?

Learning pharmacology is hard. In the UK, nearly 2000 drugs are available in over 10,000 medicinal products. The amount of information you could obtain for each one is almost limitless, as is reflected in the hefty weight of conventional pharmacology textbooks. Compounding this, universities have recently—and quite appropriately in our view—refocused the emphasis on practical prescribing in their curricula and examinations. The classic pharmacology texts that once provided students with all they needed to know (and usually much more) now appear deficient in this critically important area. Meanwhile, the prescribing manuals and formularies used in practice are generally impenetrable to students, and provide insufficient detail on the clinical pharmacology that underpins the use and understanding of drugs.

Against this backdrop, you need a place to start. You need to focus most of your attention on the most important information about the most important drugs. You need a bridge between a students' textbook and a prescribers' manual. Fundamentally, you need to know what you need to know about the drugs you are going to prescribe in practice. That is what this book seeks to provide.

What are 'the top 100 drugs'?

We analysed data from hundreds of millions of prescriptions in primary and secondary care to identify the drugs that were prescribed most often.[1] To this list we added a handful of 'emergency drugs' which, although less commonly used, are important to know about. We tested the stability of the resulting 'top 100' list over the next 2 years to confirm that it did not change significantly. We surveyed 149 foundation doctors who told us that, on average, they prescribed 41 of the top 100 drugs at least every week and another 24 at least every month. More than three-quarters said they rarely prescribed drugs that are not on the list. For the second edition, we have repeated the analysis using much larger datasets for both hospital prescriptions (electronic prescribing data from a large National Health Service [NHS] trust) and community (Prescription Cost Analysis data from NHS England).[2] This has resulted in the replacement of 11 drugs in the top 100 list; we have resisted the temptation merely to add to the list, as this would go against the ethos of the book.

How to use this book

Organisation of the book

The top 100 drugs are arranged in alphabetical order. We have generally identified them by the name of the class to which they belong: thus 'bisoprolol' is found under 'β-blockers'. We have listed common examples in order of the frequency with which they are used, with less common but still important drugs added to this where appropriate. Where a drug is effectively in a class of its own, we have identified it simply by its name: thus we use 'metformin' rather than 'biguanides'. In addition to the top 100 drugs, we have provided details of five commonly used intravenous (IV) solutions in their own section at the end of the book.

Table 1.1 Anatomy of the 'drug' pages

Drug class (or drug name, if it is in a class of its own)	
CLINICAL PHARMACOLOGY	
Common indications	A list of the **situations in which the drug is commonly used**, along with brief discussion of its **place in therapy;** in other words, where it fits in alongside other treatment options.
Spectrum of activity (antibiotics only)	For antibiotics only, a brief description of the spectrum of their antibacterial activity.
Mechanisms of action	A brief discussion of how the drug works in the indications specified
Important adverse effects	The most common and important adverse effects of the drug, with discussion of their mechanism where this aids understanding
Warnings	The situations in which the drug should be avoided (i.e. is **contraindicated**) or where extra **caution** should be used
Important interactions	The most important interactions with other drugs

To help you test and reinforce your knowledge, we have included some single-best-answer questions. The answers to these direct you to the relevant drug entries as appropriate. These also provide an opportunity to bring together information from several drugs and show how it may be integrated in practice.

Using the book

We anticipate this book being used in two main ways. One is as a 'quick reference source' for when you encounter a drug on the ward or in clinic and want to read up on it quickly. The alphabetical arrangement of the drugs aims to facilitate this. The other way you might use it is when learning about an organ system or a disease and want core information about the relevant drugs. To support this way of working, we have provided two additional tables of contents: one listing the drugs relevant to each system, and the other listing drugs used in specific indications.

In your early years of study, you will probably concentrate on learning clinical pharmacology. As you progress, you will increasingly need to supplement this with knowledge and skills in practical prescribing. Reflecting this, we have arranged the information under these two main headings in a consistent way throughout the book. We have further divided the information with standard subheadings, the purpose of which is outlined in Table 1.1. We use bold text and icons to draw out key points, as indicated in Box 1.1.

Common examples, in order of relative importance	
PRACTICAL PRESCRIBING	
Prescription	A discussion of how the drug is usually prescribed, including, as appropriate, typical starting dosage and route of administration. All dosages are for adults unless otherwise specified
Administration	A discussion of any important considerations about how the drug should be administered, beyond those already covered by the prescription
Communication	A brief discussion of the important information that should be conveyed to the patient, written in non-medical language
Monitoring	Details about how the efficacy, safety and tolerability of treatment should be monitored, as applicable
Cost	A brief mention of cost, particularly to highlight where savings can be made without affecting treatment efficacy

Clinical tip—an interesting or useful fact or tip about the drug, generally derived from clinical experience.

Box 1.1 Text features used throughout the book

Bold text is used to highlight key points for quick identification.

Underlining is used to identify drugs that are covered elsewhere in the book in more detail.

A ▲ **red triangle** is used to identify important circumstances such as co-morbidities (cautions and contraindications) or concurrent medications (interactions) in which use of the drug is risky. Although it may occasionally be used, this would be appropriate only after careful risk–benefit assessment and some extra safety measures, such as lower dosage and more intensive monitoring. As a foundation doctor, you would generally be expected to seek senior or specialist guidance in these situations.

A ✖ **red cross** is used to identify circumstances (such as co-morbidities or concurrent medications) in which we regard use of the drug to be dangerous and inappropriate.

Using the information

We provide information that we hope will inform your understanding of drugs and their practical use, but this is not a prescribing formulary. This is particularly important in relation to cautions and contraindications (which we refer to collectively as 'Warnings'). To reproduce all the points that might need to be considered in practice would be overwhelming and destroy the point of the book. Likewise, for drug doses, we will often provide a 'typical starting dose' (for adults unless otherwise specified) because we think it's useful for you to have an idea of the kind of doses you will see used in practice. However, it is not our intention that when writing real prescriptions you will look up doses in this book. The key point is this: this book is for *learning*. When you start *making decisions* for patients, you will need also to consult formularies (in the UK, the *British National Formulary* [BNF]), protocols, policies and guidance, as appropriate to the clinical context. You can practise this now – the knowledge you will acquire from this book will make the prescribing reference sources more useful and accessible.

Where next?

This book provides, in our judgement, the most important information that you need to know about drugs in order to pass your examinations and, ultimately, to become a safe and effective prescriber. However, in providing you with this 'starting point', it is not our intention to stifle your inquisitiveness. We would actively encourage you to learn more, both about the drugs in this book and others that are less commonly used. We just know, from years of experience teaching prescribers and students, that when confronted with such an overwhelming number of drugs, and all the things you could possibly know about them, it is sometimes difficult to see the wood for the trees.

Reference

1. Baker EH et al. Development of a core drug list towards improving prescribing education and reducing errors in the UK. *British Journal of Clinical Pharmacology* 2011;71:190–198.
2. Audi S et al. The 'top 100' drugs and classes in England: an updated 'starter formulary' for trainee prescribers. British Journal of Clinical Pharmacology 2018. Available online: https://doi.org/10.1111/bcp.13709 (accessed 05/09/2018).

The top 100 drugs listed by system

The top 100 drugs listed by indication

The top 100 drugs listed by indication

The top 100 drugs listed by indication

The top 100 drugs listed by indication

The top 100 drugs listed by indication

The top 100 drugs

5α-reductase inhibitors

CLINICAL PHARMACOLOGY

Common indications	In **benign prostatic enlargement,** 5α-reductase inhibitors are usually a second-line medical option after α-blockers. They improve lower urinary tract symptoms, such as difficulty passing urine, urinary retention and poor urinary flow, and reduce the need for prostate-related surgery.
Mechanisms of action	5α-reductase inhibitors reduce the size of the prostate gland. They do this by **inhibiting** the intracellular enzyme **5α-reductase,** which converts testosterone to its more active metabolite dihydrotestosterone. As dihydrotestosterone stimulates prostatic growth, inhibition of its production by 5α-reductase inhibitors reduces prostatic enlargement and improves urinary flow. However, it can take several months for this effect to become evident clinically. For this reason, an α-blocker is usually preferred for initial therapy, with a 5α-reductase inhibitor added if the response is poor or if the prostate is particularly bulky.
Important adverse effects	The most common adverse effects of 5α-reductase inhibitors relate to their antiandrogen action. These include **impotence** and **reduced libido,** which are usually transient, and breast tenderness and enlargement (**gynaecomastia**), which can affect patient adherence to treatment. An additional effect of androgen inhibition is **hair growth,** which can be exploited to advantage in treatment of male-pattern baldness. **Breast cancer** has been reported in men taking finasteride.
Warnings	Exposure of a male fetus to 5α-reductase inhibitors may cause abnormal development of the external genitalia. It is therefore important that ✖**pregnant women** do not take these drugs and are not exposed to them, e.g. by handling broken or damaged tablets or through semen during unprotected sex with a man taking these drugs.
Important interactions	There are no clinically important drug interactions.

PRACTICAL PRESCRIBING

Prescription	The usual dose for the treatment of **benign prostatic enlargement** is 5 mg orally daily.
Administration	Tablets must be prepared, stored and administered carefully. They should be swallowed whole, with or without food. Women who are, or could be, pregnant, must not touch crushed or broken tablets.
Communication	Explain to the patient that the reason he is having difficulty passing urine is because his prostate has grown and is squashing the tube coming out of the bladder. Tell him that the aim of finasteride treatment is to **reduce the bulk of the prostate gland,** which will relieve compression on the tube and make it **easier to pass urine.** However, it may take **up to 6 months** for symptoms to improve. Warn him of the **main side effects,** particularly that he may feel less keen to have sex and may be less able to get or keep an erection. It is important to point out that these problems should last for a short while only, and normal function should return as treatment continues. Explain that he may also notice some tenderness or growth in the tissue underneath his nipples. If this occurs he should see his doctor. Explain these changes are usually harmless. However, very rarely, men can get breast cancer, and this is slightly more likely on this drug. Encourage the patient to return if he is having a lot of trouble with side effects, as other treatments for his enlarged prostate could be considered. If the patient has a partner who is or could become pregnant, advise him that if she is exposed to the drug it could harm the baby. She should be advised not to handle the tablets. They should use a condom during sex.
Monitoring	Schedule a follow-up appointment in 3–6 months to review changes in lower urinary tract symptoms and the development of adverse effects. Continue check-ups every 6–12 months while treatment continues.
Cost	Finasteride is available in non-proprietary form and is inexpensive.

Clinical tip—Finasteride is a good example of the importance of **post-marketing surveillance.** In clinical trials, relatively few carefully-selected patients (hundreds to thousands) are exposed to a drug and common adverse effects are identified. After marketing, many more patients (thousands to millions) with less stringent selection criteria are exposed to the drug and less common adverse effects may emerge. In the UK, suspected adverse effects of medicines should be reported to the Medicines and Healthcare Products Regulatory Agency (**MHRA**) by health professionals or the public using the **Yellow Card scheme.** For finasteride, there were reports of breast cancer in clinical trials, but these were not statistically associated with use of the drug. Continued reports of breast cancer during post-marketing surveillance led to a review of its safety and changes in the information given to patients about breast cancer risk.

α-blockers

CLINICAL PHARMACOLOGY

Common indications	❶ As a first-line medical option to improve symptoms in **benign prostatic enlargement,** when lifestyle changes are insufficient. 5α-reductase inhibitors may be added in selected cases. Surgical treatment is also an option, particularly if there is evidence of urinary tract damage (e.g. hydronephrosis). ❷ As an add-on treatment in **resistant hypertension,** when other medicines (e.g. calcium channel blockers, angiotensin-converting enzyme (ACE) inhibitors, thiazide diuretics) are insufficient.
Mechanisms of action	Although often described using the broad term 'α-blocker,' most drugs in this class (including doxazosin, tamsulosin and alfuzosin) are highly selective for the α_1-adrenoceptor. α_1-adrenoceptors are found mainly in smooth muscle, including in blood vessels and the urinary tract (the bladder neck and prostate in particular). Stimulation induces contraction; blockade induces relaxation. α_1-blockers therefore cause **vasodilatation** and a fall in blood pressure (BP), and **reduced resistance to bladder outflow.**
Important adverse effects	Predictably from their effects on vascular tone, α-blockers can cause **postural hypotension, dizziness** and **syncope.** This is particularly prominent after the first dose (rather like with ACE inhibitors and angiotensin receptor blockers [ARBs]).
Warnings	α-blockers should not be used in patients with existing ▲**postural hypotension.**
Important interactions	In general, combining antihypertensive drugs results in additive BP lowering effects (this may well be the therapeutic aim). To avoid pronounced first-dose hypotension, it may be prudent to omit doses of one or more existing antihypertensive drugs on the day the α-blocker is started. This is particularly the case for β-blockers, which inhibit the reflex tachycardia that forms part of the compensatory response to **vasodilatation**.

---

doxazosin, tamsulosin, alfuzosin

PRACTICAL PRESCRIBING

Prescription — Doxazosin and tamsulosin are the most commonly prescribed α-blockers in the UK. They are taken orally. Doxazosin is licensed both for **benign prostatic enlargement** and **hypertension;** it is typically started at a dose of 1 mg daily and increased at 1–2 week intervals according to response. Tamsulosin is licensed for **benign prostatic enlargement** only. It also has a BP lowering effect, but this is probably less pronounced than for doxazosin. It is given in a dose of 400 micrograms daily.

Administration — Given the pronounced BP lowering effect of doxazosin, it is best to take this at bedtime, at least initially.

Communication — As appropriate, advise patients that you are offering them a treatment for their urinary symptoms or their blood pressure. Explain that it may cause dizziness on standing, particularly after the first dose. Advise them to start by taking the medicine at bedtime to minimise the impact of this (although warn them that if they need to get up in the night, they should rise from bed slowly).

Monitoring — The best guide to **efficacy** is the patient's urinary symptoms and/or BP, as applicable. For **tolerability** and **safety,** adverse effects are identified by symptom enquiry and by measuring their lying and standing BP.

Cost — Non-proprietary forms of doxazosin and tamsulosin are inexpensive. Both drugs are also available in modified-release (MR) forms which, as brand name products, are more expensive. There is little convincing evidence that the MR forms are any more effective than standard-release forms, and since they are all taken at the same frequency (daily), they do not improve convenience for the patient.

Clinical tip—Although in hypertension α-blockers are usually reserved for patients who do not respond to other drug classes, many men with hypertension also have benign prostatic enlargement. Discovering that a man with hypertension also has benign prostatic enlargement may prompt you to introduce doxazosin at an earlier stage in the treatment pathway. In doing so, you may be able to improve both conditions with a single drug. This exemplifies why the 'review of systems' is an important part of history taking.

The top 100 drugs

Acetylcholinesterase inhibitors

CLINICAL PHARMACOLOGY

Common indications	❶ Mild to moderate **Alzheimer's disease** ❷ Mild to moderate **dementia in Parkinson's disease** (rivastigmine)
Mechanisms of action	**Acetylcholine** is an important central nervous system (CNS) **neurotransmitter**, which is essential to many brain functions including **learning and memory**. A decrease in activity of the brain's cholinergic system is seen in Alzheimer's disease and in the dementia associated with Parkinson's disease. These drugs inhibit the cholinesterase enzymes that break down acetylcholine in the CNS. It is thought that by **increasing the availability of acetylcholine** for neurotransmission, they **improve cognitive function** and **reduce the rate of cognitive decline**. However, recovery of function in patients with these conditions on starting treatment is modest and not universal.
Important adverse effects	Nausea, diarrhoea and vomiting are the most common adverse effects, arising from **increased cholinergic activity in the peripheral nervous system**. These adverse effects may resolve over time. Patients with **asthma** or **chronic obstructive pulmonary disease (COPD)** may experience an exacerbation of symptoms. Less common, but serious, peripheral effects include **peptic ulcers** and **bleeding, bradycardia** and **heart block**. Central cholinergic effects may induce **hallucinations** and **altered/aggressive behaviour**. These resolve with reduction of dose or discontinuation of therapy. There is a small risk of **extrapyramidal symptoms** and **neuroleptic malignant syndrome**. These are discussed more fully in first-generation antipsychotics.
Warnings	Acetylcholinesterase inhibitors should be used with caution in patients with ▲**asthma** and ▲**COPD** and those at risk of developing ▲**peptic ulcers**. They should be avoided in patients with ✖**heart block** or ✖**sick sinus syndrome**. Rivastigmine may worsen tremor in those with ▲**Parkinson's disease**.
Important interactions	Concomitant therapy with ▲non-steroidal antiinflammatory drugs (NSAIDs) and ▲corticosteroids may increase the risk of peptic ulceration. Use alongside ▲antipsychotics may increase the risk of neuroleptic malignant syndrome. Bradycardia and/or heart block may occur when prescribed alongside other rate-limiting medications (e.g. ▲β-blockers).

donepezil, rivastigmine

PRACTICAL PRESCRIBING

Prescription	Acetylcholinesterase inhibitors should be prescribed by, or on the advice of, clinicians with experience in managing dementia or Parkinson's disease. When commencing treatment, a low dose should be used to reduce the risk of adverse effects. The starting dose is 5 mg daily for donepezil and 1.5 mg 12- hrly for rivastigmine. Dose may be titrated up after 2–4 weeks.
Administration	Generally, these drugs are available as tablets, capsules or as a liquid. In addition, rivastigmine is available as a patch, which may be useful for patients with swallowing difficulties. Donepezil should be taken at night, before bed.
Communication	You should explain to the patient and their family or caregiver that this treatment improves memory and brain function for some patients and may slow the rate of decline. You should explain that recovery of brain function is modest and that it is not a cure for their dementia. Discuss the adverse effects and explain that some may resolve with prolonged use. Ask them to report any abnormal movements or agitated/aggressive behaviour to their doctor. Explain that if these effects occur, they are reversible by reducing the dose or stopping treatment
Monitoring	Patients should be reviewed for **adverse effects** 2–4 weeks after initiation of treatment or dose adjustments. At 3 months, repeat cognitive assessment should occur to assess **treatment efficacy**. Treatment should continue only where there is a worthwhile improvement in the patient's symptoms (cognitive, functional or behavioural). Patients and their carers should be involved in any decision to change or cease treatment.
Cost	Non-proprietary formulations of acetylcholinesterase inhibitors are widely available. There are not felt to be clinically relevant differences between agents in terms of efficacy or cost-effectiveness. The drug with the lowest cost should therefore be prescribed.

Clinical tip—Vivid dreams have been reported with the use of donepezil. Where this is problematic for patients, advise them to take the drug in the morning, rather than before bed.

Acetylcysteine (N-acetylcysteine)

CLINICAL PHARMACOLOGY

Common indications	❶ As the antidote for **paracetamol poisoning.** ❷ To help prevent renal injury due to radiographic contrast material **(contrast nephropathy),** although recent evidence suggests it is not effective for this indication. ❸ To reduce the viscosity of **respiratory secretions** (acting as a mucolytic) in hospital patients. Outside hospital, orally administered carbocisteine is used.
Mechanisms of action	In therapeutic doses, <u>paracetamol</u> is metabolised mainly by conjugation with glucuronic acid and sulfate. A small amount is converted to N-acetyl-p-benzoquinone imine (NAPQI), which is hepatotoxic. Normally, this is quickly detoxified by conjugation with glutathione. However, in paracetamol poisoning, the body's supply of glutathione is overwhelmed and NAPQI is left free to cause liver damage. Acetylcysteine works mainly by **replenishing the body's supply of glutathione.** Acetylcysteine also has **antioxidant effects,** which may contribute to its effect in preventing contrast nephropathy, although this is not completely understood, and a recent large study failed to demonstrate its efficacy in this indication. If acetylcysteine is brought into contact with mucus, it **breaks disulphide bonds,** degrading the three-dimensional mucus matrix and reducing its viscosity. For patients who have tenacious respiratory secretions (e.g. in bronchiectasis), this may aid sputum clearance.
Important adverse effects	When administered intravenously in paracetamol poisoning, acetylcysteine can cause an **anaphylactoid reaction.** This is similar to an anaphylactic reaction (presenting with nausea, tachycardia, rash and wheeze), but involves histamine release independent of immunoglobulin E (IgE) antibodies. Therefore once the reaction has settled (by stopping the acetylcysteine and giving an antihistamine ± a bronchodilator), it is usually safe to restart acetylcysteine, but at a lower rate of infusion. When administered in nebulised form as a mucolytic, acetylcysteine may cause **bronchospasm.** Therefore a bronchodilator (e.g. <u>salbutamol</u>) should usually be given immediately beforehand.
Warnings	History of an anaphylactoid reaction to acetylcysteine does not contraindicate its use in future, if it is required. It is important that such reactions are not erroneously labelled as 'allergic,' which may lead to effective treatment for paracetamol poisoning being inappropriately denied. However, it is essential to obtain specialist advice if there is any doubt.
Important interactions	There are no significant adverse drug interactions with acetylcysteine.

PRACTICAL PRESCRIBING

Prescription	In the treatment of **paracetamol poisoning,** weight-adjusted doses are given as an intravenous (IV) infusion with three components (total infusion time 21 hours). You should consult the British National Formulary (BNF) and/or a local protocol for full details. Its use in the prophylaxis of **contrast nephropathy** is no longer widely recommended, but where considered appropriate a typical dose is 1200 mg orally 12-hrly for 2 days, beginning the day before the procedure. For use in tenacious **respiratory secretions,** a typical dose is 2.5–5 mL of acetylcysteine 10% solution by nebuliser every 6 hours, but you should consult local guidance if available.
Administration	Detailed instructions for the preparation and administration of acetylcysteine in paracetamol poisoning are provided in the Summary of Product Characteristics (provided with the product and also available online at www.medicines.org.uk). For use as a mucolytic, the 20% IV solution should be diluted to a 10% solution before use.
Communication	Explain to patients that you are offering treatment with a paracetamol antidote. It is given slowly through a drip over 21 hours. If it is started within about 8 hours of a single overdose, you can say that it is very effective and, provided it is administered correctly, should completely prevent serious damage to the liver. Emphasise the importance of avoiding interruptions to the treatment, while acknowledging the inconvenience of being 'tied to a drip' for the best part of a day. Mention that it occasionally causes a reaction involving a rash, nausea, or wheeziness. Patients should alert staff if they notice any of these symptoms, so that the infusion can be interrupted and treatment given.
Monitoring	In the treatment of paracetamol poisoning, patients should be monitored clinically for signs of anaphylactoid reaction. The **international normalised ratio** (INR), serum alanine aminotransferase (ALT) activity and creatinine concentration should be measured at presentation and on completion of the acetylcysteine, to track the trajectory of liver injury.
Cost	Acetylcysteine is available in non-proprietary form and is relatively inexpensive.

Clinical tip—Protocols for the use of acetylcysteine vary between countries and regions, and the UK guidelines changed substantially in 2012. When searching for information online, make sure you are referring to up-to-date information from the correct region. In clinical practice, always follow the protocol specific to the hospital in which you are working.

Activated charcoal

CLINICAL PHARMACOLOGY

Common indications	❶ A *single dose* of activated charcoal may be used to **reduce absorption of certain poisons** (including some **drugs in overdose**) from the gut. ❷ *Multiple doses* of activated charcoal may also be used to **increase the elimination of certain poisons.**
Mechanisms of action	Van der Waals (weak intermolecular) forces are responsible for the mechanism of action of activated charcoal. **Molecules are adsorbed onto the surface of the charcoal** as they travel through the gut, **reducing their absorption** into the circulation. However, activated charcoal is only useful in cases where the poison ingested is likely to be adsorbed onto it. The affinity of a substance for activated charcoal is determined by its ionic status and its solubility in water. Weakly ionic, hydrophobic substances (e.g. benzodiazepines, methotrexate) are generally well adsorbed by activated charcoal. By contrast, strongly ionic and hydrophilic substances (e.g. strong acids/bases, alcohols, lithium and iron) are not adsorbed. Activated charcoal can also **increase the elimination** of certain poisons. This may be useful for substances adsorbed by charcoal that can **readily diffuse back into the gut.** In this case, multiple doses of activated charcoal can be used to maintain a steep concentration gradient of the poison (high in the circulation, low in the gut), encouraging diffusion out of the circulation and hastening elimination of the drug. This is sometimes referred to as 'gut dialysis'. Of interest, charcoal is 'activated' during preparation through chemical processes, including blasting it with steam or hot air. These processes increase the surface area of the charcoal particles by increasing pore size. With a surface area around 1000 m^2/g, a lot of poison can be adsorbed!
Important adverse effects	**Aspiration** of activated charcoal can lead to serious complications such as **pneumonitis, bronchospasm** and **airway obstruction.** It can also precipitate **intestinal obstruction.** However, the most common adverse effects of activated charcoal are **black stools** and **vomiting.**
Warnings	Activated charcoal should not be used in patients with a **reduced level of consciousness,** unless their airway is first protected by endotracheal intubation. Caution is required when prescribing activated charcoal to patients with ▲**persistent vomiting,** as there is a risk of aspiration. Those with ▲**reduced gut motility** have an increased risk of intestinal obstruction.
Important interactions	Activated charcoal reduces the absorption of many drugs taken therapeutically as well as those taken in overdose.

PRACTICAL PRESCRIBING

Prescription	A *single dose* of activated charcoal to reduce absorption is recommended only for patients presenting **within 1 hour of ingestion of a clinically significant amount of a substance that is adsorbed by charcoal.** Later or additional doses of activated charcoal may be considered for some modified released preparations or drugs that delay gastric emptying (e.g. aspirin, opioids, tricyclic antidepressants). Activated charcoal should be prescribed on the once-only section of the drug chart at a dose of 50 g orally (or by nasogastric tube if the patient is intubated). When using *multiple doses* of activated charcoal (potential situations include significant overdose with carbamazepine, quinine, or theophylline – but seek advice), you should prescribe 50 g of activated charcoal to be administered 4-hrly. Pre-emptive treatment with an antiemetic and a laxative may be advisable.
Administration	Activated charcoal is usually mixed with 250 mL of water to form a suspension, which the patient then drinks. In patients who are unconscious but have a protected airway (i.e. following intubation), this suspension may be given via a nasogastric tube.
Communication	Advise patients that activated charcoal can help prevent absorption of the drug or poison they have taken. It may also be worth mentioning that the taste is not particularly palatable!
Monitoring	No special monitoring is necessary when a patient takes activated charcoal above that required for the overdose/poisoning situation.
Cost	A single dose of activated charcoal costs around £12.

Clinical tip—If your patient has vomited prior to presentation, but it is still felt that activated charcoal would be useful, give an antiemetic such as ondansetron (4–8 mg IV) or cyclizine (50 mg IV or IM). However, remember that if the patient is *actively vomiting*, the charcoal may not be effective (as it will not remain in the gut) and there is a risk of aspiration (see Important adverse effects, above).

Adenosine

CLINICAL PHARMACOLOGY

Common indications	As a first-line diagnostic and therapeutic agent in **supraventricular tachycardia (SVT),** usually evident on the electrocardiogram (ECG) as a regular, narrow-complex tachycardia.
Mechanisms of action	Adenosine is an agonist of adenosine receptors on cell surfaces. In the heart, activation of these G protein-coupled receptors induces several effects, including reducing the frequency of spontaneous depolarisations (automaticity) and increasing resistance to depolarisation (refractoriness). In turn, this transiently slows the sinus rate and conduction velocity and **increases atrioventricular (AV) node refractoriness.** Many forms of SVT arise from a self-perpetuating electrical (re-entry) circuit that takes in the AV node. Increasing refractoriness in the AV node **breaks the re-entry circuit,** which allows normal depolarisations from the sinoatrial (SA) node to resume control of heart rate (**cardioversion**). Where the circuit does not involve the AV node (e.g. in atrial flutter), adenosine will not induce cardioversion. However, by blocking conduction to the ventricles, it allows closer inspection of the atrial rhythm on the ECG. This may reveal the diagnosis. The duration of effect of adenosine is very short because it is rapidly taken up by cells (e.g. red cells). Its half-life in plasma is less than 10 seconds.
Important adverse effects	By interfering with the functions of the SA and AV nodes, adenosine can induce **bradycardia** and even **asystole.** Inevitably, this is accompanied by a deeply unpleasant sensation for the patient. It is said to feel like a **sinking feeling** in the chest, often accompanied by **breathlessness** and a **sense of 'impending doom.'** Fortunately, due to the drug's short-lived effect, this feeling is only brief.
Warnings	You should not administer adenosine to a patient who will not tolerate its transient bradycardic effects, including those with ✗**hypotension,** ✗**coronary ischaemia,** or ✗**decompensated heart failure.** Adenosine may induce bronchospasm in susceptible individuals, so should be avoided in patients with ✗**asthma** or ▲**COPD.** Patients who have had a ▲**heart transplant** are very sensitive to the effects of adenosine.
Important interactions	▲Dipyridamole, an antiplatelet agent, blocks cellular uptake of adenosine. This prolongs and potentiates its effect, so the dose of adenosine should be halved. Theophylline and aminophylline (systemic bronchodilators) are competitive antagonists of adenosine receptors and reduce its effect. Patients who have taken these drugs respond poorly and may require higher doses.

PRACTICAL PRESCRIBING

Prescription	Adenosine is always given intravenously. The prescription should be written in the once-only section of the drug chart. The initial dose is usually 6 mg IV. If this is ineffective, a 12-mg dose may be given. Higher doses may be given in selected cases. If using a central line, lower doses should be used (e.g. 3 mg initially).
Administration	Adenosine should be administered only by doctors experienced in its use, or under their direct supervision. **Resuscitation facilities** should be on hand. It is important that the adenosine dose reaches the heart quickly to minimise cellular uptake *en route*. This requires a **large-bore cannula** (e.g. 18 gauge [green] or bigger), sited as proximally as possible (e.g. in the antecubital fossa). Administer the dose as a **rapid injection** and then immediately follow it with a flush, e.g. 20 mL of 0.9% <u>sodium chloride</u>. The effect will usually be evident on the cardiac monitor within 10–15 seconds, and then dissipate over about 30–60 seconds.
Communication	Explain to patients that you are offering treatment with a medicine that will hopefully 'reset' their heart into a normal rhythm. Explain that it will briefly make them feel terrible, but this sensation will only last for about 30 seconds. Ensure you continue talking to the patient during its administration, offering reassurance that the unpleasant sensation will go away quickly. Observing profound bradycardia or transient asystole on the cardiac monitor will probably induce some anxiety on your part too. Try not to convey this to the patient!
Monitoring	Administration of adenosine requires very close monitoring. This *must* include a **continuous cardiac rhythm strip,** recorded for subsequent examination.
Cost	Adenosine is inexpensive.

Clinical tip—Advance preparation is invaluable in the administration of adenosine. Plan what doses you will give and draw these up away from the bedside. Use small syringes (e.g. 2 mL) for adenosine, as this will make it easier to administer rapidly. Draw up one 20 mL 0.9% sodium chloride flush for each planned dose, plus one spare. *Label all the syringes carefully.* To administer the drug, first attach a three-way tap to the cannula. Use your spare flush to check its patency. Next, replace this with a new, full 20 mL flush, and attach the first dose of adenosine to the other port. Start the continuous ECG recording, then (after warning the patient) administer the adenosine and the flush in rapid succession. Stop the ECG recording once a stable cardiac rhythm resumes, print it out and annotate it to indicate when and how much adenosine was administered.

Adrenaline (epinephrine)

CLINICAL PHARMACOLOGY

Common indications	❶ In **cardiac arrest,** adrenaline is administered as part of the Advanced Life Support (ALS) treatment algorithm for shockable and non-shockable rhythms. ❷ In **anaphylaxis,** adrenaline is a vital part of immediate management. ❸ Adrenaline may be injected directly into tissues to induce **local vasoconstriction.** For example, it is used during endoscopy to **control mucosal bleeding,** and it is sometimes mixed with local anaesthetic drugs (e.g. <u>lidocaine</u>) to **prolong local anaesthesia.**
Mechanisms of action	Adrenaline is a **potent agonist of the α_1-, α_2-, β_1- and β_2-adrenoceptors,** and correspondingly, has a multitude of sympathetic ('fight or flight') effects. These include: vasoconstriction of vessels supplying skin, mucosa and abdominal viscera (mainly α_1-mediated); increases in heart rate, force of contraction and myocardial excitability (β_1); and vasodilatation of vessels supplying the heart and muscles (β_2). These explain its use in cardiac arrest, where the **redistribution of blood flow in favour of the heart** is desirable, at least theoretically, and may improve the chances of restoring an organised rhythm. Its theoretical benefits in cardiac arrest have not been conclusively demonstrated in clinical trials; it is hoped that this will be clarified soon. Additional effects of adrenaline, mediated by β_2-receptors, are **bronchodilatation and suppression of inflammatory mediator release from mast cells.** Together with its vascular effects, these underpin its use in anaphylaxis, where widespread release of inflammatory mediators from mast cells produces generalised vasodilatation, profound hypotension and often bronchoconstriction.
Important adverse effects	Adrenaline is a dangerous drug, but its risks are balanced against the severity of the condition being treated. In cardiac arrest, restoration of output is often followed by **adrenaline-induced hypertension.** When given to conscious patients in anaphylaxis or in an attempt to produce local vasoconstriction, it often causes **anxiety, tremor, headache** and **palpitations.** It may also cause **angina, myocardial infarction** and **arrhythmias,** particularly in patients with existing heart disease.
Warnings	There are **no contraindications to its use in cardiac arrest and anaphylaxis.** When given to induce local vasoconstriction, it should be used with caution in patients with ▲**heart disease.** Combination adrenaline–anaesthetic preparations should not be used in ✖**areas supplied by an end-artery** (i.e. with poor collateral supply), such as fingers and toes, where vasoconstriction can cause tissue necrosis.
Important interactions	In patients receiving treatment with a ▲<u>β-blocker</u>, adrenaline may induce widespread vasoconstriction, because its α_1-mediated vasoconstricting effect is not opposed by β_2-mediated vasodilatation.

PRACTICAL PRESCRIBING

Prescription	In life-threatening situations, adrenaline is administered first then prescribed later. In adult **cardiac arrest** associated with a shockable rhythm (ventricular fibrillation [VF] or pulseless ventricular tachycardia), **adrenaline 1 mg IV** is given just after the third shock, and repeated every 3–5 minutes thereafter (i.e. every other cycle of cardiopulmonary resuscitation [CPR]). If the rhythm is not shockable (asystole or pulseless electrical activity), adrenaline 1 mg IV is given as soon as IV access is available, and then repeated every 3–5 minutes. In **anaphylaxis,** the dose of adrenaline is **500 micrograms IM,** repeated after 5 minutes if necessary. Take particular note of the route of administration: **do not administer IV adrenaline in anaphylaxis, unless cardiac arrest supervenes.** When **infiltrated subcutaneously** with a local anaesthetic to induce **local vasoconstriction,** a ready-mixed adrenaline–anaesthetic preparation should be used; usually this contains adrenaline at a concentration of 1:200,000 (5 micrograms/mL) along with the anaesthetic. The name 'adrenaline' is still used for prescribing in the UK, although the international non-proprietary name (epinephrine) is also printed on product packaging.
Administration	In **cardiac arrest,** adrenaline is administered from a pre-filled syringe containing a 1:10,000 (1 mg in 10 mL) solution. Administer the whole 10 mL, followed by a flush (e.g. 10 mL of 0.9% sodium chloride). In **anaphylaxis,** give 0.5 mL of a 1:1000 (1 mg in 1 mL) adrenaline solution by IM injection. Inject this into the anterolateral aspect of the thigh halfway between the knee and the hip, from where it should be rapidly absorbed. In obese patients you need to inject deeply in order to be confident of IM rather than subcutaneous (SC) administration.
Communication	In **anaphylaxis,** simultaneously with providing treatment, explain to patients that they are experiencing a severe allergic reaction and that you are giving them an injection of adrenaline to treat this.
Monitoring	In the context of **cardiac arrest** and **anaphylaxis,** intensive clinical and haemodynamic monitoring should be instituted as soon as practical.
Cost	Cost is not a consideration to decisions regarding the use of adrenaline in individual patients.

Clinical tip—The use of a local anaesthetic mixed with adrenaline often induces a mild but quite unpleasant sensation of anxiety for the patient. This only adds to the tension associated with undergoing a procedure. The use of adrenaline in this context is probably most appropriate in the operating theatre, where it can be injected while the patient is under general anaesthesia as a means of prolonging post-operative analgesia (see Lidocaine).

Aldosterone antagonists

CLINICAL PHARMACOLOGY

Common indications	❶ **Ascites and oedema due to liver cirrhosis:** spironolactone is the first-line diuretic. ❷ **Chronic heart failure:** of at least moderate severity or arising within 1 month of a myocardial infarction, usually as an addition to a β-blocker and an ACE inhibitor/angiotensin receptor blocker. ❸ **Primary hyperaldosteronism:** for patients awaiting surgery or for whom surgery is not an option.
Mechanisms of action	Aldosterone is a mineralocorticoid that is produced in the adrenal cortex. It acts on mineralocorticoid receptors in the distal tubules of the kidney to increase the activity of luminal epithelial sodium (Na^+) channels (ENaC). This increases the reabsorption of sodium and water, elevating blood pressure, with a corresponding increase in potassium excretion. Aldosterone antagonists inhibit the effect of aldosterone by **competitively binding to the aldosterone receptor.** This increases sodium and water *excretion* and potassium *retention*. Their effect is greatest when circulating aldosterone is increased, e.g. in primary hyperaldosteronism or cirrhosis.
Important adverse effects	An important adverse effect of aldosterone antagonists is **hyperkalaemia,** which can lead to muscle weakness, arrhythmias and even cardiac arrest. Spironolactone causes **gynaecomastia,** which can have a significant impact on patient adherence (see Communication). Eplerenone is less likely to cause endocrine side effects. Aldosterone antagonists can cause liver impairment and jaundice and are a cause of Stevens–Johnson syndrome (a T-cell-mediated hypersensitivity reaction) that causes a bullous skin eruption.
Warnings	Aldosterone antagonists are contraindicated in patients with ✖**severe renal impairment, ✖hyperkalaemia** and ✖**Addison's disease** (who are aldosterone deficient). Aldosterone antagonists can cross the placenta during pregnancy and appear in breast milk so should be avoided where possible in ▲**pregnant or lactating women.**
Important interactions	The combination of an aldosterone antagonist with other ▲**potassium-elevating drugs,** including ▲ACE inhibitors and ▲ARBs, increases the risk of hyperkalaemia. Nevertheless, when supported by appropriate monitoring, this may be a beneficial combination in the context of heart failure. Aldosterone antagonists should not be combined with ✖potassium supplements except in specialist practice.

spironolactone, eplerenone

PRACTICAL PRESCRIBING

Prescription	Aldosterone antagonists are only available as oral preparations. Spironolactone is used for all indications, whereas eplerenone is licensed for the treatment of heart failure only. Aldosterone antagonists should be prescribed for regular administration, generally as a single daily dose. You should tailor the dose to the specific indication as, for example, much higher doses are used to treat ascites secondary to cirrhosis than are used in heart failure. A typical starting dose of spironolactone is 100 mg daily for ascites compared with 25 mg daily for heart failure. Spironolactone is also available as a combined preparation with a thiazide or loop diuretic.
Administration	Spironolactone should generally be taken with food.
Communication	When starting treatment with spironolactone, particularly in high doses, it is important to warn men about the possibility of **growth and tenderness of tissue under the nipples** and **impotence.** Reassure them that such effects are benign and reversible, but acknowledge that they may be uncomfortable and embarrassing. Ask patients to return if they have troublesome side effects, as these may respond to dose reduction. Advise all patients that aldosterone antagonists can cause their potassium level to rise and reinforce the importance of attending for blood tests.
Monitoring	**Efficacy** should be monitored by patient report of symptoms and clinical findings, e.g. reduction in ascites, oedema and/or blood pressure. **Safety** should be monitored by checking renal function and serum potassium concentration due to the risk of renal impairment and hyperkalaemia.
Cost	Spironolactone and eplerenone are available in non-proprietary form and cost less than £10 per month.

Clinical tip—Spironolactone is a relatively weak diuretic that takes several days to start having an effect. It is therefore usually prescribed in combination with a loop or thiazide diuretic, where it both counteracts potassium wasting and potentiates the diuretic effect. For example, in the treatment of ascites due to chronic liver failure, spironolactone and furosemide are generally used together in a ratio of about 5:1 (e.g. spironolactone 200 mg with furosemide 40 mg).

Alginates and antacids

CLINICAL PHARMACOLOGY

Common indications	❶ **Gastro-oesophageal reflux disease (GORD):** for symptomatic relief of heartburn. ❷ **Dyspepsia:** for short-term relief of indigestion.
Mechanisms of action	These drugs are most often taken as compound preparations containing an alginate with one or more antacids, such as sodium bicarbonate, calcium carbonate, magnesium or aluminium salts. *Antacids* work by **buffering** stomach acids. *Alginates* act to increase the **viscosity** of the stomach contents, which reduces the reflux of stomach acid into the oesophagus. After reacting with stomach acid they form a floating **'raft',** which separates the gastric contents from the gastro-oesophageal junction to prevent mucosal damage. There is some evidence to suggest they also inhibit pepsin production. Antacids alone (usually aluminium or magnesium compounds) can be used for the short-term relief of dyspepsia.
Important adverse effects	Compound alginates cause few side effects, which vary depending on their constituents and the dose taken. Magnesium salts can cause **diarrhoea,** whereas aluminium salts can cause **constipation.**
Warnings	Compound alginates are well tolerated and are safe in pregnancy. Paediatric formulations are safe for use in infants, but compound alginates should not be given in combination with ▲**thickened milk preparations** as they can lead to excessively thick stomach contents that cause bloating and abdominal discomfort. Sodium- and potassium-containing preparations should be used with caution in patients with fluid overload or hyperkalaemia (e.g. ▲**renal failure**). Some preparations contain sucrose, which can worsen hyperglycaemia in people with diabetes mellitus.
Important interactions	The divalent cations in compound alginates can bind to other drugs, reducing their absorption. Antacids can reduce serum concentrations of many drugs, so doses should be separated by 2 hours. This applies to <u>ACE inhibitors</u>, some antibiotics (e.g. <u>cephalosporins</u>, <u>ciprofloxacin</u> and <u>tetracyclines</u>), <u>bisphosphonates</u>, <u>digoxin</u>, <u>levothyroxine</u> and <u>proton pump inhibitors (PPIs)</u>. By increasing the alkalinity of urine, antacids can increase the excretion of <u>aspirin</u> and lithium.

PRACTICAL PRESCRIBING

Prescription	Compound alginates are available as oral suspensions or chewable tablets. They may be prescribed by brand name, as they are proprietary compound products without approved compound generic names. They are usually prescribed on an as-required basis for symptomatic relief. Check the constituents of the brand chosen, particularly if prescribing for patients with renal impairment or diabetes mellitus.
Administration	They should be taken following meals, before bedtime and/or when symptoms occur. For infants, oral powder can be mixed with feeds or water.
Communication	Explain to patients that the medicine should relieve the symptoms of heartburn and acid indigestion within about 20 minutes and for several hours afterwards. However, advise them that this is only a temporary measure. Discuss **lifestyle measures** that can be taken to reduce reflux, such as eating smaller meals more often, identifying and avoiding food and drink triggers, stopping smoking and raising the head of the bed. Warn patients to return for review if symptoms persist. Advise patients to take compound alginates after mealtimes and before bed. Advise them to **leave a gap of at least 2 hours** between these medicines and other drugs that they may interact with (see Interactions).
Monitoring	Symptomatic responses should be monitored by patients and their healthcare practitioners. If there are persistent symptoms or 'red flags', such as bleeding, vomiting, dysphagia and weight loss, further investigation and specialist review are required.
Cost	Compound alginates are inexpensive. They can be purchased over the counter. If prescribing, you should prescribe the lowest-cost brand available.

Clinical tip—Compound alginates are a useful treatment in the armamentarium of the paediatrician. Around 10–20% of children suffer from GORD, and compound alginates have been shown to reduce frequency of symptoms.

Allopurinol

CLINICAL PHARMACOLOGY

Common indications	❶ To prevent recurrent attacks of **gout.** ❷ To prevent uric acid and calcium oxalate **renal stones.** ❸ To prevent **hyperuricaemia** and **tumour lysis syndrome** associated with chemotherapy.
Mechanisms of action	Allopurinol is a **xanthine oxidase inhibitor**. Xanthine oxidase metabolises xanthine (produced from purines) to uric acid. Inhibition of xanthine oxidase lowers plasma uric acid concentrations and reduces precipitation of uric acid in the joints or kidneys.
Important adverse effects	Allopurinol is generally well tolerated. However, starting allopurinol can **trigger or worsen an acute attack of gout,** possibly through effects on preformed crystals. The risk of triggering an attack may be reduced by co-prescription of an NSAID or colchicine in the initiation phase (see Prescription). The most common side effect is a **skin rash,** which may be mild or may indicate a more serious hypersensitivity reaction such as **Stevens–Johnson syndrome** or **toxic epidermal necrolysis. Allopurinol hypersensitivity syndrome** is a rare, life-threatening reaction to allopurinol that can include fever, eosinophilia, lymphadenopathy and involvement of other organs, such as the liver and skin.
Warnings	Allopurinol should not be started during ✖**acute attacks of gout,** but can be continued if a patient is already established on it, to avoid sudden fluctuations in serum uric acid levels. ✖**Recurrent skin rash** or signs of more ✖**severe hypersensitivity** to allopurinol are contraindications to therapy. Allopurinol is metabolised in the liver and excreted by the kidney. The dose should therefore be reduced in patients with severe ▲**renal impairment** or ▲**hepatic impairment.**
Important interactions	The active metabolite (mercaptopurine) of the pro-drug ▲azathioprine is metabolised by xanthine oxidase. Concurrent administration increases the risk of toxicity. Co-prescription of allopurinol with ▲ACE inhibitors or thiazides increases the risk of hypersensitivity reactions, and with amoxicillin increases the risk of skin rash.

allopurinol

PRACTICAL PRESCRIBING

Prescription	Allopurinol is taken orally. Start at a low dose (e.g. 100 mg daily) and titrate up according to serum uric acid concentrations to usual maintenance of 200–600 mg daily in 1–2 divided doses. When starting allopurinol **for gout,** an NSAID (e.g. naproxen 250 mg 12-hrly) or colchicine treatment should also be prescribed and continued for at least a month after serum uric acid levels return to normal to avoid triggering an acute attack. Although allopurinol should not be started during an acute attack of gout, patients who are already on it should continue to take it. Where allopurinol is used **as part of cancer treatment,** it should be commenced before chemotherapy.
Administration	Allopurinol should be taken after meals and patients should be encouraged to maintain good hydration with fluid intake of 2–3 litres daily.
Communication	Advise patients that the purpose of treatment is to **reduce attacks of gout** (or formation of kidney stones). Warn patients to **seek medical advice if they develop a rash.** Explain that this is usually mild and goes away on stopping the drug, but it can be a sign of a more serious allergy. Advise patients not to stop allopurinol if they get an acute attack of gout, as this could make the attack worse.
Monitoring	Serum uric acid concentrations should be checked 4 weeks after initiating allopurinol or after a change in dose. You should aim to lower uric acid concentrations to less than 300 μmol/L where possible, by increasing the dose of allopurinol as needed. Allopurinol treatment should be **stopped if a rash develops.** For mild skin rashes, treatment can be reintroduced cautiously once the rash resolves. Recurrence of the rash or signs of more severe hypersensitivity to allopurinol are contraindications to further therapy.
Cost	Allopurinol is available in a non-proprietary form and is inexpensive.

Clinical tip—Treatment with thiazide or loop diuretics increases serum uric acid concentrations and can cause gout. Low-dose aspirin inhibits renal excretion of uric acid and can trigger acute attacks of gout. Always consider drug-induced gout as a cause of new-onset joint pain in patients taking these medicines.

Aminosalicylates

CLINICAL PHARMACOLOGY

Common indications	❶ Mesalazine is used first-line in the treatment of mild-moderate **ulcerative colitis (UC);** sulfasalazine is an alternative but has largely been replaced by mesalazine for this indication. Corticosteroids are also used. ❷ Sulfasalazine is one of several options for the management of **rheumatoid arthritis,** in which it is used as a disease-modifying antirheumatic drug (DMARD), usually as part of combination therapy.
Mechanisms of action	In ulcerative colitis, mesalazine and sulfasalazine both exert their therapeutic effects by releasing **5-aminosalicylic acid (5-ASA).** The precise mechanism of action of 5-ASA is unknown, but it has both **antiinflammatory and immunosuppressive effects,** and appears to act topically on the gut rather than systemically. For this reason, 5-ASA preparations are designed to delay delivery of the active ingredient to the colon. The oral form of mesalazine comprises a tablet with a coating that resists gastric breakdown, instead releasing 5-ASA further down the gut. Sulfasalazine consists of a molecule of 5-ASA linked to sulfapyridine. In the colon, bacterial enzymes break this link and release the two molecules. Sulfapyridine does not contribute to its therapeutic effect in ulcerative colitis, but it does cause side effects, and for this reason it has largely been replaced by mesalazine for this indication. By contrast, sulfapyridine is probably the active component of sulfasalazine in rheumatoid arthritis, though its mechanism is unclear. Mesalazine has no role in rheumatoid arthritis.
Important adverse effects	Mesalazine generally causes fewer side effects than sulfasalazine. Most commonly, these are **gastrointestinal upset** (e.g. nausea, dyspepsia) and **headache.** Both drugs can cause rare but serious blood abnormalities (e.g. **leucopenia, thrombocytopenia**) and **renal impairment.** In men, sulfasalazine may induce a reversible decrease in the number of sperm (**oligospermia**). It can also cause a **serious hypersensitivity reaction,** comprising fever, rash and liver abnormalities.
Warnings	Mesalazine and sulfasalazine are salicylates, like aspirin. Patients who have ✖**aspirin hypersensitivity** should not take these drugs.
Important interactions	Mesalazine tablets with a pH-sensitive coating (e.g. Asacol® MR) may interact with drugs that alter gut pH. For example, PPIs increase gastric pH and so may cause the coating to be broken down prematurely. Lactulose lowers stool pH and may prevent 5-ASA release in the colon.

PRACTICAL PRESCRIBING

Prescription	In patients with mild-moderate rectal or rectosigmoid **ulcerative colitis,** a mesalazine enema or suppository is generally recommended in the first instance. In an acute attack, this is taken once or 12-hrly for 4–6 weeks to induce remission. If the disease is more proximal, or the patient would prefer not to take the drug rectally, an oral formulation may be used. Drug choice (and therefore dosage regimen) is likely to be dictated by local policies. Decisions regarding choice of therapy in **rheumatoid arthritis** should be taken by a specialist.
Administration	The Asacol® foam enema, a common mesalazine preparation, requires thorough mixing before administration, by shaking the can vigorously for two 15-second periods. An applicator is then attached, and this is inserted as far as possible into the rectum. The can must be upside-down when the dome is pressed and released to deliver a dose. The applicator should then be removed and disposed of cleanly, and the patient should wash their hands. For suppositories, patients should empty their bowels first if necessary, insert the suppository, and then avoid opening their bowels for at least an hour if possible. Tablet forms of mesalazine should be swallowed whole, not chewed or crushed.
Communication	Explain to patients the aim of treatment as appropriate for the indication. Ensure they understand how to take the medicine, particularly if it is a rectal preparation (see Administration and Clinical tip). In patients taking the drug orally, ask them to report any unexplained bleeding, bruising, or infective symptoms to a doctor as soon as possible, since this could be a sign of a blood count abnormality that may require urgent assessment.
Monitoring	The best guide to **efficacy** in ulcerative colitis is the patient's symptoms. In rheumatoid arthritis, this may be supplemented by disease activity scores and measurement of acute phase reactant concentrations (C-reactive protein, erythrocyte sedimentation rate). For **safety,** renal function should be checked in patients receiving oral mesalazine, and full blood count (FBC) and liver profile monitored in patients receiving sulfasalazine.
Cost	Mesalazine is available in several branded forms which vary in price. Choice is likely to be dictated by local formulary agreements.

Clinical tip—Administration of the rectal forms of mesalazine is not easy, particularly for patients with active proctitis. Give patients written advice and ensure they understand this. For those using a foam enema, consider supplying (or advising them to obtain) a water-based lubricant to facilitate insertion of the applicator. Similarly, insertion of suppositories can be made easier by greasing their tip with a little petroleum jelly.

Amiodarone

CLINICAL PHARMACOLOGY

Common indications	Amiodarone is used in a wide range of **tachyarrhythmias,** including atrial fibrillation (AF), atrial flutter, supraventricular tachycardia (SVT), ventricular tachycardia (VT) and refractory ventricular fibrillation (VF). It is generally used only when other therapeutic options (drugs or electrical cardioversion) are ineffective or inappropriate.
Mechanisms of action	Amiodarone has many effects on myocardial cells, including **blockade of sodium, calcium and potassium channels,** and **antagonism of α- and β-adrenergic receptors.** These effects reduce spontaneous depolarisation (automaticity), slow conduction velocity and increase resistance to depolarisation (refractoriness), including in the atrioventricular (AV) node. By interfering with AV node conduction, amiodarone reduces the ventricular rate in AF and atrial flutter. Through its other effects, it may also increase the chance of conversion to, and maintenance of, sinus rhythm. In SVT involving a self-perpetuating ('re-entry') circuit that includes the AV node, amiodarone may break the circuit and restore sinus rhythm. Amiodarone's effects in suppressing spontaneous depolarisations make it an option for both treatment and prevention of VT, and for improving the chance of successful defibrillation in refractory VF.
Important adverse effects	In acute use, compared with other antiarrhythmic drugs, amiodarone causes relatively little myocardial depression. It can cause **hypotension** during IV infusion, although this is probably an effect of the solvent with which it is formulated, rather than the drug itself. When taken chronically, amiodarone has many side effects, several of which are serious. These include effects on the lungs (**pneumonitis**), heart (**bradycardia, AV block**), liver (**hepatitis**) and skin (**photosensitivity** and **grey discolouration**). Due to its iodine content (am*IOD*arone) and structural similarities to thyroid hormone, it may cause **thyroid abnormalities,** including hypo- and hyperthyroidism. Amiodarone has an extremely long half-life. After discontinuation, it may take months to be completely eliminated.
Warnings	Amiodarone is a potentially dangerous drug that should be used only when the risk–benefit balance justifies this. It should generally be avoided in patients with ▲**severe hypotension,** ▲**heart block** and ▲**active thyroid disease.**
Important interactions	Amiodarone interacts with many drugs – too many to list here. Notably, it increases plasma concentrations of ▲digoxin, ▲diltiazem and ▲verapamil. This may increase the risk of bradycardia, AV block and heart failure. The doses of these drugs should be halved if amiodarone is started.

PRACTICAL PRESCRIBING

Prescription	A decision to prescribe amiodarone, whether for acute or long-term use, always requires senior involvement and should not be taken independently by a foundation doctor. One exception is in **cardiac arrest,** in which it is given for VF or pulseless VT immediately after the third shock in the Advanced Life Support (ALS) algorithm. The dose is 300 mg IV, followed by 20 mL of 0.9% sodium chloride or 5% glucose as a flush. In this instance, it should be administered first and prescribed later.
Administration	In cardiac arrest, amiodarone is given as a bolus injection. It is often provided in a pre-filled syringe to facilitate easy administration. It should be given through the 'best' IV cannula available. Outside cardiac arrests, if continuous or repeated IV infusions are anticipated, these should be given via a **central line.** This is because peripheral IV administration can cause significant phlebitis.
Communication	As appropriate, explain to patients that you are offering a treatment aimed at correcting their fast or irregular heart rhythm. Explain that it has several important and potentially serious side effects, and it is being used only because their condition is serious and no other treatments are suitable or effective. In long-term use, ask the patient to report any symptoms of breathlessness, persistent cough, jaundice, restlessness, weight loss, tiredness or weight gain. Advise patients not to drink grapefruit juice, as this can increase the risk of side effects, and to minimise exposure of their skin to direct sunlight due to the risk of photosensitivity.
Monitoring	The **efficacy** of treatment is best judged by monitoring the patient's heart rate and rhythm. For **safety,** IV infusion should be accompanied by continuous cardiac monitoring. In long-term therapy, baseline tests should include renal, liver and thyroid profiles, and a chest X-ray. The liver and thyroid profiles should then be repeated 6-monthly.
Cost	Amiodarone is inexpensive.

Clinical tip—While foundation doctors should never initiate amiodarone independently, they may need to re-write prescriptions for ongoing therapy. Always confirm whether it is appropriate to continue amiodarone and, if you are in any doubt, consult a senior colleague. When writing the prescription, do not blindly copy the preceding dose. This may have been a **loading dose** (which seeks to achieve therapeutic concentrations rapidly), whereas you probably need to prescribe a **maintenance dose.** Again, never hesitate to seek advice. If you find yourself prescribing amiodarone on a discharge prescription, always confirm with a senior colleague whether this is appropriate. If the acute problems have resolved, it may be possible to stop it.

Angiotensin-converting enzyme (ACE) inhibitors

CLINICAL PHARMACOLOGY

Common indications	❶ **Hypertension:** for the first- or second-line treatment of hypertension, to reduce the risk of stroke, myocardial infarction and death from cardiovascular disease. ❷ **Chronic heart failure:** for the first-line treatment of all grades of heart failure, to improve symptoms and prognosis. ❸ **Ischaemic heart disease:** to reduce the risk of subsequent cardiovascular events such as myocardial infarction and stroke. ❹ **Diabetic nephropathy** and **chronic kidney disease (CKD) with proteinuria:** to reduce proteinuria and progression of nephropathy.
Mechanisms of action	ACE inhibitors block the action of ACE, to **prevent the conversion of angiotensin I to angiotensin II.** Angiotensin II is a vasoconstrictor and stimulates aldosterone secretion. Blocking its action reduces peripheral vascular resistance (afterload), which lowers blood pressure (BP). It particularly dilates the efferent glomerular arteriole, which reduces intraglomerular pressure and slows the progression of CKD. Reducing the aldosterone level promotes sodium and water excretion. This can help to reduce venous return (preload), which has a beneficial effect in heart failure.
Important adverse effects	Common side effects include **hypotension** (particularly after the **first dose**), **persistent dry cough** (due to increased levels of bradykinin, which is usually inactivated by ACE) and **hyperkalaemia** (because a lower aldosterone level promotes potassium retention). They can cause or worsen **renal failure.** This is particularly relevant in patients with renal artery stenosis, who rely on constriction of the efferent glomerular arteriole to maintain glomerular filtration. If detected early, these adverse effects are usually reversible on stopping the drug. Rare but important idiosyncratic side effects of ACE inhibitors include **angioedema** and other **anaphylactoid reactions.**
Warnings	ACE inhibitors should be avoided in patients with ✖**renal artery stenosis** or ✖**acute kidney injury;** in women who are, or could become, ▲**pregnant;** and those who are ▲**breastfeeding.** Although ACE inhibition is potentially valuable in some forms of ▲**CKD,** lower doses should be used and the effect on renal function monitored closely.
Important interactions	Due to the risk of hyperkalaemia, avoid prescribing ACE inhibitors with other ▲**potassium-elevating drugs,** including potassium supplements and potassium-sparing diuretics, except under specialist advice for advanced heart failure. In combination with diuretics they may be associated with profound first-dose hypotension. The combination of an ▲NSAID and an ACE inhibitor particularly increases the risk of nephrotoxicity.

PRACTICAL PRESCRIBING

Prescription	ACE inhibitors are taken orally. The starting dose varies according to the indication, generally being lower in heart failure than in other indications. A common choice is ramipril 1.25 mg daily in heart failure or nephropathy, or 2.5 mg daily in most other indications. This is **titrated up** to a maximum of 10 mg daily over a period of weeks, according to the patient's response, side effects and renal function.
Administration	ACE inhibitors can be taken with or without food. It is best to take the **first dose before bed** to reduce symptomatic hypotension.
Communication	Explain to patients that you are offering treatment with a medicine to improve blood pressure and reduce strain on their heart. Advise patients about common side effects such as a **dry cough,** and about the possibility of **dizziness** as a result of low blood pressure, particularly after the first dose. Mention that, very rarely, this medicine can cause effects similar to severe **allergic reactions;** they should stop taking it and seek urgent medical advice if they develop facial swelling or stomach pains. Make sure they understand the need for **blood test monitoring**, explaining that ACE inhibitors can interfere with their kidney function and upset potassium balance. Advise them to **avoid** taking over-the-counter **antiinflammatories** (e.g. ibuprofen) due to the risk of kidney damage.
Monitoring	Monitor **efficacy** clinically: for example, reduced **symptoms** of breathlessness in heart failure or improved **blood pressure** control in hypertension. For **safety,** check **electrolytes** and **renal function** before starting treatment. Repeat these 1–2 weeks into treatment and after increasing the dose. Biochemical changes can be tolerated provided they are within certain limits. In the absence of other causes, the ACE inhibitor should be stopped if the serum creatinine concentration rises more than 30% or the estimated glomerular filtration rate (eGFR) falls more than 25%. If serum potassium rises above 5.0 mmol/L, stop other potassium-elevating and nephrotoxic drugs (see Important interactions). If, despite this, it remains above 5.0 mmol/L, reduce the dose of ACE inhibitor. If it exceeds 6.0 mmol/L, stop the ACE inhibitor and seek expert advice.
Cost	Most ACE inhibitors are available as non-proprietary products, which are inexpensive. There is generally no reason to use a branded product, which can be significantly more expensive.

Clinical tip— Profound hypotension may occur following the first dose of an ACE inhibitor, particularly in patients on other diuretics, such as loop diuretics, and those with restricted salt and water intake. You should start at a low dose and titrate up gradually. In addition, it can sometimes be advisable to omit the diuretic dose that precedes the first dose of the ACE inhibitor.

Angiotensin receptor blockers

CLINICAL PHARMACOLOGY

Common indications	Angiotensin receptor blockers (ARBs) are generally used when ACE inhibitors are not tolerated due to cough. The indications are the same: ❶ **Hypertension:** for the first- or second-line treatment of hypertension, to reduce the risk of stroke, myocardial infarction and death from cardiovascular disease. ❷ **Chronic heart failure:** for the first-line treatment of all grades of heart failure, to improve symptoms and prognosis. ❸ **Ischaemic heart disease:** to reduce the risk of subsequent cardiovascular events such as myocardial infarction and stroke. ❹ **Diabetic nephropathy** and **chronic kidney disease (CKD) with proteinuria:** to reduce proteinuria and progression of nephropathy.
Mechanisms of action	ARBs have similar effects to ACE inhibitors, but instead of inhibiting the conversion of angiotensin I to angiotensin II, ARBs **block the action of angiotensin II on the angiotensin type 1 (AT₁) receptor.** Angiotensin II is a vasoconstrictor and stimulates aldosterone secretion. Blocking its action reduces peripheral vascular resistance (afterload), which lowers blood pressure. It particularly dilates the efferent glomerular arteriole, which reduces intraglomerular pressure and slows the progression of CKD. Reducing the aldosterone level promotes sodium and water excretion. This can help to reduce venous return (preload), which has a beneficial effect in heart failure.
Important adverse effects	ARBs can cause **hypotension** (particularly after the **first dose**), **hyperkalaemia** and **renal failure.** The mechanism is the same as for ACE inhibitors. Patients most at risk of renal failure are those with renal artery stenosis, who rely on constriction of the efferent glomerular arteriole to maintain glomerular filtration. Unlike ACE inhibitors, ARBs are less likely to cause a dry cough, as they do not inhibit ACE, and therefore do not affect bradykinin metabolism. For the same reason, they are less likely to cause angioedema.
Warnings	ARBs should be avoided in patients with ✖**renal artery stenosis** or ✖**acute kidney injury;** in women who are, or could become, ▲**pregnant;** and those who are ▲**breastfeeding.** Although ARB therapy is potentially valuable in some forms of ▲**CKD,** lower doses should be used and the effect on renal function monitored closely.
Important interactions	Due to the risk of hyperkalaemia, avoid prescribing ARBs with other ▲**potassium-elevating drugs,** including potassium supplements and potassium-sparing diuretics, except under specialist advice for advanced heart failure. In combination with other diuretics they may be associated with profound first-dose hypotension. The combination of NSAIDs with ARBs increases the risk of nephrotoxicity

losartan, candesartan, irbesartan

PRACTICAL PRESCRIBING

Prescription	ARBs are taken **orally.** The starting dose varies according to the indication, generally being lower in heart failure than in other indications. A common choice is losartan 12.5 mg daily in heart failure or 50 mg daily in other indications. This is **titrated up** to the maximum recommended dose over a period of weeks, according to the patient's response, side effects and renal function.
Administration	ARBs can be taken with or without food. It is best to take **the first dose before bed** to reduce symptomatic hypotension.
Communication	Explain to patients that you are offering treatment with a medicine to improve their blood pressure and reduce strain on their heart. If the patient has previously been unable to tolerate an ACE inhibitor due to cough, explain that the new treatment does not cause this side effect. Advise patients about the possibility of **dizziness** due to low blood pressure, particularly after the first dose. Make sure they understand the need for **blood test monitoring,** explaining that ARBs can interfere with their kidney function and upset potassium balance. Advise them to **avoid taking** over-the-counter anti-inflammatories (e.g. ibuprofen) due to the risk of kidney damage.
Monitoring	Monitor **efficacy** clinically: for example, reduced **symptoms** of breathlessness in heart failure or improved **blood pressure** control in hypertension. For **safety,** check **electrolytes** and **renal function** before starting treatment. Repeat this 1–2 weeks into treatment and after increasing the dose. Biochemical changes can be tolerated provided they are within certain limits. In the absence of other causes, the ARB should be stopped if the serum creatinine concentration rises more than 30% or the eGFR falls more than 25%. If serum potassium rises above 5.0 mmol/L, stop other potassium-elevating and nephrotoxic drugs (see Important interactions). If, despite this, it remains above 5.0 mmol/L, reduce the dose of the ARB. If it exceeds 6.0 mmol/L, stop the ARB and seek expert advice.
Cost	Losartan is available in non-proprietary form and is inexpensive; the equivalent brand name form costs about twice as much. There is no compelling reason to choose a branded product over a non-proprietary one.

Clinical tip—The incidence of angioedema related to ACE inhibitor treatment is five times higher (about 1%) in black people of African or Caribbean origin. The exact mechanism by which ACE inhibitors lead to angioedema is not completely understood but is thought to relate to altered bradykinin metabolism. ARBs do not affect levels of bradykinin and are less likely to cause angioedema. ARBs, therefore may be preferable to ACE inhibitors in this group.

Antidepressants, selective serotonin reuptake inhibitors

CLINICAL PHARMACOLOGY

Common indications	❶ As first-line treatment for **moderate-to-severe depression,** and in **mild depression** if psychological treatments alone are insufficient. ❷ **Panic disorder.** ❸ **Obsessive compulsive disorder.**
Mechanisms of action	Selective serotonin reuptake inhibitors (SSRIs) preferentially **inhibit neuronal reuptake of 5-HT** from the synaptic cleft, thereby increasing its availability for neurotransmission. This appears to be the mechanism by which SSRIs improve mood and physical symptoms in depression and relieve symptoms of panic and obsessive disorders. SSRIs differ from <u>tricyclic antidepressants</u> in that they do not inhibit noradrenaline uptake and cause less blockade of other receptors. The efficacy of the two drug classes in the treatment of depression is similar. However, SSRIs are generally preferred as they have fewer adverse effects and are less dangerous in overdose.
Important adverse effects	Common adverse effects include **GI upset,** changes in **appetite** and **weight** (loss or gain), and **hypersensitivity** reactions, including skin rash. **Hyponatraemia** is an important adverse effect, particularly in the elderly, and may present with confusion and reduced consciousness. **Suicidal thoughts and behaviour** may be increased in patients on SSRIs. They may **lower the seizure threshold** (the evidence for this is conflicting). Some (e.g. citalopram) can **prolong the QT interval,** predisposing to arrhythmias. SSRIs also increase the risk of **bleeding.** At high doses, in overdose, or in combination with other **serotonergic drugs** (e.g. other antidepressants, <u>tramadol</u>), SSRIs can cause **serotonin syndrome.** This triad of autonomic hyperactivity, altered mental state and neuromuscular excitation usually responds to treatment withdrawal and supportive therapy. **Sudden withdrawal** of SSRIs can cause GI upset, neurological and influenza-like symptoms and sleep disturbance.
Warnings	Caution is required in patients at heightened risk of adverse effects, including in ▲**epilepsy** and ▲**peptic ulcer disease.** In ▲**young people,** SSRIs have poor efficacy and are associated with an increased risk of self-harm and suicidal thoughts, so should only be prescribed by specialists. As SSRIs are metabolised by the liver, dose reduction may be required in people with ▲**hepatic impairment.**
Important interactions	SSRIs should not be given with ✖**monoamine oxidase inhibitors** and other ▲**serotonergic drugs** (e.g. <u>tramadol</u>), as together they may precipitate serotonin syndrome. Gastroprotection should be considered for patients taking SSRIs with <u>aspirin</u> or <u>NSAIDs</u>, due to an increased risk of bleeding. Bleeding risk is also increased where SSRIs are co-prescribed with <u>anticoagulants</u>. They should not be combined with other ▲**drugs that prolong the QT interval,** such as <u>antipsychotics</u>.

citalopram, fluoxetine, sertraline, escitalopram

PRACTICAL PRESCRIBING

Prescription	SSRIs are prescribed for oral administration. They should be started at a low dose to be taken regularly, usually once a day. A typical starting prescription might be for citalopram 20 mg daily. The dose is increased as necessary according to response. Lower starting and maximum doses are prescribed for elderly patients.
Administration	Citalopram is available as tablets and as oral drops, which can be mixed with water or other drinks. As the oral drops have greater bioavailability than tablets, they are prescribed at different doses. For example, one 20 mg citalopram tablet is equivalent to 16 mg citalopram in four oral drops.
Communication	Advise patients that treatment should **improve symptoms** over a few weeks, particularly sleep and appetite. Discuss referring them for **psychological therapy,** which may offer more long-term benefits than drug treatment. Explain that they should carry on with drug treatment for **at least 6 months** after they feel better to stop the depression from coming back (2 years for recurrent depression). Warn them **not to stop treatment suddenly** as this may cause a tummy upset, flu-like **withdrawal symptoms** and sleeplessness. When the time comes to stop treatment, they should reduce the dose slowly over at least 4 weeks (fluoxetine has the lowest risk of withdrawal symptoms). While patients may find some of the more common adverse effects unpleasant, they may tolerate them in favour of relieving depressive symptoms. Discussing at an early stage what side effects are expected may encourage patients to persist with treatment, at least until the full antidepressant effects are realised.
Monitoring	Symptoms should be reviewed 1–2 weeks after starting treatment and regularly thereafter. If no effect has been seen at 4 weeks, you should consider changing the dose or drug; otherwise, the dose should not be adjusted until after 6–8 weeks of therapy.
Cost	Most SSRIs are available in non-proprietary form and are inexpensive.

Clinical tip—Citalopram and sertraline appear to have fewer interactions than other SSRIs. You should therefore consider choosing these drugs when prescribing antidepressants for patients with multiple co-morbidities who are taking lots of other drugs.

Antidepressants, tricyclics and related drugs

CLINICAL PHARMACOLOGY

Common indications	❶ As second-line treatment for **moderate-to-severe depression** where first-line <u>selective serotonin reuptake inhibitors</u> (SSRIs) are ineffective. ❷ As a treatment option for **neuropathic pain,** although they are not licensed for this indication.
Mechanisms of action	Tricyclic antidepressants **inhibit neuronal reuptake of 5-HT and noradrenaline** from the synaptic cleft, thereby increasing their availability for neurotransmission. This appears to be the mechanism by which they improve mood and physical symptoms in moderate-to-severe (but not mild) depression and probably accounts for their effect in modifying neuropathic pain. Tricyclic antidepressants also **block a wide array of receptors,** including muscarinic, histamine (H$_1$), α-adrenergic (α$_1$ and α$_2$) and dopamine (D$_2$) receptors. This accounts for the extensive adverse-effects profile that limits their clinical utility.
Important adverse effects	Blockade of **antimuscarinic** receptors causes dry mouth, constipation, urinary retention and blurred vision. Blockade of H$_1$- and α$_1$-receptors causes **sedation** and **hypotension.** Cardiac adverse effects (multiple mechanisms) include **arrhythmias** and **ECG changes** (including prolongation of the QT and QRS durations). In the brain, more serious effects include **convulsions, hallucinations** and **mania.** Blockade of dopamine receptors can cause **breast changes** and **sexual dysfunction** and rarely causes **extrapyramidal symptoms** (tremor and dyskinesia). Tricyclic antidepressants are **dangerous in overdose,** causing severe hypotension, arrhythmias, convulsions, coma and respiratory failure, which can be fatal. **Sudden withdrawal** of tricyclic antidepressants can cause gastrointestinal upset, neurological and influenza-like symptoms and sleep disturbance.
Warnings	Caution is required in patients at heightened risk of adverse effects, including ▲**elderly** patients, and those with ▲**epilepsy** or ▲**cardiovascular disease.** People with ▲**prostatic hypertrophy** or ▲**glaucoma,** and those prone to ▲**constipation,** may have their condition worsened by the drugs' antimuscarinic effects.
Important interactions	Tricyclic antidepressants should not be given with ✖**monoamine oxidase inhibitors** as both drug classes increase 5-HT and noradrenaline levels at the synapse and together they can precipitate hypertension and hyperthermia or serotonin syndrome (see <u>Antidepressants, selective serotonin reuptake inhibitors</u>). Tricyclic antidepressants can augment antimuscarinic, sedative or hypotensive adverse effects of other drugs.

PRACTICAL PRESCRIBING

Prescription	**Depression:** tricyclic antidepressants have similar efficacy to other classes of antidepressant (e.g. SSRIs), but have more adverse effects and are more dangerous in overdose. They are therefore reserved for patients in whom SSRIs are ineffective and should only be prescribed by a healthcare professional with relevant mental health training. In fact, a switch to a second SSRI is often trialled *before* considering a switch to tricyclic antidepressants where initial SSRI treatment is ineffective. Lofepramine appears to have fewer side effects, including sedation, than other tricyclics.
	Neuropathic pain: amitriptyline is used at a much lower dose (e.g. starting dose 10 mg at night) for this indication than for depression (where starting dose is 75 mg daily).
Administration	Tricyclic antidepressants are available as tablets and in oral solution. When prescribing for depression, particularly for people who are at risk of suicide, it is good practice to **supply a small quantity** of medication at a time (e.g. enough for 2 weeks) to reduce the risk of serious overdose.
Communication	Advise patients that treatment will **improve symptoms** over a few weeks, particularly sleep and appetite. Discuss referring them for **psychological therapy,** which may offer more long-term benefits than drug treatment. Explain that they should carry on with drug treatment for **at least 6 months** after they feel better to stop the depression from coming back (2 years for recurrent depression). Warn them **not to stop treatment suddenly** as this may cause flu-like **withdrawal symptoms** and sleeplessness. When the time comes to stop treatment, they should reduce the dose slowly over at least 4 weeks. While patients may find some of the more common side effects unpleasant, they may tolerate them in favour of relieving depressive symptoms. Discussing at an early stage what side effects are expected may encourage patients to persist with treatment, at least until the full antidepressant effects are realised.
Monitoring	Symptoms should be reviewed 1–2 weeks after starting treatment and regularly thereafter. If no effect has been seen at 4 weeks, you should consider changing the dose or drug; otherwise, the dose should not be adjusted until after 6–8 weeks of therapy.
Cost	Tricyclic antidepressants are available as non-proprietary preparations and are inexpensive.

Clinical tip—In our experience, patients admitted to hospital often have their antidepressants stopped abruptly, either because they are thought to be contributing to their presentation, or because they are overlooked. Take care not to do this, to avoid precipitating a withdrawal reaction.

Antidepressants, venlafaxine and mirtazapine

CLINICAL PHARMACOLOGY

Common indications	❶ As an option for treatment of **major depression** where first-line <u>selective serotonin reuptake inhibitors</u> (SSRIs) are ineffective or not tolerated. ❷ **Generalised anxiety disorder** (venlafaxine).
Mechanisms of action	*Venlafaxine* is a serotonin and noradrenaline reuptake inhibitor (SNRI), interfering with uptake of these neurotransmitters from the synaptic cleft. *Mirtazapine* is an antagonist of inhibitory pre-synaptic α_2-adrenoceptors. **Both drugs increase availability of monoamines for neurotransmission,** which appears to be the mechanism whereby they improve mood and physical symptoms in moderate-to-severe (but not mild) depression. Venlafaxine is a weaker antagonist of muscarinic and histamine (H_1) receptors than <u>tricyclic antidepressants</u>, whereas mirtazapine is a potent antagonist of histamine (H_1) but not muscarinic receptors. They therefore have fewer antimuscarinic side effects than tricyclic antidepressants, although mirtazapine commonly causes sedation.
Important adverse effects	Common adverse effects of both drugs include **gastrointestinal (GI) upset** (e.g. dry mouth, nausea, change in weight and diarrhoea or constipation) and **neurological effects** (e.g. headache, abnormal dreams, insomnia, confusion and convulsions). Less common but serious adverse effects include **hyponatraemia** and **serotonin syndrome** (see <u>Antidepressants, selective serotonin reuptake inhibitors</u>). **Suicidal thoughts and behaviour** may increase. Venlafaxine prolongs the QT interval and can increase the risk of ventricular arrhythmias. **Sudden drug withdrawal** can cause GI upset, neurological and influenza-like symptoms and sleep disturbance. Venlafaxine is associated with a greater risk of withdrawal effects than other antidepressants.
Warnings	As with many centrally acting medications, the ▲**elderly** are at particular risk of adverse effects. A dose reduction should be considered in people with ▲**hepatic** or ▲**renal impairment.** Venlafaxine should be used with caution (if at all) in patients at risk of ▲**arrhythmias** (e.g. due to ischaemic heart disease).
Important interactions	The combination of these drugs with drugs from other antidepressant classes can increase the risk of adverse effects (including serotonin syndrome, see <u>Antidepressants, selective serotonin reuptake inhibitors</u>) and should, in general, be avoided.

venlafaxine, mirtazapine

PRACTICAL PRESCRIBING

Prescription	Venlafaxine and mirtazapine are only available for oral administration. They should be prescribed only by healthcare professionals with expertise in mental health and used in conjunction with psychological therapies. As with other antidepressants, treatment is started at a low dose and titrated up according to response. Typical starting doses are venlafaxine 37.5 mg orally 12-hrly (titrated to a maximum of 375 mg daily) and mirtazapine 15 mg orally daily (titrated to a maximum of 45 mg daily).
Administration	Mirtazapine should be taken at night to minimise (or benefit from) its sedative effects.
Communication	Advise patients that treatment should **improve symptoms** over a few weeks, particularly sleep and appetite. Discuss referring them for **psychological therapy,** which may offer more long-term benefits than drug treatment. Explain that they should carry on with drug treatment for **at least 6 months** after they feel better to stop the depression from coming back (2 years for recurrent depression). Warn them **not to stop treatment suddenly** as this may cause flu-like **withdrawal symptoms** and sleeplessness. When the time comes to stop treatment, they should reduce the dose slowly over at least 4 weeks. Warn patients taking *mirtazapine* to seek medical advice for symptoms of infection, such as sore throat, so that a blood test can be taken to check for blood disorders. While patients may find some of the more common side effects unpleasant, they may tolerate them in favour of relieving depressive symptoms. Discussing at an early stage what side effects are expected may encourage patients to persist with treatment, at least until the full antidepressant effects are realised.
Monitoring	Symptoms should be reviewed 1–2 weeks after starting treatment and regularly thereafter. If no effect has been seen at 4 weeks, you should consider changing the dose or drug; otherwise, the dose should not be adjusted until after 6–8 weeks of therapy.
Cost	Both drugs are available in non-proprietary form and are relatively inexpensive.

Clinical tip—Perhaps counterintuitively, there is some evidence to suggest that the sedative effects of mirtazapine are *less severe* at *higher* doses than at lower doses. In theory, this may be because at low dose the antihistamine effects of mirtazapine predominate. By contrast, at higher doses, augmented monoamine transmission counteracts the sedating effects of H_1 receptor antagonism. However, as it is not proven that this phenomenon occurs at clinical doses (15–45 mg), we would not advise increasing the dose of mirtazapine to overcome sedation or somnolence.

Antiemetics, dopamine D₂-receptor antagonists

CLINICAL PHARMACOLOGY

Common indications	Prophylaxis and treatment of **nausea and vomiting** in a wide range of conditions, but particularly in the context of **reduced gut motility.**
Mechanisms of action	Nausea and vomiting are triggered by gut irritation, drugs, motion and vestibular disorders, as well as higher stimuli (sights, smells, emotions). The various pathways converge on a 'vomiting centre' in the medulla, which receives inputs from the chemoreceptor trigger zone, the solitary tract nucleus (which is innervated by the vagus nerve), the vestibular system and higher neurological centres. Dopamine, via D₂ receptors, is relevant in two respects. First, **the D₂ receptor is the main receptor in the chemoreceptor trigger zone** (CTZ), which is the area responsible for sensing emetogenic substances in the blood. D₂-receptor antagonists are therefore effective in nausea and vomiting caused by CTZ stimulation (e.g. by emetogenic drugs). Second, dopamine is an important neurotransmitter in the gut, where it promotes relaxation of the stomach and lower oesophageal sphincter and inhibits gastroduodenal coordination. D₂-receptor antagonists therefore have a **prokinetic effect,** promoting gastric emptying, which contributes to their antiemetic action in conditions associated with reduced gut motility (e.g. due to opioids or diabetic gastroparesis).
Important adverse effects	**Diarrhoea** is a common side effect. Metoclopramide can induce **extrapyramidal syndromes** (movement abnormalities) via the same mechanism as <u>antipsychotics</u>. In short-term treatment, this is most likely to take the form of an **acute dystonic reaction** such as an oculogyric crisis. Domperidone tends not to cause extrapyramidal symptoms because it does not cross the blood–brain barrier (note that the CTZ is largely outside the blood–brain barrier). Domperidone is associated with an increased risk of **QT-interval prolongation** and **arrhythmias**.
Warnings	To reduce the risk of extrapyramidal effects, metoclopramide should be prescribed for no more than 5 days. It should be avoided in ✘**neonates,** ▲**children** and ▲**young adults,** who are at increased risk of adverse effects. Domperidone is contraindicated in patients with ✘**cardiac conduction abnormalities** and severe ▲**hepatic impairment**. Both drugs are avoided in ▲**intestinal obstruction** and ✘**perforation** their prokinetic effects. Metoclopramide should be avoided in ▲**Parkinson's disease**, but domperidone may be used as it does not cross the blood–brain barrier.
Important interactions	The risk of extrapyramidal side effects is increased when metoclopramide is prescribed with ▲<u>antipsychotics</u>. It should not be combined with ✘<u>dopaminergic agents for Parkinson's disease</u>, as it will antagonise their effects. Domperidone should not be prescribed alongside other **drugs that prolong the QT interval,** such as <u>antipsychotics</u>, <u>quinine</u> and <u>selective serotonin reuptake inhibitors</u> or those which inhibit **cytochrome P450 (CYP) inhibitors** (e.g. <u>amiodarone</u>, <u>diltiazem</u>, <u>macrolides</u>, <u>fluconazole</u>, protease inhibitors) as these may increase the risk of adverse effects. If in doubt, check the BNF.

metoclopramide, domperidone

PRACTICAL PRESCRIBING

Prescription	The starting dose for both metoclopramide and domperidone is 10 mg 8-hrly. Metoclopramide can be prescribed for IM or IV injection; the dose remains the same. The route of administration, and whether it is prescribed on a regular or as-required basis, depends on the clinical situation. For example, the oral route is clearly inappropriate for a patient who is actively vomiting. Neither drug should be prescribed for more than a week (5 days for metoclopramide). When treating gastroparesis, metoclopramide is preferred owing to its better safety profile.
Administration	Intravenous injections of metoclopramide should be given slowly (over at least 3 minutes for a standard 10-mg dose).
Communication	Explain to patients that you are offering an antisickness medicine. Outline the risk of movement disorders by explaining that although most individuals are able to take it without significant side effects, a minority experience movement abnormalities, which can be significant. Ask your patient to stop taking the medicine and seek medical attention if they notice any side effects of this type.
Monitoring	Resolution of symptoms is the best guide to efficacy. Prolonged use is not recommended (see Clinical tip), but where it is unavoidable, you should monitor the patient for extrapyramidal features, as these may be subtle (e.g. an increased tendency to falls) and their relationship to the drug may not be obvious to patients or other healthcare professionals.
Cost	Non-proprietary preparations of these drugs are inexpensive

Clinical tip—Despite general recommendations to limit duration of D_2-receptor antagonist therapy, patients with gastroparesis may require long-term prokinetic treatment (i.e. greater than 5 days). To minimize exposure to metoclopramide, it should be used at the lowest effective dose (e.g. 5 mg 8-hrly). It may be alternated with erythromycin, which also has prokinetic properties. It is also good practice to have regular trials of treatment suspension ('drug holidays') to ensure it is still needed.

Antiemetics, histamine H₁-receptor antagonists

CLINICAL PHARMACOLOGY

Common indications	Prophylaxis and treatment of **nausea and vomiting,** particularly in the context of **motion sickness** or **vertigo.** Other drugs in this class are used in the treatment of allergies (see <u>Antihistamines (H₁-receptor antagonists)</u>).
Mechanisms of action	Nausea and vomiting are triggered by gut irritation, drugs, motion and vestibular disorders, as well as higher stimuli (sights, smells, emotions). The various pathways converge on a 'vomiting centre' in the medulla, which receives inputs from the chemoreceptor trigger zone (CTZ), the solitary tract nucleus (which is innervated by the vagus nerve), the vestibular system and higher neurological centres. Histamine (H₁) and acetylcholine (muscarinic) receptors predominate in the **vomiting centre** and in its communication with the **vestibular system.** Drugs such as cyclizine block both receptors. This makes them useful treatments for nausea and vomiting in a wide range of conditions (e.g. drug-induced, post-operative, radiotherapy), particularly when associated with motion or vertigo.
Important adverse effects	The most common adverse effect is **drowsiness.** Cyclizine is the least sedating drug in this class and is therefore usually preferred. Due to their anticholinergic effects they may cause **dry throat and mouth.** This is usually undesirable, but in patients with copious mucosal secretions it may be beneficial. After IV injection they may cause transient **tachycardia,** which the patient may notice as **palpitations.** Along with their central anticholinergic effects (excitation or depression) this may make for a rather unpleasant experience.
Warnings	Due to their sedating effect, these drugs should be avoided in patients at risk of ▲**hepatic encephalopathy.** They should also be avoided in patients susceptible to anticholinergic side effects, such as those with ▲**prostatic enlargement** (who may develop urinary retention).
Important interactions	Sedation may be greater when combined with other sedative drugs (e.g. <u>benzodiazepines</u>, <u>opioids</u>). Anticholinergic effects may be more pronounced in patients taking <u>ipratropium</u> or <u>tiotropium</u>.

PRACTICAL PRESCRIBING

Prescription	A typical prescription might be for cyclizine 50 mg 8-hrly as required. It may be given orally, IV or IM; no dosage adjustment is required when switching between routes. The route of administration, and whether it is prescribed on a regular or as-required basis, depends on the clinical situation. For example, the oral route is clearly inappropriate for a patient who is actively vomiting. As IM injections are painful and rapid IV injections are unpleasant (see Adverse effects), we would suggest that *slow* IV injection is the best choice when oral administration is inappropriate.
Administration	Intravenous injections of cyclizine should be given slowly (over about 2 minutes).
Communication	Explain to patients that you are offering an antisickness medicine. Although it is generally effective, it does not work for everyone and a second or different medicine may be necessary. Ask patients to let you know if they do not achieve satisfactory relief. Advise that it may cause drowsiness and impair the ability to perform tasks such as driving, which they should therefore avoid.
Monitoring	Resolution of symptoms is the best guide to efficacy.
Cost	The antihistamine antiemetics are relatively inexpensive.

Clinical tip—H_1-receptor antagonists are commonly used in the treatment and prophylaxis of motion sickness. Hyoscine hydrobromide (an antimuscarinic drug) is a useful alternative. It is widely used as an over-the-counter remedy for this indication and is effective. It can also be usefully administered transdermally using a patch, applied behind the ear a few hours before departure. One 1.5-mg patch can be left in place for up to 72 hours, over which time the average amount absorbed is 1 mg.

Antiemetics, serotonin 5-HT₃-receptor antagonists

CLINICAL PHARMACOLOGY

Common indications	Prophylaxis and treatment of **nausea and vomiting,** particularly in the context of general anaesthesia and chemotherapy.
Mechanisms of action	Nausea and vomiting are triggered by gut irritation, drugs, motion and vestibular disorders, as well as higher stimuli (sights, smells, emotions). The various pathways converge on a 'vomiting centre' in the medulla, which receives inputs from the chemoreceptor trigger zone (CTZ), the solitary tract nucleus (which is innervated by the vagus nerve), the vestibular system and higher neurological centres. 5-HT plays an important role in two of these pathways. First, **there is a high density of 5-HT₃ receptors in the CTZ,** which are responsible for sensing emetogenic substances in the blood (e.g. drugs). Second, **5-HT is the key neurotransmitter released by the gut** in response to emetogenic stimuli. Acting on 5-HT₃ receptors, it stimulates the vagus nerve, which in turn activates the vomiting centre via the solitary tract nucleus. Of note, 5-HT is not involved in communication between the vestibular system and the vomiting centre. Thus 5-HT₃ antagonists are effective against nausea and vomiting as a result of CTZ stimulation (e.g. drugs) and visceral stimuli (gut infection, radiotherapy), but not in motion sickness.
Important adverse effects	Adverse effects are rare with these medications, although constipation, diarrhoea and headaches can occur.
Warnings	There is a small risk that 5-HT₃ antagonists may prolong the QT interval, although this is usually evident only at high doses (e.g. >16 mg ondansetron). Nevertheless, they should be avoided in patients with a ▲**prolonged QT interval.** If there is clinical suspicion, review an ECG before prescribing.
Important interactions	Avoid 5-HT₃ antagonists when patients are taking ▲**drugs that prolong the QT interval,** such as <u>antipsychotics</u>, <u>quinine</u> and <u>selective serotonin reuptake inhibitors</u>. If in doubt, check the BNF.

PRACTICAL PRESCRIBING

Prescription	A typical starting dose for ondansetron is 4–8 mg 12-hrly, orally or IV. The dosing regimens differ for each indication, with higher doses generally reserved for chemotherapy-induced nausea and vomiting. Oral, rectal and injectable preparations are available. The route of administration, and whether it is prescribed on a regular or as-required basis, depends on the clinical indication. As IM injections are painful, the IV route is usually preferable if oral/rectal administration is inappropriate. Where drugs are used to prevent nausea (e.g. before an anaesthetic), oral doses should be taken an hour before symptoms are anticipated. Intravenous doses can be given immediately before the treatment or procedure.
Administration	There are no special considerations in relation to administration.
Communication	Explain to patients that you are offering an antisickness medicine. This is unlikely to cause any significant side effects. Although it is generally effective, it does not work for everyone and a second or different medicine may be necessary. Ask patients to let you know if they do not achieve satisfactory relief.
Monitoring	Resolution of symptoms is the best guide to efficacy.
Cost	Non-proprietary formulations are available with costs that now compare favourably with other antiemetics

Clinical tip—Morning sickness is an unpleasant manifestation of early pregnancy that can be severe enough to require hospitalisation. It can be difficult to treat as drugs administered during the first trimester of pregnancy may cause spontaneous abortion and fetal abnormalities. Although ondansetron is not licensed for morning sickness, a retrospective study of 608,385 women in Denmark found no evidence of adverse fetal outcomes related to taking ondansetron in pregnancy. Ondansetron may therefore be an option for severe morning sickness (e.g. hyperemesis gravidarum) where the benefits outweigh potential risks.

Antifungal drugs

CLINICAL PHARMACOLOGY

Common indications	❶ Treatment of **local fungal infections,** including of the oropharynx, vagina or skin. They may be applied topically (nystatin, clotrimazole) or taken orally (fluconazole). ❷ Systemic treatment of **invasive or disseminated fungal infections.** Specialist treatment is required for these infections, which will not be discussed further in this book.
Mechanisms of action	Fungal cell membranes contain ergosterol. As ergosterol is not seen in animal or human cells it is a target for antifungal drugs. **Polyene antifungals** (e.g. *nystatin*) bind to ergosterol in fungal cell membranes, creating a polar pore which allows intracellular ions to leak out of the cell. This can kill or slow growth of the fungi. **Imidazole** (e.g. *clotrimazole*) and **triazole antifungals** (e.g. *fluconazole*) inhibit ergosterol synthesis, impairing cell membrane synthesis, cell growth and replication. Resistance to antifungals is relatively infrequent but can occur during long-term treatment in immunosuppressed patients. Mechanisms include alteration of membrane synthesis to exclude ergosterol, changes in target enzymes or increased drug efflux.
Important adverse effects	Nystatin and clotrimazole are used topically at the site of infection, so have few adverse effects apart from occasional **local irritation** where applied. Fluconazole is taken orally and so has systemic adverse effects. The most common are **gastrointestinal upset** (including nausea, vomiting, diarrhoea and abdominal pain), **headache, hepatitis** and **hypersensitivity** causing skin rash. Rare but potentially life-threatening reactions include: **severe hepatic toxicity; prolonged QT interval** predisposing to **arrhythmias;** and severe hypersensitivity, including **cutaneous reactions** and **anaphylaxis.**
Warnings	Topically administered nystatin and clotrimazole have no major contraindications. Fluconazole should be prescribed with caution in patients with ▲**liver disease** because of the risk of hepatic toxicity. A dose reduction is required in ▲**moderate renal impairment.** It should be avoided in ✖**pregnancy** due to the risk of fetal malformation.
Important interactions	There are no significant drug interactions with topical nystatin or clotrimazole. Fluconazole inhibits cytochrome P450 (CYP) enzymes, causing an increase in plasma concentrations and risk of adverse effects when prescribed with ▲**drugs that are metabolised by CYP enzymes,** including <u>carbamazepine</u>, phenytoin, <u>warfarin</u>, <u>diazepam</u>, <u>simvastatin</u> and <u>sulphonylureas</u>. It may reduce the antiplatelet actions of <u>clopidogrel</u>, a pro-drug which requires activation by liver metabolism. It also increases the risk of serious arrhythmias if prescribed with ▲**drugs that prolong the QT interval,** such as <u>amiodarone</u>, <u>antipsychotics</u>, <u>quinine</u>, <u>quinolone</u> and <u>macrolide</u> antibiotics, and <u>SSRIs</u>.

PRACTICAL PRESCRIBING

Prescription	Nystatin is administered topically as an oral suspension for **oropharyngeal candidiasis** (thrush) at a dose of 100,000 units four times daily for 7 days or until 48 hours after lesions have resolved. Clotrimazole is used to treat fungal infections of the skin and genital tract, such as **tinea** (ringworm, including athlete's foot) and **candida** (thrush). For skin or mucosal infections, clotrimazole 1% cream (contains 1 g clotrimazole in 100 g cream) is applied two to three times daily until 1–2 weeks after infection has resolved. Clotrimazole is also formulated as a pessary for vaginal candidiasis.
	Oral fluconazole is prescribed as a single dose of 150 mg for **vaginal candidiasis.** For **other mucosal infections,** e.g. of the oropharynx, oesophagus and airways, it is prescribed at 50 mg daily for a more prolonged course (e.g. 1–2 weeks). Treatment duration may be longer for **fungal skin infections.** Fluconazole is also available as an IV preparation for invasive or disseminated fungal infection.
Administration	Oral nystatin should be administered after food and held in the mouth to allow good contact with the lesions. If the patient wears dentures, they should remove them to expose affected areas to treatment.
Communication	Advise patients that, with correct application, treatment should improve symptoms. For skin infections, encourage them to continue treatment for 1–2 weeks after symptoms resolve. Warn patients treated with a prolonged course of fluconazole to seek medical advice if they experience any unusual symptoms such as nausea, loss of appetite, lethargy or dark urine which could indicate liver poisoning.
Monitoring	Efficacy can be monitored clinically. For fluconazole, liver enzymes should be measured before and during prolonged courses of treatment, particularly where high doses are used, to monitor for hepatic toxicity.
Cost	Nystatin, clotrimazole and fluconazole are inexpensive in standard formulations.

Clinical tip—Elderly hospital inpatients are particularly susceptible to oral candida infection. They are commonly treated with <u>antibiotics</u> and systemic or inhaled <u>corticosteroids</u>, which predispose to oral candidiasis, and with <u>antimuscarinic</u> drugs that reduce saliva (natural defence mechanism). A sore mouth can reduce appetite and delay recovery. Take a torch on your ward round to check for oral candida infection. Encourage mouth care and prescribe nystatin to promote recovery.

Antihistamines (H₁-receptor antagonists)

CLINICAL PHARMACOLOGY

Common indications	❶ As a first-line treatment for **allergies,** particularly **hay fever** (seasonal allergic rhinitis). ❷ To aid relief of itchiness (**pruritus**) and hives (**urticaria**) due, for example, to insect bites, infections (e.g. chickenpox) and drug allergies. ❸ As an adjunctive treatment in **anaphylaxis,** after administration of adrenaline and other life-saving measures. Other drugs in this class may be used for **nausea and vomiting** (see Antiemetics, histamine H₁-receptor antagonists).
Mechanisms of action	The term 'antihistamine' is generally used to mean an antagonist of the H₁ receptor. H₂-receptor antagonists have different uses and are discussed separately. Histamine is released from storage granules in mast cells in response to antigen binding to IgE on the cell surface. Mainly via H₁ receptors, histamine induces the features of immediate-type (type 1) hypersensitivity: increased capillary permeability causing oedema formation (wheal), vasodilatation causing erythema (flare) and itch as a result of sensory nerve stimulation. When histamine is released in the nasopharynx, as in hay fever, it causes nasal irritation, sneezing, rhinorrhoea, congestion, conjunctivitis and itch. In the skin, it causes urticaria. Widespread histamine release, as in anaphylaxis, produces generalised vasodilatation and vascular leakage, with consequent hypotension. Antihistamines work in these conditions by antagonism at the H₁ receptor, blocking the effects of excess histamine. In anaphylaxis, their effect is too slow to be life-saving, so adrenaline is the more important first-line treatment.
Important adverse effects	The 'first-generation' antihistamines (e.g. chlorphenamine) cause **sedation.** This is because histamine, via H₁ receptors, has a role in the brain in maintaining wakefulness. Newer 'second-generation' antihistamines (including loratadine, cetirizine and fexofenadine) do not cross the blood–brain barrier, so tend not to have this effect. They have few adverse effects.
Warnings	Commonly used antihistamines, including those mentioned above, are safe in most patients. Sedating antihistamines (e.g. chlorphenamine) should be avoided in ▲**severe liver disease,** as they may precipitate hepatic encephalopathy.
Important interactions	The antihistamines mentioned here are not subject to any major drug interactions.

cetirizine, loratadine, fexofenadine, chlorphenamine

PRACTICAL PRESCRIBING

Prescription	Cetirizine (10 mg tablets), loratadine (10 mg tablets) and chlorphenamine (4 mg tablets and 2 mg/5 mL oral solution) may be purchased without prescription. Cetirizine and loratadine are taken orally on a once daily basis. Chlorphenamine is taken orally every 4–6 hours. In **anaphylaxis,** chlorphenamine 10 mg IV or IM may be administered, but this must not be prioritised over <u>adrenaline</u> and other life-saving measures (e.g. fluid resuscitation).
Administration	There are no special considerations for the administration for cetirizine and loratadine. Although oral chlorphenamine may be taken throughout the day, some patients prefer to reserve it for use in the evening when its sedating effect may be desirable.
Communication	As appropriate, explain to patients that you are offering a treatment to help relieve their allergic symptoms or their itchy rash/hives. In hay fever, the tablets should improve sneezing, itchiness and runniness, but tend not to help with nasal congestion. In the cases of cetirizine and loratadine, you can say that you do not anticipate any side effects. For chlorphenamine, you should mention that it may make them feel sleepy or lose concentration. They should therefore avoid taking it if they need to drive or carry out any other activity that requires concentration. They should also avoid combining it with alcohol, which may exacerbate the effect.
Monitoring	Clinical assessment of allergic symptoms, physical signs (e.g. rash) and enquiry about side effects is the best form of monitoring.
Cost	Non-proprietary antihistamines listed here are inexpensive. Patients who pay for their prescriptions will generally save money if they buy them directly from a pharmacy. There is no reason to use the more expensive brand name products.

Clinical tip—It may be useful to advise patients that larger pack sizes can be obtained if they buy them from the pharmacy counter, rather than off the shelf or from a non-pharmacy retailer. These may be more convenient and economical.

Antimotility drugs

CLINICAL PHARMACOLOGY

Common indications	As a symptomatic treatment for **diarrhoea,** usually in the context of irritable bowel syndrome (IBS) or viral gastroenteritis.
Mechanisms of action	Loperamide is an opioid that is pharmacologically similar to pethidine. However, unlike pethidine, is does not penetrate the central nervous system (CNS), so has no analgesic effects. It is an **agonist of the opioid μ-receptors in the gut.** This increases non-propulsive contractions of the gut smooth muscle but reduces propulsive (peristaltic) contractions. As a result, **transit of bowel contents is slowed and anal sphincter tone is increased.** Slower gut transit also allows more time for water absorption, which (in the context of watery diarrhoea) has a desirable effect in hardening the stool. Other opioids (e.g. codeine phosphate) have similar effects but, unless analgesia is also required, there is little reason to prefer them over loperamide.
Important adverse effects	Loperamide is a safe drug with few *direct* adverse effects. These are mostly **GI effects** predictable from its mechanism of action (e.g. constipation, abdominal cramping and flatulence). *Indirectly,* adverse effects may arise from use in inappropriate situations (see Warnings). Where CNS-penetrating opioids are used (e.g. codeine phosphate), there is a risk of opioid toxicity and dependence (see Opioids, weak).
Warnings	Loperamide should be avoided in ▲**acute ulcerative colitis (UC)** where inhibition of peristalsis may increase the risk of megacolon and perforation. For the same reason, it should be avoided where there is a possibility of ▲*Clostridium difficile* **colitis,** including in patients who develop diarrhoea in association with broad-spectrum antibiotic use (see Clinical tip). It should not be used in ▲**acute bloody diarrhoea (dysentery)** because this may signify bacterial infection. Particularly worrying in this context is *Escherichia coli*, certain strains of which can cause haemolytic–uraemic syndrome (HUS). Use of antimotility drugs appears to increase the risk of HUS.
Important interactions	There are no clinically significant interactions.

loperamide, codeine phosphate

PRACTICAL PRESCRIBING

Prescription	Loperamide may be purchased over the counter without prescription. In acute 'simple' diarrhoea, the usual dose is 4 mg, followed by 2 mg with each loose stool, generally to a maximum of 8 mg (four tablets) per day.
Administration	Loperamide is usually taken as a capsule or tablet. A syrup form is available, which may be useful in children (over 4 years old) with acute viral gastroenteritis.
Communication	You should ensure your patient is aware that the only purpose of loperamide is to help settle the diarrhoea. It does nothing for the underlying cause. Make sure patients know to stop taking it if they develop constipation, abdominal pain, or (in acute diarrhoea) they find they need to take it for more than 5 days.
Monitoring	The best means of monitoring is to enquire about stool frequency and abdominal symptoms.
Cost	Loperamide is available in non-proprietary form and is inexpensive. Patients who pay for their prescriptions will probably save money if they buy it over the counter rather than on prescription.

Clinical tip—Because of the risks of inhibiting peristalsis in the context of *C. difficile* colitis, it is generally unwise to prescribe an antimotility drug for a patient who develops diarrhoea while in hospital. You should at least wait until you have a better idea of its aetiology, such as a positive viral polymerase chain reaction (PCR) and/or negative *C. difficile* toxin test. Make sure you explain this to patients, who may be frustrated that while in hospital they cannot get a medicine that, if they were at home, they would simply buy from the chemist.

Antimuscarinics, bronchodilators

CLINICAL PHARMACOLOGY

Common indications	❶ In **chronic obstructive pulmonary disease (COPD)**, *short-acting antimuscarinics* are used to relieve breathlessness, e.g. brought on by exercise or during exacerbations. *Long-acting antimuscarinics* (LAMAs) are used to prevent breathlessness and exacerbations. ❷ In **asthma**, *short-acting antimuscarinics* are used to help relieve breathlessness during acute exacerbations (added to a short-acting β₂ agonist, e.g. salbutamol). *LAMAs* (tiotropium) can be added to high-dose inhaled corticosteroids and long-acting β₂ agonists (LABA) as maintenance treatment in patients who have had one or more severe asthma exacerbations in the past year.
Mechanisms of action	Antimuscarinic drugs bind to the muscarinic receptor, where they act as a **competitive inhibitor of acetylcholine.** *Stimulation* of the muscarinic receptor brings about a wide range of parasympathetic 'rest and digest' effects. In *blocking* the receptor, antimuscarinics have the opposite effects: they increase heart rate and conduction; **reduce smooth muscle tone,** including in the respiratory tract and bladder; and **reduce secretions** from glands in the respiratory and GI tracts. In the eye, they cause relaxation of the pupillary constrictor and ciliary muscles, causing pupillary dilatation and preventing accommodation, respectively.
Important adverse effects	After inhalation, antimuscarinic bronchodilators are rapidly absorbed from the lungs into the circulation where they are inactivated by hydrolysis. This occurs at different rates for different drugs, being particularly rapid for aclidinium. Adverse effects can include irritation of the **respiratory tract** with nasopharyngitis, sinusitis and cough, **GI** disturbance including dry mouth and constipation, urinary retention, blurred vision and headaches. However, the incidence of antimuscarinic adverse effects is lower with inhaled than oral/IV antimuscarinics and particularly low for aclidinium due to its rapid metabolism.
Warnings	Antimuscarinics should be used with caution in patients susceptible to ▲**angle-closure glaucoma,** in whom they can precipitate a dangerous rise in intraocular pressure. They should be used with caution in patients with or at risk of ▲**arrhythmias** or ▲**urinary retention**. However, in practice, most patients can take these drugs by inhalation without major problems.
Important interactions	Interactions are not generally a problem due to low systemic absorption.

ipratropium, tiotropium, glycopyrronium, aclidinium

PRACTICAL PRESCRIBING

Prescription	**Short-acting antimuscarinics** such as ipratropium are prescribed to be taken four times daily or as needed when the patient feels breathless. They are prescribed at a standard dose (e.g. ipratropium 40 micrograms) by inhalation for stable patients, but at a much higher dose (250–500 micrograms 6-hrly) by nebulisation during an acute attack. **Long-acting antimuscarinics** (e.g. tiotropium, glycopyrronium, aclidinium) are prescribed for regular administration once or twice daily.
Administration	Inhaled medication comes in a range of inhaler devices, with the choice of medicine often being directed by the device that best suits the patient. Medication for nebulisation comes as a liquid, which is put into the chamber below a mask covering the mouth and nose of the patient. Gas (usually <u>oxygen</u>) is bubbled through the liquid, vaporising the medicine for the patient to inhale. In patients with ▲**chronic type 2 (hypercapnic) respiratory failure,** who are at risk of carbon dioxide retention, medical air is used as the driving gas.
Communication	Explain to patients that you are offering a treatment to open up their airways, which should improve their breathing. They should understand that this treats the symptoms, not the disease. Ensure they are clear on how and when to take the inhaler (e.g. for acute symptoms, pre-emptively before exercise or regularly for long-acting medication). Discuss possible side effects, such as dry mouth, and advise them to chew gum or suck sweets (which should be sugar-free; see <u>Antimuscarinics, genitourinary uses</u>), or keep a bottle of water with them to relieve these.
Monitoring	You should check if the treatment has worked by asking patients about symptoms and reviewing peak flow measurements (asthma). You should enquire about side effects, particularly dry mouth. You should **check their inhaler technique** every time they are reviewed and correct it as necessary to optimise potential treatment benefits.
Cost	Ipratropium is available in non-proprietary form and is inexpensive. Long-acting antimuscarinics are newer medicines, with most drugs and inhaler devices remaining under patent protection. They are therefore relatively expensive.

Clinical tip—There is no advantage in prescribing short-acting antimuscarinics more than four times daily as this increases adverse effects without increasing benefits. By contrast, <u>β₂ agonists</u> can be administered much more frequently (e.g. 2-hrly) if needed.

Antimuscarinics, cardiovascular and gastrointestinal uses

CLINICAL PHARMACOLOGY

Common indications	❶ Atropine is used as a first-line treatment in the management of severe or symptomatic **bradycardia** to increase heart rate. ❷ Antimuscarinics (particularly hyoscine butylbromide) are a first-line pharmacological treatment option for **irritable bowel syndrome (IBS),** where they are used for their antispasmodic effect. ❸ In the care of the dying patient, antimuscarinics (e.g. hyoscine butylbromide) may have a role in reducing **copious respiratory secretions.**
Mechanisms of action	Antimuscarinic drugs bind to the muscarinic receptor, where they act as a **competitive inhibitor of acetylcholine.** *Stimulation* of the muscarinic receptor brings about a wide range of parasympathetic 'rest and digest' effects. In *blocking* the receptor, antimuscarinics have the opposite effects: they **increase heart rate and conduction; reduce smooth muscle tone and peristaltic contraction,** including in the gut and urinary tract; and **reduce secretions** from glands in the respiratory tract and gut. In the eye they cause relaxation of the pupillary constrictor and ciliary muscles, causing pupillary dilatation and preventing accommodation, respectively.
Important adverse effects	Predictably from their antagonism of parasympathetic 'rest and digest' effects, antimuscarinics can cause **tachycardia, dry mouth** and **constipation.** By reducing detrusor muscle activity, they can cause **urinary retention** in patients with benign prostatic enlargement. The ocular effects may cause **blurred vision,** especially for near objects. Some antimuscarinics (including atropine) have central effects, which may precipitate **drowsiness** and **confusion,** particularly in the elderly.
Warnings	Antimuscarinics should be used with caution in patients susceptible to ▲**angle-closure glaucoma,** in whom they can precipitate a dangerous rise in intraocular pressure. They should generally be avoided in patients at risk of ▲**arrhythmias** (e.g. those with significant cardiac disease), unless the indication for use is bradycardia.
Important interactions	Adverse effects are more pronounced when they are combined with other drugs that have antimuscarinic effects, such as tricyclic antidepressants.

atropine, hyoscine butylbromide, glycopyrronium

PRACTICAL PRESCRIBING

Prescription	For **bradycardia,** atropine is usually preferred and is given IV in incremental doses (e.g. 500 micrograms every 1–2 mins) until an acceptable heart rate is restored (to a maximum of 3 mg). Glycopyrronium is an alternative. It does not penetrate the brain so causes less drowsiness, but it tends not to be so readily available on general wards. For **IBS,** an antimuscarinic is taken orally on a regular basis: hyoscine butylbromide (Buscopan®) 10 mg 8-hrly is a common choice. This is available without prescription. For **the control of respiratory secretions,** hyoscine butylbromide or hyoscine hydrobromide is usually given subcutaneously, either by injection or as part of a continuous subcutaneous infusion. Note that hyoscine butylbromide and hyoscine hydrobromide have quite different doses – take care that both you and the nursing staff are clear on which one you are using, and that the dose is correct.
Administration	In general, IV administration of atropine should be performed only by, or under direct supervision of, an individual experienced in its use. To facilitate rapid administration in emergencies, atropine is provided in pre-filled disposable syringes. It is a good idea to familiarise yourself with these devices before you need to use them for real. The concentration of atropine in pre-filled syringes may be 100, 200 or 300 micrograms/mL – be sure to check this before administration.
Communication	Depending on the clinical context, it may be appropriate to warn patients about common adverse effects of antimuscarinics, such as dry mouth and blurred vision.
Monitoring	When using antimuscarinics to increase heart rate, high-intensity monitoring (including continuous cardiac rhythm monitoring) is required. It is essential that this is continued after restoration of normal heart rate, as the effect of the drug may be transient. For other indications, enquiry about symptoms is the best form of monitoring. The dose is titrated to achieve the optimal balance between beneficial and adverse effects.
Cost	Antimuscarinics are relatively inexpensive.

Clinical tip—When treating bradycardia, some practitioners recommend that the initial dose of atropine should be no less than 600 micrograms. This is because, paradoxically, low-dose atropine may transiently *slow* the heart rate before the more predictable positive chronotropic effect supervenes.

Antimuscarinics, genitourinary uses

CLINICAL PHARMACOLOGY

Common indications	To reduce urinary frequency, urgency and urge incontinence in **overactive bladder,** as a first-line pharmacological treatment if bladder training is ineffective.
Mechanisms of action	Antimuscarinic drugs bind to muscarinic receptors, where they act as a **competitive inhibitor of acetylcholine.** Contraction of the smooth muscle of the bladder is under parasympathetic control. Blocking muscarinic receptors therefore **promotes bladder relaxation,** increasing bladder capacity. In patients with overactive bladder, this may **reduce urinary frequency, urgency and urge incontinence.** Antimuscarinics help in overactive bladder through **antagonism of the M_3 receptor,** which is the main muscarinic receptor subtype in the bladder. Solifenacin is more selective for the M_3 receptor, which may reduce side effects.
Important adverse effects	Predictably from their antimuscarinic action, **dry mouth** is a very common side effect of these drugs. Other classic antimuscarinic side effects such as **tachycardia, constipation** and **blurred vision** are also common. Urinary retention may occur if there is bladder outflow obstruction.
Warnings	Antimuscarinics are contraindicated in ✗**urinary tract infection.** Urinalysis is therefore an important part of assessment before prescribing treatment for overactive bladder. Neurological side effects (drowsiness and confusion) can be particularly problematic in the ▲**elderly** and especially patients with ▲**dementia.** Antimuscarinics should be used with caution in patients susceptible to ▲**angle-closure glaucoma,** in whom they can precipitate a dangerous rise in intraocular pressure. They should be used with caution in patients at risk of ▲**arrhythmias** (e.g. those with significant cardiac disease) and, for obvious reasons, those at risk of ▲**urinary retention.**
Important interactions	Adverse effects are more pronounced when combined with other drugs that have antimuscarinic effects, such as ▲tricyclic antidepressants.

PRACTICAL PRESCRIBING

Prescription	You should prescribe antimuscarinics for **urge incontinence** only after an adequate trial of bladder retraining. Where they are indicated, an immediate-release form of oxybutynin or tolterodine is recommended for first-line therapy. A typical prescription would be for oxybutynin 5 mg orally every 8 or 12 hours. Other formulations (e.g. MR tablets, transdermal patches) and other antimuscarinics should be reserved for use when an immediate-release preparation is ineffective or poorly tolerated.
Administration	Immediate-release antimuscarinics should be taken at roughly equal intervals, with or without food. MR forms should be taken at a similar time each day and swallowed whole, not chewed.
Communication	Explain to patients that you are offering a treatment with a medicine that relaxes the bladder. This will hopefully reduce how often they need to pass water, the urgency with which they need to get to the toilet, and the chance of accidents. Explain that dry mouth is a very common side effect, affecting more than one in ten patients (see Clinical tip). When prescribing for elderly patients it may be prudent to mention that the medicine may cause drowsiness and confusion, and to stop taking it if this occurs.
Monitoring	You should arrange to review your patient within a month of starting therapy to review response and side effects.
Cost	Immediate-release oxybutynin is available in non-proprietary form and is relatively inexpensive. Other preparations are more expensive and should be reserved for second-line use.

Clinical tip—Dry mouth is a very common side effect of antimuscarinic therapy. Patients may find that chewing gum or sucking sweets helps to alleviate this. This may be worth mentioning in your communication with patients, but it is important to say that they should use sugar-free products, because dry mouth increases the risk of tooth decay. For the same reason, good dental care is important for all patients who require antimuscarinic treatment on a long-term basis.

Antipsychotics, first-generation (typical)

CLINICAL PHARMACOLOGY

Common indications	❶ Urgent treatment of severe **psychomotor agitation** that is causing dangerous or violent behaviour, or to calm patients to permit assessment. ❷ **Schizophrenia,** particularly when the metabolic side effects of second-generation (atypical) antipsychotics are likely to be problematic. ❸ **Bipolar disorder,** particularly in acute episodes of mania or hypomania. ❹ **Nausea and vomiting,** particularly in the palliative care setting.
Mechanisms of action	Antipsychotic drugs **block post-synaptic dopamine D₂ receptors.** There are three main dopaminergic pathways in the brain. The *mesolimbic/mesocortical pathway* runs between the midbrain and the limbic system/frontal cortex. D₂ blockade in this pathway is probably the main determinant of antipsychotic effect, but this is incompletely understood. The *nigrostriatal pathway* connects the substantia nigra with the corpus striatum of the basal ganglia. The *tuberohypophyseal pathway* connects the hypothalamus with the pituitary gland. Activity in these pathways explains some of the drugs' adverse effects. D₂ receptors are also found in the *chemoreceptor trigger zone*, where blockade accounts for their use in nausea and vomiting. All antipsychotics, but particularly chlorpromazine, have some sedative effect. This may be beneficial in the context of acute psychomotor agitation.
Important adverse effects	**Extrapyramidal effects**—movement abnormalities that arise from D₂ blockade in the *nigrostriatal pathway*—are the main drawback of first-generation antipsychotics. They take several forms: **acute dystonic reactions** are involuntary parkinsonian movements or muscle spasms; **akathisia** is a state of inner restlessness; and **neuroleptic malignant syndrome** is a rare but life-threatening side effect characterised by rigidity, confusion, autonomic dysregulation and pyrexia. These all tend to occur early in treatment. By contrast, **tardive dyskinesia** is a late adverse effect (*tardive*, late), occurring after months or years of therapy. This comprises movements that are pointless, involuntary and repetitive (e.g. lip smacking). It is disabling and may not resolve on stopping treatment. Other adverse effects include **drowsiness, hypotension, QT-interval prolongation** (and consequent **arrhythmias**), **erectile dysfunction,** and symptoms arising from **hyperprolactinaemia** due to *tuberohypophyseal* D₂ blockade (e.g. menstrual disturbance, galactorrhoea and breast pain).
Warnings	▲**Elderly** patients are particularly sensitive to antipsychotics, so start with lower doses. Antipsychotics should ideally be avoided in ▲**dementia,** as they may increase the risk of death and stroke. They should be avoided if possible in ▲**Parkinson's disease** due to their extrapyramidal effects.
Important interactions	Consult the BNF when prescribing for a patient taking antipsychotics as there is an extensive list of interactions. Prominent among these are ▲**drugs that prolong the QT interval** (e.g. amiodarone, macrolides).

haloperidol, chlorpromazine, prochlorperazine

PRACTICAL PRESCRIBING

Prescription	**Regular treatment** is required to treat **schizophrenia** and should only be started or adjusted under the guidance of a psychiatrist. A **single dose** may be used to control **acute or violent behaviour.** Haloperidol is a common first-line choice. The dosage depends on the clinical context and you will require guidance from a clinician experienced in its use. For example, an elderly patient may be markedly sedated by as little as 0.5 mg IM, whereas a young patient with extreme agitation may need 5 mg or more to achieve an adequate response. For the control of **nausea**, haloperidol is used in regular small oral or SC doses (e.g. 1.5 mg at night) or as a component of a continuous SC infusion.
Administration	For regular administration, typical antipsychotics can be taken orally (tablet and liquid) or given by slow-release IM ('depot') injection. In emergencies, haloperidol is usually given by rapid-acting IM injection and occasionally IV for rapid control of symptoms, although it is not licensed by this route. Intravenous haloperidol should only be administered by clinicians capable of managing neurological and cardiac side effects including arrhythmias such as torsade de pointes (a form of ventricular tachycardia), which are more likely when antipsychotics are given by injection or in high dose.
Communication	Adherence is a significant issue when treating psychiatric disorders, both because of the underlying disease and adverse effects of treatment. Good communication with your patient about the aims and benefits of treatment, as well as its potential side effects, is therefore very important. It is also important to emphasise that patients should report that they are taking antipsychotics to other healthcare professionals involved in their care, as many other medicines can interfere with the way they work.
Monitoring	The aim of treatment with antipsychotics is control of symptoms, so frequent reviews of symptoms and signs are important. The antipsychotic effects may take several weeks to become established and the dose may need to be adjusted to obtain the optimum balance between beneficial and adverse effects. When using high doses for acute control of psychotic/violent behaviour the dose–response relationship is unpredictable, so you should ensure that appropriate monitoring is available to detect neurological, respiratory and cardiovascular effects.
Cost	Typical antipsychotics are relatively old drugs and are available in inexpensive non-proprietary forms. Branded products, including oral solutions and depot injections, are more expensive.

Clinical tip—Chlorpromazine and haloperidol are also licensed for the treatment of intractable hiccups, as is metoclopramide. This can be a very distressing condition which is difficult to treat. A variety of non-pharmacological manoeuvres (e.g. Valsalva manoeuvre, breath holds, sipping ice-cold water) may be tried first. In our experience, they rarely work in intractable cases. However, we have found chlorpromazine (e.g. 25 mg orally) to be effective.

Antipsychotics, second-generation (atypical)

CLINICAL PHARMACOLOGY

Common indications	❶ Urgent treatment of severe **psychomotor agitation** leading to dangerous or violent behaviour, or to calm such patients to permit assessment. ❷ **Schizophrenia,** particularly when extrapyramidal side effects have complicated the use of <u>first-generation (typical) antipsychotics</u>, or when negative symptoms are prominent. ❸ **Bipolar disorder,** particularly in acute episodes of mania or hypomania.
Mechanisms of action	Antipsychotic drugs **block post-synaptic dopamine D_2 receptors.** There are three main dopaminergic pathways in the brain. The *mesolimbic/mesocortical pathway* runs between the midbrain and the limbic system/frontal cortex. D_2 blockade in this pathway probably explains the drugs' antipsychotic effects, but this is incompletely understood. The *nigrostriatal pathway* connects the substantia nigra with the corpus striatum of the basal ganglia. The *tuberohypophyseal pathway* connects the hypothalamus with the pituitary gland. Activity in these pathways explains some of the drugs' adverse effects. As compared with first-generation antipsychotics, second-generation agents seem more efficacious in 'treatment-resistant' schizophrenia (particularly clozapine) and against negative symptoms, and have a lower risk of extrapyramidal symptoms. This may be because of a higher affinity for **other receptors** (particularly 5-HT_{2A}), and a characteristic of **'looser' binding** to D_2 receptors (in the case of clozapine and quetiapine).
Important adverse effects	Most antipsychotics cause some degree of **sedation.** Blocking dopamine in the *nigrostriatal pathway* may produce movement abnormalities called **extrapyramidal effects.** These are more common with <u>first-generation antipsychotics</u>, where they are discussed more fully. **Metabolic disturbance,** including weight gain, diabetes mellitus and lipid changes, is a common problem with second-generation antipsychotics. Antipsychotics can **prolong the QT interval** and thus cause **arrhythmias.** Risperidone has particular effects on dopaminergic transmission in the *tuberohypophyseal pathway,* which regulates secretion of prolactin. This can cause **breast symptoms** (in both women and men) and **sexual dysfunction.** Clozapine causes a severe deficiency of neutrophils **(agranulocytosis)** in about 1% of patients, and rarely causes **myocarditis.**
Warnings	Antipsychotics should be used with caution in patients with ▲**cardiovascular disease.** Clozapine must not be used in patients with ✖**severe heart disease** or a history of ✖**neutropenia.**
Important interactions	Sedation may be more pronounced when used with other sedating drugs. They should not be combined with other ▲<u>dopamine-blocking antiemetics</u> and ▲**drugs that prolong the QT interval** (e.g. <u>amiodarone, quinine, macrolides, selective serotonin reuptake inhibitors</u>).

quetiapine, olanzapine, risperidone, clozapine

PRACTICAL PRESCRIBING

Prescription	Decisions to start treatment with a second-generation antipsychotic drug should be taken by a specialist. They may be used both for treatment of acute symptoms and for prevention of subsequent attacks. Options include daily oral treatment or intermittent slow-release IM ('depot') injections. Clozapine is considered when other agents have proved ineffective or intolerable. You are most likely to encounter these drugs in patients already established on treatment: for example, when they are admitted to hospital. In this situation you should not usually stop them, but must check carefully that the acute illness is not caused by the antipsychotic; that it does not present a contraindication to antipsychotic treatment; and that any new drugs introduced do not interact with the antipsychotic.
Administration	Oral antipsychotic medications are best taken at bedtime.
Communication	When you encounter patients established on antipsychotic treatment, it is worth reminding them that they should always inform any healthcare professional involved in their care what treatment they are on. This is particularly important for antipsychotics, as many other medicines can interfere with the way they work. Patients taking clozapine should know about the need for regular blood test monitoring and of the need to report infective symptoms immediately.
Monitoring	Assessment of symptoms and signs is the best form of monitoring for treatment efficacy. For most antipsychotics, blood tests (typically FBC, renal and liver profiles) are required at the start of treatment and periodically thereafter; an intensive monitoring programme is required for clozapine due to the risk of agranulocytosis. Monitoring for metabolic and cardiovascular side effects is important for second-generation antipsychotics. This includes measurement of weight, lipid profile and fasting blood glucose at baseline and intermittently during treatment.
Cost	Non-proprietary forms of quetiapine, olanzapine and risperidone are available and are substantially less expensive than their brand name counterparts.

Clinical tip—When you see a patient in hospital who is taking an antipsychotic drug, always check the QT interval on their ECG. Most antipsychotics can lengthen this to some extent (which presents a risk of dangerous arrhythmias), and this may be exacerbated by drugs administered for the acute problem (e.g. macrolide antibiotics for infection).

Antiviral drugs

CLINICAL PHARMACOLOGY

Common indications	❶ **Treatment of acute episodes of herpesvirus infections,** including herpes simplex (e.g. cold sores, genital ulcers, encephalitis) and varicella-zoster (e.g. chickenpox, shingles). ❷ **Suppression of recurrent herpes simplex attacks** where these are occurring at a frequency of 6 or more per year.
Mechanisms of action	The herpesvirus family includes herpes simplex 1 and 2 and varicella-zoster. These viruses contain double-stranded deoxyribonucleic acid (DNA), which requires a herpes-specific DNA polymerase for the virus to replicate. Aciclovir enters herpes-infected cells and **inhibits the herpes-specific DNA polymerase**, stopping further viral DNA synthesis and therefore replication.
Important adverse effects	Common adverse effects of aciclovir include **headache, dizziness, gastrointestinal disturbances** and **skin rash**. Intravenous (IV) aciclovir commonly causes inflammation or **phlebitis** at the injection site. Aciclovir is relatively water insoluble. During high-dose IV therapy, delivery of a high concentration of aciclovir into the renal tubules can cause precipitation, leading to crystal-induced **acute renal failure.** The risk of this can be minimised by ensuring good hydration and slowing the rate of infusion.
Warnings	Aciclovir has no major contraindications. It does cross the placenta and is expressed in breast milk, so caution is advised in ▲**pregnant women** and women who are ▲**breastfeeding**. However, as infections such as viral encephalitis, varicella pneumonia and genital herpes carry significant risks to the mother and fetus, the benefits of treatment in such circumstances are likely to outweigh its risks. Aciclovir is **excreted by the kidneys**; the dose and/or frequency of administration should therefore be reduced in patients with ▲**severe renal impairment** to prevent accumulation of the drug and subsequent toxicity.
Important interactions	There are no clinically important drug interactions with aciclovir.

PRACTICAL PRESCRIBING

Prescription	**Acute episodes of oral and genital herpes simplex** can be treated with aciclovir topically (five times a day for 5–10 days) or orally (200 mg five times a day). Treatment should ideally be started during the prodromal phase. In **recurrent infections**, suppressive treatment (400 mg 12-hrly) may be given. **Herpes simplex encephalitis** requires high-dose IV therapy (10–15 mg/kg 8-hrly). Treatment may be started empirically for patients presenting with encephalitic features, then later stopped if analysis of cerebrospinal fluid shows no evidence of herpesviruses, and clinical suspicion of herpes infection is low. In confirmed cases, or if clinical suspicion is high, treatment should be continued for 14–21 days.
Administration	Topical aciclovir should be applied liberally to the lesion five times a day. Tablets are taken with water, with or without food. Intravenous aciclovir should be given by infusion over at least 1 hour to minimise tubular precipitation. Care should be taken to ensure the cannula is properly sited in a vein, as extravasation causes tissue damage.
Communication	Explain to patients that aciclovir is an antiviral medicine that works by **stopping the virus from growing**, that the treatment does not clear the virus from the body completely and that **recurrent infections are common**. This is particularly true for cold sores and genital infections, but these usually become less frequent and less severe after a couple of years. For patients with cold sores, advise them to apply aciclovir cream to the sore **as soon as they notice symptoms** such as tingling, and to wash their hands before and after use to prevent spread of infection. If the cold sore has not healed after 10 days they should return to see their doctor. For genital infections, advise patients to start a 5-day course of treatment as soon as they experience tingling or numbness. If aciclovir is prescribed for **suppressive treatment,** explain that while aciclovir may reduce both the frequency of infections and the **risk of passing on the virus** to sexual partners, it does not prevent these altogether. Warn all patients of common side effects such as headache, dizziness and stomach upset.
Monitoring	Efficacy can be monitored clinically. In patients receiving high-dose IV treatment, **renal function** should be monitored for safety.
Cost	Aciclovir is inexpensive. Topical aciclovir is available over the counter.

Clinical tip—The treatment of other viral infections such as **hepatitis** and **human immunodeficiency virus (HIV)** should be initiated and monitored by specialists only. However, you should be aware of the potential for drug–drug interactions and drug toxicity in patients receiving antiretroviral treatment. Whenever initiating or adjusting concomitant medicines in patients established on antiretrovirals, consider consulting a specialist pharmacist for advice on interactions. A useful reference is the University of Liverpool HIV Drug Interactions website www.hiv-druginteractions.org.

Antiplatelet drugs, ADP-receptor antagonists

CLINICAL PHARMACOLOGY

Common indications	❶ For treatment of **acute coronary syndrome (ACS)**, usually in combination with <u>aspirin</u>, where rapid inhibition of platelet aggregation can prevent or limit arterial thrombosis and reduce subsequent mortality. ❷ To prevent occlusion of **coronary artery stents**, usually in combination with <u>aspirin</u>. ❸ For long-term secondary prevention of thrombotic arterial events in patients with **cardiovascular, cerebrovascular and peripheral arterial disease,** alone or in combination with <u>aspirin</u>.
Mechanisms of action	Thrombotic events occur when platelet-rich thrombus forms in atheromatous arteries and occludes the circulation. These drugs **prevent platelet aggregation** and reduce the risk of arterial occlusion by binding irreversibly to **adenosine diphosphate (ADP) receptors** ($P2Y_{12}$ subtype) on the surface of platelets. As this process is independent of the cyclooxgenase (COX) pathway, its actions are synergistic with those of aspirin.
Important adverse effects	The most common adverse effect is **bleeding,** which can be serious, particularly if gastrointestinal, intracranial or following a surgical procedure. **Gastrointestinal upset,** including dyspepsia, abdominal pain and diarrhoea, is also common. Rarely, antiplatelet agents can affect platelet numbers as well as function, causing **thrombocytopenia.**
Warnings	Antiplatelet drugs should not be prescribed for people with significant ✘**active bleeding** and may need to be stopped 7 days before ▲**elective surgery** and other procedures (see Clinical tip). They should be used with caution in patients with ▲**renal and hepatic impairment,** especially where patients otherwise have an increased risk of bleeding.
Important interactions	Clopidogrel is a **pro-drug** that requires metabolism by hepatic cytochrome P450 (CYP) enzymes to its active form to have an antiplatelet effect. Its efficacy may be reduced by ▲**CYP inhibitors** by *inhibiting its activation.* Relevant examples include <u>omeprazole</u>, <u>ciprofloxacin</u>, <u>erythromycin</u>, some <u>antifungals</u> and some <u>selective serotonin reuptake inhibitors</u>. Where gastroprotection with a proton pump inhibitor (see <u>Aspirin</u>) is required for patients taking clopidogrel, <u>lansoprazole</u> or <u>pantoprazole</u> are preferred over omeprazole as they are considered less likely to inhibit clopidogrel activation. Prasugrel is also a pro-drug but is less susceptible to interactions. Ticagrelor is not a pro-drug, but interacts with ▲**CYP inhibitors** (which may increase the risk of toxicity) and **inducers** (which may reduce efficacy). Co-prescription with other ▲**antiplatelet drugs,** ▲**anticoagulants** (e.g. <u>heparin</u>) or ▲<u>NSAIDs</u> increases the risk of bleeding.

clopidogrel, ticagrelor, prasugrel

PRACTICAL PRESCRIBING

Prescription	Clopidogrel is the most commonly used example in this class. It is available only as an oral preparation. Low doses of clopidogrel require up to a week to reach their full antiplatelet effect. When rapid effect is needed you should prescribe a **loading dose,** normally 300 mg orally for ACS, in the once-only section of the drug chart before commencing a regular **maintenance dose** of 75 mg orally daily. It is good practice to write the indication and intended duration of antiplatelet therapy as additional instructions on the inpatient and discharge prescriptions. This is of particular importance following the insertion of a **drug-eluting coronary stent.** In this context, dual antiplatelet therapy should be continued for **12 months** to reduce the risk of stent thrombosis and should not be discontinued prematurely without prior discussion with a cardiologist.
Administration	Clopidogrel can be given with or without food.
Communication	Advise patients that the purpose of treatment is to reduce the risk of heart attacks or strokes and to prolong life. In those who are taking clopidogrel following the insertion of a drug-eluting stent, emphasise the importance of continuing treatment as directed, usually for 12 months, to make sure that the stent stays open and does not block and cause a heart attack. Before starting therapy, check that the patient does not have any active bleeding. Explain that if bleeding does occur while on treatment it might take longer than usual to stop. Patients should report any unusual or sustained bleeding to their doctor.
Monitoring	Clinical monitoring for adverse effects is most appropriate.
Cost	Clopidogrel is available as an inexpensive non-proprietary preparation.

Clinical tip—Clopidogrel acts irreversibly. It therefore takes the lifespan of a platelet (around 7 to 10 days) for its antiplatelet effect to wear off. Clopidogrel should be stopped 7 days before elective surgery or other invasive procedures, unless the risk of stopping clopidogrel exceeds the risk of continuing. Thus in patients who have had a drug-eluting coronary artery stent inserted within the last 12 months, surgery should be delayed if possible. In emergency cases, patients taking clopidogrel may require platelet infusion to help stop bleeding.

Antiplatelet drugs, aspirin

CLINICAL PHARMACOLOGY

Common indications	❶ For treatment of **acute coronary syndrome (ACS)** and **acute ischaemic stroke,** where rapid inhibition of platelet aggregation can prevent or limit arterial thrombosis and reduce subsequent mortality. ❷ For long-term secondary prevention of thrombotic arterial events in patients with **cardiovascular, cerebrovascular** and **peripheral arterial disease.** Historically, aspirin was used to control **mild-to-moderate pain and fever**, although other <u>NSAIDs</u> are now usually preferred for this indication.
Mechanisms of action	Thrombotic events occur when platelet-rich thrombus forms in atheromatous arteries and occludes the circulation. Aspirin **irreversibly inhibits cyclooxygenase** (COX) to reduce production of the pro-aggregatory factor thromboxane from arachidonic acid, **reducing platelet aggregation** and the risk of arterial occlusion. The antiplatelet effect of aspirin occurs at **low doses** and lasts for the lifetime of a platelet (which does not have a nucleus to allow synthesis of new COX) and thus only wears off as new platelets are made.
Important adverse effects	The most common adverse effect of aspirin is **gastrointestinal irritation.** More serious effects include **peptic ulceration** and **haemorrhage** and hypersensitivity reactions including **bronchospasm.** In regular high-dose therapy aspirin causes **tinnitus.** Aspirin is life-threatening in **overdose.** Features include hyperventilation, hearing changes, metabolic acidosis and confusion, followed by convulsions, cardiovascular collapse and respiratory arrest.
Warnings	Aspirin should not be given to ✘**children aged under 16 years** due to the risk of **Reye's syndrome,** a rare but life-threatening illness that principally affects the liver and brain. It should not be taken by people with ✘**aspirin hypersensitivity,** i.e. who have had bronchospasm or other allergic symptoms triggered by exposure to aspirin or another <u>NSAID</u>. However, aspirin is not *routinely* contraindicated in asthma. Aspirin should be avoided in the ✘**third trimester of pregnancy** when prostaglandin inhibition may lead to premature closure of the ductus arteriosus. Aspirin should be used with caution in people with ▲**peptic ulceration** (e.g. prescribe gastroprotection) or ▲**gout,** as it may trigger an acute attack.
Important interactions	Aspirin acts synergistically with other antiplatelet agents, which although therapeutically beneficial can lead to increased risk of bleeding. Thus although it may be given with ▲**antiplatelet drugs** (e.g. <u>clopidogrel</u>) and ▲**anticoagulants** (e.g. <u>heparin</u>, <u>warfarin</u>) in some situations (e.g. ACS), caution is required.

PRACTICAL PRESCRIBING

Prescription	Aspirin is available for oral or rectal (higher doses) administration. In **ACS,** prescribe aspirin initially as a once-only *loading dose* of 300 mg followed by a regular dose of 75 mg daily. For **acute ischaemic stroke,** prescribe aspirin 300 mg daily for 2 weeks. For **long-term prevention of thrombosis** after an acute event prescribe low-dose aspirin 75 mg daily. Much higher doses of aspirin are required for the treatment of **pain,** with a maximum daily dose of 4 g, taken in divided doses. **Gastroprotection** (e.g. omeprazole 20 mg daily, see <u>Proton pump inhibitors</u>) should be considered for patients taking low-dose aspirin who are at increased risk of gastrointestinal complications. Risk factors include age >65 years, previous peptic ulcer disease, co-morbidities (such as cardiovascular disease, diabetes), and concurrent therapy with other drugs with GI side effects, particularly <u>NSAIDs</u> and <u>prednisolone</u>.
Administration	To minimise gastric irritation, aspirin should be taken after food. Enteric-coated tablets may help further, but are associated with slower absorption and are therefore not suitable for use in medical emergencies or for rapid pain relief.
Communication	Advise patients that the purpose of low-dose aspirin treatment is to prevent heart attacks or strokes and to prolong life. Warn them to watch out for indigestion or bleeding symptoms and report these to their doctor if they occur.
Monitoring	Enquiry about side effects is the most appropriate form of monitoring.
Cost	Aspirin is inexpensive, available off-patent and over the counter.

Clinical tip—In the UK, aspirin is not recommended or licensed for use in primary prevention of cardiovascular disease (i.e. in patients who have not previously had an event). The reason is that large-scale randomised-controlled trials and meta-analyses have found that the absolute risk of serious vascular events in this group is low (around 1/500), and any potential benefits of low-dose aspirin are offset by the increased risk of serious bleeding (around 1/1000).

Azathioprine

CLINICAL PHARMACOLOGY

Common indications	❶ Maintenance of remission of **Crohn's disease** and **ulcerative colitis (UC).** ❷ As a disease-modifying agent in **rheumatoid arthritis** and **autoimmune conditions** not responding to corticosteroids or other standard treatments. ❸ To **prevent organ rejection** in **transplant recipients.**
Mechanisms of action	Azathioprine is a pro-drug. This means that it is not itself pharmacologically active, but on metabolism it is converted to substances that are. The main metabolite is **6-mercaptopurine,** which is further metabolised to active substances. These inhibit **synthesis of purines** (notably the nucleosides adenine and guanine) and therefore **inhibit DNA and ribonucleic acid (RNA) replication.** Whereas most cells can 'salvage' or 'recycle' purines, lymphocytes are dependent on purine synthesis, and so are particularly affected by azathioprine metabolites. Metabolism and elimination of azathioprine and its metabolites involves the enzymes **xanthine oxidase** and **thiopurine methyltransferase (TPMT).** The activity of the latter is reduced or absent in some individuals.
Important adverse effects	The most serious dose-related adverse effect of azathioprine is **bone marrow suppression,** which results most significantly in leukopenia and an increased risk of infection. A reduction in dose or temporary break in therapy may resolve this. TPMT phenotyping may identify those at risk (see Warnings). **Nausea** is common and may be reduced by dividing the daily dose. **Hypersensitivity reactions,** which may manifest as **diarrhoea** and **vomiting, rash, fever, myalgia, hypotension** and **pancreatitis,** may occur. Other rare but serious adverse effects include **veno-occlusive disease, hepatotoxicity** and an increased risk of some tumours, such as **lymphoma**.
Warnings	TPMT phenotyping should be performed before starting therapy. Azathioprine should not be prescribed for patients with ✖**absent TPMT activity**. Those with ▲**reduced TPMT activity** should be treated only by a specialist. **Hypersensitivity reactions** may be serious and should prompt cessation of therapy. Dosage should be reduced ▲**hepatic** and ▲**renal impairment**. Azathioprine is teratogenic in animal studies, although the effects in humans are less clear. In general, treatment should not be initiated in ▲**pregnancy** but may continue in those already established on treatment where the benefits outweigh the risks of stopping (e.g. transplant recipients).
Important interactions	The risk of infection is increased if used with other immunosuppressants, such as <u>corticosteroids</u>, although co-prescription may be unavoidable in the conditions indicated. Azathioprine should not be prescribed with **xanthine oxidase inhibitors** such as ✖<u>allopurinol</u>, as they reduce azathioprine metabolism and increase the risk of toxicity. The **risk of leukopenia** is increased when prescribed with other drugs that are myelosuppressive or have effects on purine synthesis (e.g. ▲<u>trimethoprim</u>). Azathioprine may reduce the effect of ▲<u>warfarin</u>, necessitating dosage adjustment.

azathioprine

PRACTICAL PRESCRIBING

Prescription	Azathioprine is an immunosuppressive therapy with significant adverse effects. Treatment should only be initiated by, or on the advice of, a specialist. It is prescribed on a weight basis at 1–3 mg/kg daily in divided doses. The dose is adjusted to response. Treatment may be started at a high dose in some conditions to induce remission, then reduced to lower doses for maintenance therapy.
Administration	**Oral** treatment is preferred. **Intravenous** preparations are available but are an irritant to blood vessels. Where IV use is unavoidable, the drug should be diluted (e.g. to 100–250 mL) and given by infusion (e.g. over 60 min).
Communication	Explain to patients that azathioprine treatment should lead to an **improvement in symptoms** (e.g. of stool frequency in UC). Explain that it may take some time to reach maximal effect. Warn patients to seek **urgent medical advice** if they develop sore throat or fever (infection), bruising or bleeding (low platelet count) or rash, diarrhoea, vomiting or abdominal pain (hypersensitivity). Give advice on potential complications in the event of **pregnancy** and advise patients to discuss treatment plans with their specialist and or an obstetrician should they wish to conceive.
Monitoring	For safety, **full blood counts** should be monitored weekly for the first 4 weeks after initiation or dose alteration and 3-monthly thereafter. Patients and doctors should look out for signs and symptoms of bone marrow suppression and hypersensitivity.
Cost	Azathioprine is relatively inexpensive.

Clinical tip—As a junior doctor you should not initiate treatment with immunosuppressants, but you will see plenty of patients taking these medications in other clinical contexts, e.g. when they are admitted with acute medical conditions. Never unilaterally stop immunosuppressants, although you may temporarily withhold a dose if you suspect a serious adverse reaction. Contact the specialty team who initiated the drug (e.g. nephrology if it was prescribed following renal transplant) urgently to discuss its ongoing risks and benefits.

β-blockers

CLINICAL PHARMACOLOGY

Common indications	**❶ Ischaemic heart disease:** to improve symptoms and prognosis associated with **angina** and **acute coronary syndrome (ACE).** **❷ Chronic heart failure:** bisoprolol and carvedilol are used to improve prognosis. **❸ Atrial fibrillation (AF):** to reduce the ventricular rate and, in paroxysmal AF, to maintain sinus rhythm. **❹ Supraventricular tachycardia (SVT):** as an option in patients without circulatory compromise to restore sinus rhythm. **❺ Hypertension:** although not indicated for initial therapy, β-blockers may be used when other medicines (e.g. <u>calcium channel blockers</u>, <u>ACE inhibitors</u>, <u>thiazide diuretics</u>) are insufficient or inappropriate.
Mechanisms of action	β_1-adrenoreceptors are located mainly in the heart, whereas β_2-adrenoreceptors are found mostly in smooth muscle of blood vessels and airways. Via the β_1-receptor, **β-blockers reduce force of contraction and speed of conduction in the heart.** This relieves myocardial ischaemia by reducing cardiac work and oxygen demand, and increasing myocardial perfusion. They improve prognosis in heart failure, probably by 'protecting' the heart from chronic sympathetic stimulation. They slow the ventricular rate in AF mainly by **prolonging the refractory period of the atrioventricular (AV) node.** Through the same effect they may terminate SVT if this is due to a self-perpetuating ('re-entry') circuit that takes in the AV node. In hypertension, β-blockers lower BP through a variety of means, one of which is by **reducing renin secretion** from the kidney, since this is mediated by β_1-receptors.
Important adverse effects	β-blockers commonly cause fatigue, cold extremities, headache and GI disturbance (e.g. nausea). They can cause sleep disturbance and nightmares. They may cause **impotence** in men.
Warnings	In patients with ✖**asthma,** β-blockers can cause life-threatening bronchospasm and should be avoided. This effect is mediated by blockade of β_2-adrenoreceptors in the airways. β-blockers are usually safe in **COPD,** although it is prudent to choose a β-blocker that is relatively β_1-selective (e.g. bisoprolol, metoprolol), rather than non-selective (e.g. propranolol, carvedilol). When used in ▲**heart failure,** β-blockers should be started at a very low dose and increased slowly, as they may initially impair cardiac function. They should be avoided in patients with ▲**haemodynamic instability** and are contraindicated in ✖**heart block.** β-blockers generally require dosage reduction in significant ▲**hepatic failure.**
Important interactions	β-blockers must not be used with ✖<u>non-dihydropyridine calcium channel blockers</u> (e.g. <u>verapamil</u>, <u>diltiazem</u>), except in specialist practice. This combination can cause heart failure, bradycardia and even asystole.

bisoprolol, atenolol, propranolol, metoprolol, carvedilol

PRACTICAL PRESCRIBING

Prescription	β-blockers are usually prescribed orally as part of the patient's regular medication. Dosage varies according to the drug and the indication – the starting dose in heart failure is lower than that for ischaemic heart disease or hypertension. It is generally best to start at the lowest dosage listed in the BNF for that indication. Intravenous preparations (e.g. of metoprolol) are available for use when rapid effect is necessary.
Administration	Orally administered β-blockers should be taken at equal intervals (e.g. roughly the same time each day for once-daily drugs such as bisoprolol); the exact time is not important. Intravenous preparations should be prescribed and administered only by those experienced in their use, and only in a well-monitored environment.
Communication	Explain to patients the rationale for treatment as appropriate for the situation. Discuss common side effects, including **impotence** where relevant. Warn patients with heart failure about the risk of initial deterioration in their symptoms, and advise them to seek medical attention if this occurs. Warn patients with obstructive airways disease to stop treatment and seek medical advice if they develop any breathing difficulty.
Monitoring	The best guide to dosage adjustment is the patient's symptoms (e.g. chest pain) and heart rate (in ischaemic heart disease, aim for a resting heart rate of around 55–60 beats/min).
Cost	The commonly used β-blockers are available in non-proprietary forms, which are generally inexpensive.

Clinical tip—When starting a β-blocker acutely, such as in ACS, it is usually best to select a drug with a relatively short half-life, e.g. oral metoprolol (typical starting dose 12.5 mg 8-hrly; later increased to 25 mg 8-hrly). This will be more responsive to dosage adjustment and can be stopped quickly if necessary. Once the patient is stable, it can be converted to a once-daily preparation (e.g. bisoprolol), which will be more convenient for long-term use.

β₂-agonists

CLINICAL PHARMACOLOGY

Common indications	❶ **Asthma:** short-acting β₂-agonists are used to relieve breathlessness. Long-acting β₂ agonists (LABAs) are used as treatment for chronic asthma when <u>inhaled corticosteroids</u> alone are insufficient, but must *always* be given in combination with <u>inhaled corticosteroids</u>. ❷ **Chronic obstructive pulmonary disease (COPD):** short-acting β₂-agonists (SABAs) are used to relieve breathlessness. LABAs are an option for second-line therapy of COPD, to improve symptoms and reduce exacerbations. ❸ **Hyperkalaemia:** nebulised salbutamol may be used as an additional treatment to lower serum potassium concentration (along with <u>insulin</u> and <u>glucose</u>; and <u>calcium gluconate</u> to stabilise the myocardium).
Mechanisms of action	β₂-receptors are found in smooth muscle of the bronchi, gut, uterus and blood vessels. Stimulation of this G protein-coupled receptor activates a signalling cascade that leads to **smooth muscle relaxation.** This improves airflow in constricted airways, reducing the symptoms of breathlessness. Like insulin, β₂-agonists also **stimulate Na⁺/K⁺-adenosine triphosphatase (ATPase) pumps** on cell surface membranes, thereby **causing a shift of K⁺ from the extracellular to intracellular compartment.** This makes them a useful adjunct in the treatment of **hyperkalaemia,** particularly when IV access is difficult. However, their effect is less reliable than other therapies, so they should not be used in isolation. β₂ agonists are classified as short-acting (salbutamol, terbutaline) or long-acting (o.g. salmeterol, formoterol) according to their duration of effect.
Important adverse effects	Activation of β₂-receptors in other tissues accounts for the common 'fight or flight' adverse effects of **tachycardia, palpitations, anxiety** and **tremor.** They also promote glycogenolysis, and so may increase the serum glucose concentration. At high doses, serum lactate levels may also rise. Long-acting β₂ agonists can cause **muscle cramps**.
Warnings	Long-acting β₂ agonists should be used in asthma only if an <u>inhaled corticosteroid</u> is also part of therapy. This is because, without a steroid, LABAs are associated with increased asthma deaths. Care should be taken when prescribing β₂-agonists for patients with ▲**cardiovascular disease,** in whom tachycardia may provoke angina or arrhythmias. This is especially pertinent in the treatment of hyperkalaemia, when high doses may be necessary.
Important interactions	<u>β-blockers</u> may reduce the effectiveness of β₂-agonists. Concomitant use of high-dose nebulised β₂-agonists with theophylline and <u>corticosteroids</u> can lead to hypokalaemia, so serum potassium concentrations should be monitored.

salbutamol, terbutaline, salmeterol, formoterol, indacaterol

PRACTICAL PRESCRIBING

Prescription	Inhaled short-acting β_2-agonists are prescribed for 'as required' administration. A common choice in adults is salbutamol 100–200 micrograms inhaled as required. In asthma and COPD exacerbations requiring hospital treatment, nebulised therapy is more often used (e.g. salbutamol 2.5 mg nebulised 4-hrly; see Clinical tip), although inhalation via a spacer (e.g. 10 doses of salbutamol 100 micrograms inhaled) is reasonable provided the exacerbation is not life threatening. LABAs are used for maintenance therapy and are therefore prescribed regularly (usually 12-hrly). To assure co-administration with a steroid in asthma, they may be prescribed as part of a combination inhaler (e.g. Symbicort® or Seretide®, usually prescribed by brand name). These combinations are also used in COPD, where they can improve convenience.
Administration	Inhaled medication is administered by a range of devices, with choice of medicine often being directed by the device that best suits the patient. Drugs are delivered in **aerosol** (metered dose inhaler [MDI]) or **dry powder** form. Provision of a **spacer with MDIs** can improve airway deposition and treatment efficacy and reduce oral adverse effects. Patients should be trained how to use their **inhalers** and **technique** should be checked and corrected at every consultation.
Communication	Explain to patients that the aim of treatment is to make their airways relax and therefore improve their breathing. Make sure that they understand that this treats the symptoms, not the disease. Consequently, if they find themselves needing to use the inhaler very frequently, then they should seek medical advice, or increase their other treatment (e.g. inhaled corticosteroid) in accordance with a written action plan. Make sure that they are clear on how and when to take the inhaler (e.g. for acute symptoms, pre-emptively before exercise or regularly for long-acting medication). Explain that multiple doses in a short time period may make them feel shaky and anxious.
Monitoring	Patients with asthma can monitor their disease severity through their symptoms and by serial measurements of peak expiratory flow rate. They may be able to adjust their own treatment with guidance from their action plan. Likewise, symptom severity and exacerbation rates are the main indicators of effect in COPD.
Cost	Non-proprietary versions of short-acting β_2-agonists are relatively inexpensive. However, LABAs, particularly as part of combination inhalers, are costly. Together, Seretide® and Symbicort® prescriptions cost National Health Service (NHS) England more than £300m per annum.

Clinical tip—When prescribing nebuliser therapy, you should always indicate whether the nebuliser should be driven by oxygen or air. In general, <u>oxygen</u> should be used in asthma, whereas medical air should be used in COPD, due to the risk of CO_2 retention.

Benzodiazepines

CLINICAL PHARMACOLOGY

Common indications	❶ In the first-line management of **seizures** and **status epilepticus.** ❷ In the first-line management of **alcohol withdrawal reactions.** ❸ As a common choice for **sedation for interventional procedures,** if general anaesthesia is unnecessary or undesirable. ❹ For *short-term* treatment of severe, disabling or distressing **anxiety** or **insomnia,** although non-pharmacological treatment (or treatment of the underlying cause, if applicable) is invariably preferable.
Mechanisms of action	The target of benzodiazepines is the γ-aminobutyric acid type A (GABA$_A$) receptor. The GABA$_A$ receptor is a chloride channel that opens in response to binding by gamma-aminobutyric acid (GABA), the main inhibitory neurotransmitter in the brain. Opening the channel allows chloride to flow into the cell, making the cell more resistant to depolarisation. **Benzodiazepines facilitate and enhance binding of GABA to the GABA$_A$ receptor.** This has a widespread depressant effect on synaptic transmission. The clinical manifestations of this include reduced anxiety, sleepiness, sedation and anticonvulsive effects. Ethanol ('alcohol') also acts on the GABA$_A$ receptor, and in chronic excessive use the patient becomes tolerant to its presence. Abrupt cessation then provokes the excitatory state of **alcohol withdrawal.** This can be treated by introducing a benzodiazepine, which can then be withdrawn in a gradual and more controlled way.
Important adverse effects	Predictably, benzodiazepines cause dose-dependent **drowsiness, sedation** and **coma.** There is relatively little cardiorespiratory depression in **benzodiazepine overdose** (in contrast to opioid overdose), but loss of airway reflexes can lead to **airway obstruction** and **death.** If used repeatedly for more than a few weeks, a state of **dependence** can develop. Abrupt cessation then produces a **withdrawal reaction** similar to that seen with alcohol.
Warnings	The ▲**elderly** are more susceptible to the effects of benzodiazepines and so should receive a lower dose. Benzodiazepines are best avoided in patients with significant ▲**respiratory impairment** or ▲**neuromuscular disease** (e.g. myasthenia gravis). Benzodiazepines should also be avoided in ▲**liver failure** as they may precipitate hepatic encephalopathy; if their use is essential (e.g. for alcohol withdrawal), lorazepam may be the best choice, as it depends less on the liver for its elimination.
Important interactions	The effects of benzodiazepines are additive to those of other sedating drugs, including alcohol and opioids. Most depend on cytochrome P450 (CYP) enzymes for elimination, so concurrent use with ▲**CYP inhibitors** (e.g. amiodarone, diltiazem, macrolides, fluconazole, protease inhibitors) may increase their effects.

diazepam, temazepam, lorazepam, chlordiazepoxide, midazolam

PRACTICAL PRESCRIBING

Prescription	The effects of the various benzodiazepines are similar. What distinguishes them is their *duration of action*, and this dictates how they are used. For **seizures,** a long-acting drug is preferred, usually lorazepam (initial dose 4 mg IV) or diazepam (10 mg IV). Diazepam can also be given rectally for seizures, but you must use the rectal solution (rather than suppositories) to ensure rapid absorption. For **alcohol withdrawal,** oral chlordiazepoxide (also long-acting) is the traditional choice, but diazepam and lorazepam are probably equally acceptable; the dosage regimen depends on a patient's symptoms and usual alcohol intake. In **sedation for interventional procedures,** a short-acting drug is best, as this allows rapid recovery after completion of the procedure or inadvertent over-sedation. Midazolam is most appropriate here, but it should only be used by individuals skilled in safe sedation practice, and in an appropriately equipped and monitored environment. For **insomnia** and **anxiety,** use an intermediate-acting drug at the lowest effective dose (e.g. temazepam 10 mg orally) for the shortest possible period (generally no longer than 2 weeks).
Administration	Diazepam is available as a water-based solution and an oil-in-water emulsion. The solution is more irritant to veins. Intravenous administration of benzodiazepines, whether for seizures or sedation, should be undertaken only where facilities and expertise exist to deal with over-sedation (including airway management).
Communication	When treating **insomnia** and **anxiety,** advise your patient that pharmacological therapy is only a short-term measure. Discuss with patients the risk of dependence, advising that this can be minimised by avoiding daily use if possible and taking the drug for the shortest possible period. Advise patients that they should not drive or operate complex or heavy machinery after taking the drug, and caution them that sometimes sleepiness may persist the following day.
Monitoring	Close monitoring of the patient's clinical status and vital signs are essential following IV or high-dose oral administration of a benzodiazepine, including the settings of **seizures, alcohol withdrawal** and **sedation.** In **insomnia** and **anxiety,** enquiry about symptoms and side effects is the best form of monitoring.
Cost	Benzodiazepines are generally inexpensive.

Clinical tip—Flumazenil is a specific antagonist of benzodiazepines. However, use of this drug is rarely indicated. Specifically, it should *not* be given to reverse benzodiazepine-induced sedation when this forms part of a mixed or uncertain overdose. In this context, flumazenil may precipitate seizures which—having now blocked the benzodiazepine receptor—will be difficult to treat.

Bisphosphonates

CLINICAL PHARMACOLOGY

Common indications	❶ Alendronic acid is used as the first-line drug treatment option for patients at risk of **osteoporotic fragility fractures.** ❷ Pamidronate and zoledronic acid are used in the treatment of **severe hypercalcaemia of malignancy** after appropriate IV rehydration. ❸ For patients with **myeloma** and **breast cancer with bone metastases,** pamidronate and zoledronic acid reduce the risk of pathological fractures, cord compression and the need for radiotherapy or surgery. ❹ Bisphosphonates are used as first-line treatment of metabolically active **Paget's disease,** with the aim of reducing bone turnover and pain.
Mechanisms of action	Bisphosphonates reduce bone turnover by inhibiting the action of osteoclasts, the cells responsible for bone resorption. Bisphosphonates have a similar structure to naturally occurring pyrophosphate: hence they are readily incorporated into bone. As bone is resorbed, bisphosphonates accumulate in osteoclasts, where they inhibit activity and promote apoptosis. The net effect is reduction in bone loss and improvement in bone mass.
Important adverse effects	Common side effects include **oesophagitis** (when taken orally) and **hypophosphataemia.** A rare but serious adverse effect of bisphosphonates is **osteonecrosis of the jaw,** which is more likely with high-dose IV therapy. Good dental care is important to minimise the risk of this. Another rare but important adverse effect is **atypical femoral fracture,** particularly in patients on long-term treatment.
Warnings	Bisphosphonates are renally excreted and should be avoided in ✖**severe renal impairment.** They are contraindicated in the context of ✖**hypocalcaemia.** Oral administration is contraindicated in patients with active ✖**upper gastrointestinal disorders.** Because of the risk of jaw osteonecrosis, care should be exercised in prescribing bisphosphonates for ▲**smokers** and patients with major ▲**dental disease.**
Important interactions	Bisphosphonates bind calcium. Their absorption is therefore reduced if taken with <u>calcium</u> salts (including milk), as well as <u>antacids</u> and <u>iron</u> salts (see Administration).

alendronic acid, disodium pamidronate, zoledronic acid

PRACTICAL PRESCRIBING

Prescription	For **osteoporosis,** alendronic acid is prescribed orally, 70 mg once weekly. For severe **hypercalcaemia** and **bone metastases,** pamidronate or zoledronic acid are prescribed as slow IV infusions, in single or divided doses. Calcium-lowering effects may not become apparent for 3–4 days and are maximal at 7–10 days, so re-prescription should not be considered before 1 week. For **Paget's disease,** risedronate is given orally and pamidronate as an IV infusion.
Administration	Oral bisphosphonates are poorly absorbed, but this can be enhanced by correct administration. For example, alendronic acid tablets should be swallowed whole at least 30 minutes before breakfast or other medications, and taken with plenty of water. The patient should remain upright for 30 minutes after taking to reduce oesophageal irritation.
Communication	Explain to patients that you are recommending a medicine to help strengthen the bones to prevent fractures and/or lower calcium levels in the blood to improve symptoms. Explain that the tablets can cause inflammation of the gullet. To minimise this risk, give clear advice on how to take the tablets and ask them to report any symptoms of oesophageal irritation. Advise patients to see their dentist before and during bisphosphonate treatment. Emphasise the dose and frequency of bisphosphonate treatment to avoid overdosing errors.
Monitoring	In **osteoporosis,** check and replace calcium and vitamin D before treatment. Monitor efficacy using dual-energy X-ray absorptiometry (DEXA) scans every 1–2 years to check whether bone density is stable or increasing. For **hypercalcaemia,** monitor efficacy by symptom enquiry and reduction in calcium levels. In the treatment of **myeloma, bone metastases** and **Paget's disease,** enquire about symptoms (e.g. bone pain) and bone complications (e.g. pathological fracture). For **safety,** be alert to symptoms of oesophagitis, osteonecrosis of the jaw and atypical femoral fractures, and monitor calcium and phosphate.
Cost	Alendronic acid is the cheapest bisphosphonate; non-proprietary preparations cost around £1 a month. Pamidronate costs around £200 a month for Paget's disease and zoledronic acid (currently branded preparations only) costs around £175 a month for bone metastases.

Clinical tip—Fragility fractures cause significant morbidity and mortality. After hip fracture, 30% die within 1 year and 50% are left with loss of function. Bisphosphonates reduce recurrent fracture by 50%. You can assume a diagnosis of osteoporosis in women aged >75 years who have had a fragility fracture, and start treatment with a bisphosphonate without need for further investigation for osteoporosis: i.e. do not do a DEXA scan.

Calcium and vitamin D

CLINICAL PHARMACOLOGY

Common indications	❶ Calcium and vitamin D are used in **osteoporosis** to ensure positive calcium balance when dietary intake and/or sunlight exposure are insufficient. Other treatments, such as bisphosphonates, may be given to reduce the risk of fragility fractures. ❷ Calcium and vitamin D are used in **chronic kidney disease (CKD)** to treat and prevent secondary hyperparathyroidism and renal osteodystrophy. ❸ Calcium (as *calcium gluconate*) is used in **severe hyperkalaemia** to prevent life-threatening arrhythmias. Other treatments, e.g. insulin with glucose, are given to lower the potassium concentration. ❹ Calcium is used in **hypocalcaemia** that is symptomatic (e.g. paraesthesia, tetany, seizures) or severe (<1.9 mmol/L). ❺ Vitamin D is used in the prevention and treatment of **vitamin D deficiency,** including rickets (in children) and osteomalacia (adults).
Mechanisms of action	Calcium is essential for normal function of muscle, nerves, bone and clotting. Calcium homeostasis is controlled by parathyroid hormone and vitamin D, which increase serum calcium levels and bone mineralisation, and calcitonin, which reduces serum calcium levels. In **osteoporosis** there is a loss of bone mass, which increases the risk of fracture. Restoring positive calcium balance, either by dietary means or by administering calcium and vitamin D, may reduce the rate of bone loss; whether this prevents fractures is less clear. In severe **CKD,** impaired phosphate excretion and reduced activation of vitamin D cause hyperphosphataemia and hypocalcaemia. This stimulates secondary hyperparathyroidism, which leads to a range of bone changes called renal osteodystrophy. Treatment may include oral calcium supplements to bind phosphate in the gut, and alfacalcidol to provide vitamin D that does not depend on renal activation. In **hyperkalaemia,** calcium raises the myocardial threshold potential, reducing excitability and the risk of arrhythmias. It has no effect on the serum potassium level. The rationale for the use of calcium in **hypocalcaemia** and vitamin D in **vitamin D deficiency** is self-explanatory.
Important adverse effects	Oral calcium is usually well tolerated, but may cause **dyspepsia** and **constipation.** When administered IV for the treatment of hyperkalaemia, calcium gluconate can cause **cardiovascular collapse** if administered too fast, and **local tissue damage** if accidentally given into subcutaneous tissue.
Warnings	Calcium and vitamin D should be avoided in ✖**hypercalcaemia.**
Important interactions	Oral calcium reduces the absorption of many drugs, including iron, bisphosphonates, tetracyclines and levothyroxine. Administered IV, calcium must not be allowed to mix with ✖sodium bicarbonate due to the risk of precipitation.

calcium carbonate, calcium gluconate, colecalciferol, alfacalcidol

PRACTICAL PRESCRIBING

Prescription	In **osteoporosis,** you should aim to supplement dietary intake with 1–1.2 g of calcium and 800 units of vitamin D per day. Various combined preparations of calcium and vitamin D are available; a common choice is Adcal-D3® two tablets daily (each tablet contains calcium 600 mg and colecalciferol 400 units). In **severe hyperkalaemia,** you should prescribe 10 mL of calcium gluconate 10% for administration by slow IV injection. Repeat doses may be required if ECG changes persist. Given the urgency of the situation, it is acceptable to administer the treatment first and write the prescription later. You should **seek expert guidance** for the management of severe or symptomatic hypocalcaemia; vitamin D deficiency; and in the use of calcium and vitamin D in severe CKD.
Administration	**Oral calcium** preparations should usually be chewed then swallowed. Doses should be separated from potentially interacting medicines (see Important interactions) by about 4 hours. These preparations may also interact with certain foods, including spinach, bananas and whole cereals; about 2 hours' separation is required if these have been consumed. **Calcium gluconate** should be administered by slow IV injection over 5–10 minutes into a large vein. Make sure the cannula is working by first flushing it with sodium chloride 0.9%, to avoid accidental subcutaneous administration ('extravasation').
Communication	Explain to patients the rationale for treatment as appropriate for the clinical indication. Advise them to seek medical advice if they develop side effects such as abdominal pain and limb pain, as these may be a sign of high calcium levels, requiring a blood test.
Monitoring	Patients with severe hyperkalaemia require continuous cardiac monitoring. You should repeat a 12-lead ECG after administration of calcium gluconate to confirm resolution of initial ECG abnormalities (e.g. normalisation of PR interval and QRS duration). For any patient receiving calcium or vitamin D supplements, check serum calcium levels at regular intervals or if they develop symptoms of hypercalcaemia.
Cost	Oral calcium and vitamin D preparations are relatively inexpensive on an individual patient basis, but at a population level they account for substantial healthcare spending. Calcium gluconate is inexpensive.

Clinical tip—Hyperkalaemia is common among hospital inpatients and is potentially life threatening. Calcium gluconate is the first-line emergency treatment for severe hyperkalaemia associated with ECG abnormalities. As such, you should know its dose by heart (10 mL of calcium gluconate 10% IV over 5–10 minutes).

Calcium channel blockers

CLINICAL PHARMACOLOGY

Common indications	❶ Amlodipine and, to a lesser extent, nifedipine are used for the first- or second-line treatment of **hypertension,** to reduce the risk of stroke, myocardial infarction and death from cardiovascular disease. ❷ All calcium channel blockers can be used to control symptoms in people with **stable angina;** β-blockers are the main alternative. ❸ Diltiazem and verapamil are used to control cardiac rate in people with **supraventricular arrhythmias,** including supraventricular tachycardia, atrial flutter and atrial fibrillation.
Mechanisms of action	Calcium channel blockers decrease calcium ion (Ca^{2+}) entry into vascular and cardiac cells, reducing intracellular calcium concentration. This causes **relaxation and vasodilation in arterial smooth muscle,** lowering arterial pressure. In the heart, calcium channel blockers **reduce myocardial contractility.** They **suppress cardiac conduction,** particularly across the atrioventricular (AV) node, slowing ventricular rate. Reduced cardiac rate, contractility and afterload reduce **myocardial oxygen demand,** preventing angina. Calcium channel blockers can broadly be divided into two classes. *Dihydropyridines*, including amlodipine and nifedipine, are relatively selective for the vasculature, whereas *non-dihydropyridines* are more selective for the heart. Of the *non-dihydropyridines*, verapamil is the most cardioselective, whereas diltiazem also has some effects on blood vessels.
Important adverse effects	Common adverse effects of *amlodipine* and *nifedipine* include **ankle swelling, flushing, headache** and **palpitations,** which are caused by vasodilatation and compensatory tachycardia. *Verapamil* commonly causes **constipation** and less often, but more seriously, can cause **bradycardia, heart block** and **cardiac failure.** As *diltiazem* has mixed vascular and cardiac actions, it can cause any of these adverse effects.
Warnings	*Verapamil* and *diltiazem* should be used with caution in patients with ▲**poor left ventricular function** as they can precipitate or worsen heart failure. They should generally be avoided in people with ▲**AV nodal conduction delay** in whom they may provoke complete heart block. *Amlodipine* and *nifedipine* should be avoided in patients with ✖**unstable angina** as vasodilatation causes a reflex increase in contractility and tachycardia, which increases myocardial oxygen demand. In patients with ✖**severe aortic stenosis,** amlodipine and nifedipine should be avoided as they can provoke collapse.
Important interactions	Non-dihydropyridine calcium channel blockers (*verapamil* and *diltiazem)* should not be prescribed with ✖β-blockers except under close specialist supervision. Both drug classes are negatively inotropic and chronotropic, and together may cause heart failure, bradycardia, and even asystole.

amlodipine, nifedipine, diltiazem, verapamil

CAL PRESCRIBING

Prescription	Calcium channel blockers are generally taken orally; of the examples in this book, only verapamil is available for IV administration in the acute management of arrhythmias. Amlodipine has a plasma half-life of 35–50 hours and is suitable for once-daily administration. By contrast, the half-lives of nifedipine (2–3 hours), verapamil (2–8 hours) and diltiazem (6–8 hours) are relatively short. Diltiazem and nifedipine are available in standard-release preparations that are taken 8-hrly, and modified release (MR) preparations taken 12-hrly or daily. These may need to be prescribed by brand name (see Clinical tip). Example treatment regimens are: for **hypertension,** amlodipine 5–10 mg orally daily; for **angina,** diltiazem MR 90 mg orally 12-hrly; and for **supraventricular arrhythmias,** verapamil 40–120 mg orally 8-hrly.
Administration	MR and long-acting preparations should be **swallowed whole,** and not crushed or chewed as this will interfere with the slow release of the drug.
Communication	Explain to patients why the calcium channel blocker has been prescribed, depending on indication. As appropriate, discuss other measures to **reduce cardiovascular risk,** including smoking cessation. Discuss **common side effects,** particularly ankle oedema if relevant.
Monitoring	Treatment efficacy can be judged by regular blood pressure monitoring for hypertension, enquiry about chest pain for angina and by pulse rate from examination or ECG. A 24-hour tape can be performed to review arrhythmias.
Cost	Amlodipine is available in non-proprietary form and is inexpensive. For diltiazem and nifedipine, only the longer-acting preparations are licensed to treat hypertension. These are more expensive.

Clinical tip—The different longer-acting preparations of nifedipine and diltiazem may not be 'bioequivalent' (i.e. pharmaceutically interchangeable). You should therefore request a specific brand when prescribing either of these drugs.

Carbamazepine

CLINICAL PHARMACOLOGY

Common indications	❶ Seizure prophylaxis in **epilepsy.** Epilepsy is classified by seizure type, which, in turn, guides antiepileptic drug choice. Carbamazepine is a first-line option for prophylaxis of generalised tonic-clonic seizures and focal seizures (with or without secondary generalisation). It is *not* recommended in absence or myoclonic seizures. ❷ **Trigeminal neuralgia,** as a first-line option to control pain and reduce frequency and severity of attacks.
Mechanisms of action	The mechanism of action of carbamazepine is incompletely understood. It appears to **inhibit neuronal sodium channels,** stabilising resting membrane potentials and reducing neuronal excitability. This may inhibit spread of seizure activity in epilepsy and control neuralgic pain by blocking synaptic transmission in the trigeminal nucleus.
Important adverse effects	The most common dose-related adverse effects are **GI upset** (e.g. nausea and vomiting) and **neurological effects** (particularly dizziness and ataxia). Carbamazepine **hypersensitivity** affects about 10% of people taking the drug and most commonly manifests as a mild maculopapular skin rash. **Antiepileptic hypersensitivity syndrome** affects around 1 in 5000 people taking carbamazepine, usually within 2 months of starting treatment. It can occur with a variety of other antiepileptic drugs, including lamotrigine and phenytoin, and rarely there is cross-sensitivity between drugs. Clinical features include severe skin reactions (e.g. Stevens–Johnson syndrome, toxic epidermal necrolysis), fever and lymphadenopathy with systemic (e.g. haematological, hepatic, renal) involvement and mortality of about 10%. Other common adverse effects include **oedema** and **hyponatraemia** due to an antidiuretic hormone-like effect.
Warnings	Carbamazepine exposure *in utero* is associated with neural tube defects, cardiac and urinary tract abnormalities and cleft palate. Women with epilepsy planning ▲**pregnancy** should discuss treatment with a specialist and start taking high-dose folic acid supplements before conception. Prior ✘**antiepileptic hypersensitivity syndrome** is a contraindication to carbamazepine and related drugs, due to potential cross-sensitivity. Carbamazepine should be prescribed with caution in patients with ▲**hepatic,** ▲**renal or** ▲**cardiac disease,** due to increased risk of toxicity.
Important interactions	Carbamazepine induces cytochrome P450 (CYP) enzymes, reducing plasma concentration and efficacy of ▲**drugs that are metabolised by CYP enzymes** (e.g. warfarin, oestrogens and progestogens). Carbamazepine is itself metabolised by these enzymes, so its concentration and adverse effects are increased by ▲**CYP inhibitors** (e.g. macrolides). Complex interactions occur with ▲**other antiepileptic drugs** (e.g. see Lamotrigine), due to altered drug metabolism. The efficacy of antiepileptic drugs is reduced by ▲**drugs that lower the seizure threshold** (e.g. antipsychotics, tramadol).

PRACTICAL PRESCRIBING

Prescription	Carbamazepine is only available for oral or rectal administration. It is usually **started at a low dose,** e.g. 100–200 mg once or twice daily, to limit dose-related adverse effects. As tolerance develops to adverse effects, the dose is **increased gradually** to a usual maximum of 1.6 g/day in divided doses. Treatment should not be stopped suddenly, but should be withdrawn gradually under medical supervision, due to risk of disease recurrence.
Administration	Oral carbamazepine is available as immediate- or modified-release tablets, chewable tablets and oral suspension. As carbamazepine bioavailability differs between formulations, switching between them is best avoided. For patients with **epilepsy,** you should seek to **avoid brand switching**. This is because loss of seizure control and/or worsening of side effects have been reported in patients who change brands, due to differing absorption characteristics. Use of rectal suppositories should be limited to short periods when oral administration is not possible as rectal irritation may occur with prolonged use.
Communication	Explain to patients that the aim of treatment is to reduce seizure frequency, not to 'cure' epilepsy. Warn patients to look out for signs of severe hypersensitivity, including skin rashes; bruising, bleeding, a high temperature or mouth ulcers (blood toxicity); and reduced appetite or abdominal pain (liver toxicity). If any of these occur they should seek urgent medical advice. For women, discuss contraception and pregnancy (see Valproate). Advise patients that they must not drive unless they have been seizure-free for 12 months, and for 6 months after changing or stopping treatment.
Monitoring	Treatment **efficacy** is monitored by comparing seizure frequency before and after starting treatment or dose adjustment. The most useful way to monitor **safety** is by asking the patient to report any unusual symptoms immediately (as above). Routine measurement of full blood count and liver enzymes is unlikely to coincide with unpredictable hypersensitivity reactions and so is not recommended. **Plasma carbamazepine concentrations** are not routinely measured, but may be useful in selected cases. Blood should be taken immediately before the next dose, when carbamazepine concentrations should be 4–12 mg/L. Time to steady-state plasma concentrations (and appropriate sampling for repeat measurements) is 1–2 weeks after starting treatment or a dose change.
Cost	Carbamazepine in any oral formulation is inexpensive.

Clinical tip—Neuropathic pain can be difficult to manage, with little evidence to guide choice between agents. Trigeminal neuralgia is, to an extent, an exception to this. It therefore stands alone in having a clear first-line choice (carbamazepine), the effectiveness of which has been well demonstrated. By contrast, the effectiveness of carbamazepine in other neuropathic pain syndromes has not been well studied. What little evidence there is generally suggests that gabapentin/pregabalin and the tricyclic antidepressants are preferable.

Cephalosporins and carbapenems

CLINICAL PHARMACOLOGY

Common indications	❶ Oral cephalosporins are second- and third-line options for treatment of **urinary** and **respiratory tract infections.** ❷ Parenteral cephalosporins and carbapenems are reserved for infections that are **very severe** or **complicated,** or caused by **antibiotic-resistant organisms.**
Spectrum of activity	Cephalosporins and carbapenems have a **broad** spectrum of action. For cephalosporins, progressive structural modification has led to successive 'generations' (first to fifth), with increasing activity against Gram-negative bacteria including *Pseudomonas aeruginosa* and variable activity against Gram-positive bacteria including *Staphylococcus aureus.* Cephalosporins and carbapenems are naturally more **resistant to β-lactamases** than penicillins due to fusion of the β-lactam ring with a dihydrothiazine ring (*cephalosporins*) or a unique hydroxyethyl side chain (*carbapenems*).
Mechanisms of action	Cephalosporins and carbapenems are derived from naturally occurring antimicrobials produced by fungi and bacteria. Like penicillins, their **bactericidal** effect is due to their **β-lactam ring.** During bacterial cell growth, cephalosporins and carbapenems inhibit enzymes responsible for cross-linking peptidoglycans in bacterial cell walls. This weakens cell walls, preventing them from maintaining an osmotic gradient, resulting in **bacterial cell swelling, lysis** and **death.**
Important adverse effects	**Gastrointestinal (GI) upset,** such as nausea and diarrhoea, is common. Less frequently, **antibiotic-associated colitis** occurs. Broad-spectrum antibiotics kill normal gut flora, allowing overgrowth of toxin-producing *Clostridium difficile*. This debilitating colitis can be complicated by colonic perforation and death. **Hypersensitivity,** including immediate and delayed reactions, may occur (see Penicillins). As cephalosporins and carbapenem share structural similarities to penicillins, cross-reactivity can occur in penicillin-allergic patients. There is a risk of **neurological toxicity,** including **seizures,** particularly where carbapenems are prescribed in high dose or to patients with renal impairment.
Warnings	Cephalosporins and carbapenems should be used with caution in people ▲**at risk of *C. difficile* infection,** particularly those in hospital and the elderly. The main contraindication is history of ✖**allergy** to a penicillin, cephalosporin or carbapenem, particularly if there was an ✖**anaphylactic reaction.** *Carbapenems* should be used with caution in patients with ▲**epilepsy.** Dose reduction is required in patients with ▲**renal impairment.**
Important interactions	Cephalosporins and carbapenems can enhance the anticoagulant effect of warfarin by killing normal gut flora that synthesise vitamin K. Cephalosporins may increase nephrotoxicity of aminoglycosides. Carbapenems reduce plasma concentration and efficacy of ▲valproate.

cefalexin, cefotaxime, meropenem, ertapenem

PRACTICAL PRESCRIBING

Prescription	*Cephalosporins* are usually prescribed for 6–12-hrly administration. Only certain cephalosporins (e.g. cefalexin) are orally active. Intravenous cephalosporins are used at high dose for severe infections (e.g. cefotaxime 2 g IV 6-hrly for bacterial meningitis). *Carbapenems* are only available for IV administration (e.g. meropenem 1–2 g IV 8-hrly). The indication, review date and duration of treatment should be documented on all inpatient antibiotic prescriptions to aid antibiotic stewardship.
Administration	*Cephalosporins* can be administered orally, as tablets, capsules or oral suspension, or by injection, which can be IV, as bolus injection or infusion, or IM. *Carbapenems* can be administered as IV injection or infusion. Ertapenem is a carbapenem that is administered once daily. This facilitates outpatient administration of IV antibiotic therapy and allows patients needing prolonged treatment to be at home.
Communication	Explain to patients that the aim of treatment is to get rid of infection and improve symptoms. Before prescribing, always check with patients personally or get collateral history to ensure they do not have an **allergy** to any form of penicillin or other β-lactam antibiotics. Warn them to seek medical advice if a rash or other unexpected symptoms develop. If an allergy develops during treatment, give the patient written and verbal advice not to take this antibiotic class in the future and make sure that the allergy is clearly documented in the patient's medical records.
Monitoring	Check that infection resolves by symptoms, signs (e.g. resolution of pyrexia) and blood tests (e.g. falling C-reactive protein and white cell count).
Cost	The costs of IV antibiotic therapy include drugs, administration time and equipment, complications (e.g. *C. difficile* infection), and need for inpatient stay. Where clinically appropriate, costs can be reduced by limiting duration of antibiotic therapy, IV-to-oral antibiotic switch during recovery and outpatient administration of IV antibiotics.

Clinical tip—Individual hospitals have antibiotic policies to protect valuable antibiotics from the development of resistance and reduce the risk of hospital-acquired infection. In many hospitals, IV cephalosporins and carbapenems can only be prescribed with the approval of a microbiologist. As antibiotic-associated colitis seems to occur more commonly with second- and third-generation cephalosporins, their use is now particularly restricted. Always get to know and follow your local antibiotic guidelines and seek microbiology advice where these do not cover a specific clinical situation.

Chloramphenicol

CLINICAL PHARMACOLOGY

Common indications	❶ **Bacterial conjunctivitis** using *eye drops* or *ointment*. ❷ **Otitis externa** using *ear drops*. Due to its toxicity, systemic (oral or IV) chloramphenicol is rarely used. In the UK, it is restricted to the treatment of life-threatening infection, and only where other, safer antibiotic classes cannot be used due to allergy or bacterial resistance. This may include occasional cases of epiglottitis (*Haemophilus influenzae*) and typhoid fever (*Salmonella* spp.).
Spectrum of activity	Chloramphenicol has **broad activity** against many Gram-positive, Gram-negative, aerobic and anaerobic organisms.
Mechanisms of action	Chloramphenicol binds to bacterial ribosomes, inhibiting protein synthesis. It is thus **bacteriostatic** (stopping bacterial growth), which helps the immune system to clear microorganisms. In high concentrations and with highly susceptible organisms it can be bactericidal (killing). The most common **mechanism of bacterial resistance** to chloramphenicol is production of acetyltransferase enzymes that directly inactivate the drug. Other mechanisms include target modification, decreased membrane permeability and increased expression of efflux pumps. Bacteria share antibiotic resistance genes by 'horizontal transfer' in plasmids. However, many bacteria remain sensitive to chloramphenicol, probably due to its **restricted use** over recent decades.
Important adverse effects	The most common adverse effects to *topical administration* are transient **stinging, burning** and **itching** when applied. *Systemic administration*, which is rare in developed-world practice, carries a significant risk of bone marrow toxicity. This takes two distinct forms: (i) **Dose-related bone marrow suppression** is more likely with high-dose therapy, or when the drug accumulates due to impaired hepatic metabolism. It occurs during treatment and is reversed on drug withdrawal. (ii) **Aplastic anaemia** is idiosyncratic; it has an unpredictable relationship with dose and may be delayed. It is a rare but life-threatening reaction to systemic therapy only. **Grey baby syndrome** is circulatory collapse occurring in exposed **neonates** who are unable to metabolise and excrete the drug. **Optic and peripheral neuritis** may occur with prolonged systemic administration.
Warnings	It is contraindicated in people with previous ✖**hypersensitivity reactions** to chloramphenicol, and a personal or family history of ✖**bone marrow disorders**. *Systemic chloramphenicol* is contraindicated in the ✖**third trimester of pregnancy,** ✖**breastfeeding** and in ✖**children <2 years** because of the risk of grey baby syndrome; *topical* preparations should also be avoided unless essential. Chloramphenicol is metabolised by the liver, and so dose adjustment and monitoring are required in ▲**hepatic impairment**.
Important interactions	Chloramphenicol has no important interactions when administered topically.

PRACTICAL PRESCRIBING

Prescription	Chloramphenicol is prescribed for **topical administration** as eye or ear drops or eye ointment. In these preparations, the amount of chloramphenicol is expressed as a percentage, which refers to the mass in grams of drug in 100 mL of diluent (e.g. 0.5 g/100 mL for a 0.5% solution). For **eye infections**, drug application needs to be frequent as tears and blinking remove the drug. Eye **drops** (0.5%) should be prescribed initially as one drop every 2 hours (when awake), with frequency reduced to 3–4 times daily as infection is controlled. Eye **ointment** (1%) stays in the eye for longer, so should be applied 3–4 times daily. Treatment should be continued for 48 hours after healing. For **otitis externa**, 3–4 ear drops (5–10%, higher concentration than eye drops as less risk of systemic absorption) are administered to the affected ear 2–3 times daily for up to 1 week. You should not prescribe systemic chloramphenicol without expert guidance.
Administration	Eye drops (optic) and ear drops (otic) are formulated differently. **Ear drops should not be put into the eye**, where they can cause injury with burning, stinging and blurred vision. Eye drops can be used safely in the ear, but may be less effective due to lower drug concentrations in eye preparations.
Communication	For **eye drops or ointment**, advise patients that **transient blurred vision** may occur and that they should not drive until vision is clear. Soft contact lenses may be damaged by eye drop preservatives and all **contact lenses should be avoided** during ocular infections. Advise patients to **ensure that eye drops/ointment are not contaminated** by microbes that could make the infection worse. They should check the preparation is sealed when they receive it, wash hands before use, take care not to touch the bottle or tube with hands, eye or skin, and discard any remaining drug at the end of the course. If patients obtain chloramphenicol **over the counter** for a self-diagnosed eye infection they should **seek medical advice** if there is no improvement after 2 days or if symptoms worsen, as this may indicate an incorrect diagnosis or superinfection with resistant organisms.
Monitoring	Monitoring during systemic therapy should be guided by a specialist. **Full blood count** should be monitored closely and the drug stopped if any signs of myelosuppression are evident.
Cost	Chloramphenicol eye and ear drops are inexpensive and can be sold directly to the public from pharmacies.

Clinical tip—Systemic chloramphenicol is not currently first-line treatment for any indication in the UK. However, as multidrug resistance to antibiotics evolves, 'older', more toxic, antibiotics may increasingly be needed. You will need to demonstrate continued professional development in antimicrobial prescribing to adapt to such changes.

Corticosteroids (glucocorticoids), inhaled

CLINICAL PHARMACOLOGY

Common indications	**❶ Asthma:** to treat airways inflammation and control symptoms where asthma is not adequately controlled by occasional use of a short-acting β₂-agonist alone. **❷ Chronic obstructive pulmonary disease (COPD):** to control symptoms and prevent exacerbations in patients who have severe airflow obstruction on spirometry and/or recurrent exacerbations. Inhaled corticosteroids are usually prescribed in combination with a long-acting β₂ agonist (LABA).
Mechanisms of action	Corticosteroids pass through the plasma membrane and interact with receptors in the cytoplasm. The activated receptor then passes into the nucleus to modify the transcription of a large number of genes. Pro-inflammatory interleukins, cytokines and chemokines are downregulated, while antiinflammatory proteins are upregulated. In the airways, **this reduces mucosal inflammation, widens the airways and reduces mucus** secretion. This **improves symptoms and reduces exacerbations** in asthma and COPD.
Important adverse effects	The main adverse effects of inhaled corticosteroids occur locally in the airway, where their immunosuppressive effect can cause **oral candidiasis** (thrush infection). They can also cause a **hoarse voice.** In COPD, there is some evidence they may increase the risk of **pneumonia.** Very little is absorbed into the blood, so there are few systemic adverse effects unless taken at a very high dose when systemic side effects including adrenal suppression, growth retardation (children) and osteoporosis may occur.
Warnings	High-dose inhaled corticosteroids, particularly fluticasone, should be used with caution in COPD patients with a ▲**history of pneumonia** and in ▲**children,** where there is potential for growth suppression.
Important interactions	There are no clinically significant adverse drug interactions with inhaled corticosteroids.

beclometasone, budesonide, fluticasone

PRACTICAL PRESCRIBING

Prescription	A variety of inhaler devices are available. Selecting the device that best suits the patient is important, and this may dictate drug choice. Inhaled corticosteroids should usually be prescribed for **twice-daily administration,** with dose depending on the drug chosen and nature and severity of illness. For example, beclometasone (e.g. as Clenil Modulite® MDI) 100 micrograms, two puffs 12-hrly would be an option for initiation of treatment in asthma. Brand name prescribing may be necessary as different preparations of the same drug may have different potencies depending on how they are deposited in the airway.
Administration	Drugs are delivered in **aerosol** (metered-dose inhaler, MDI) or **dry powder** form. Provision of a **spacer with MDIs** can improve airway deposition and treatment efficacy and reduce oral adverse effects. The patient should be trained how to use their **inhaler** and **technique** should be checked and corrected at every consultation.
Communication	Explain to patients that you are offering a steroid inhaler to 'dampen down' inflammation in the lung. Reassure them that hardly any of the steroid is absorbed into the body, so, except in very high-dose treatment, there are unlikely to be any serious side effects (or weight gain). Advise them to rinse their mouth and gargle after taking the inhaler to prevent development of a sore mouth or hoarse voice. Show patients how to use the device and check and correct their technique as necessary every time you see them.
Monitoring	Patients with asthma can monitor their disease severity through symptoms and serial peak expiratory flow rate measurements. They may be able to adjust their own treatment with guidance from a written 'action plan.' Likewise, symptom severity and exacerbation rates are the main indicators of effect in COPD. In general, a review after 3–6 months of therapy should be undertaken to see if therapy should be maintained, intensified or reduced.
Cost	In general, inhalers that contain corticosteroids only are relatively cheap, whereas combination inhalers are more expensive.

Clinical tip—Poorly controlled airway inflammation in asthma can lead to airways remodelling and fixed airflow obstruction. As inflammation is generally steroid-responsive, patients with **asthma** should be strongly encouraged to **take sufficient inhaled corticosteroids to control symptoms and prevent disease progression.** By contrast, airways inflammation in COPD is poorly responsive to steroids and, although inhaled corticosteroids can improve lung function and reduce exacerbations, they do not prevent disease progression.

Corticosteroids (glucocorticoids), systemic

CLINICAL PHARMACOLOGY

Common indications	❶ To treat **allergic** or **inflammatory disorders,** e.g. anaphylaxis, asthma. ❷ Suppression of **autoimmune disease,** e.g. inflammatory bowel disease, inflammatory arthritis. ❸ In the treatment of some **cancers** as part of chemotherapy or to reduce tumour-associated swelling. ❹ Hormone replacement in **adrenal insufficiency** or **hypopituitarism.**
Mechanisms of action	These corticosteroids exert mainly glucocorticoid effects. They bind to cytosolic glucocorticoid receptors, which then translocate to the nucleus and bind to glucocorticoid-response elements, which regulate gene expression. Corticosteroids are most commonly prescribed to **modify the immune response**. They **upregulate antiinflammatory genes** and **downregulate pro-inflammatory genes** (e.g. cytokines, tumour necrosis factor α). Direct actions on inflammatory cells include suppression of circulating monocytes and eosinophils. Their **metabolic effects** include increased gluconeogenesis from increased circulating amino and fatty acids, released by catabolism (breakdown) of muscle and fat. These drugs also have **mineralocorticoid effects**, stimulating Na^+ and water retention and K^+ excretion in the renal tubule.
Important adverse effects	**Immunosuppression** increases the risk and severity of infection and alters the host response. **Metabolic** effects include diabetes mellitus and osteoporosis. Increased catabolism causes proximal muscle weakness, skin thinning with easy bruising and gastritis. **Mood** and **behavioural changes** include insomnia, confusion, psychosis and suicidal ideas. Hypertension, hypokalaemia and oedema can result from **mineralocorticoid** actions. 　Corticosteroid treatment suppresses pituitary adrenocorticotropic hormone (ACTH) secretion, switching off the stimulus for normal adrenal cortisol production. In *prolonged treatment*, this causes **adrenal atrophy,** preventing endogenous cortisol secretion. If corticosteroids are withdrawn suddenly, an acute **Addisonian crisis** with Cardiovascular collapse may occur. Slow withdrawal is required to allow recovery of adrenal function. Symptoms of **chronic glucocorticoid deficiency** that occur during treatment withdrawal include fatigue, weight loss and arthralgia.
Warnings	Corticosteroids should be prescribed with caution in people with ▲**infection** and in ▲**children** (in whom they can suppress growth).
Important interactions	Corticosteroids increase the risk of peptic ulceration and GI bleeding when used with <u>NSAIDs</u> and enhance hypokalaemia in patients taking β_2-agonists, theophylline, <u>loop</u> or <u>thiazide diuretics</u>. Their efficacy may be reduced by ▲**Cytochrome P450 inducers** (e.g. phenytoin, <u>carbamazepine</u>, rifampicin). Corticosteroids reduce the immune response to vaccines.

prednisolone, hydrocortisone, dexamethasone

PRACTICAL PRESCRIBING

Prescription	Different corticosteroids have different antiinflammatory potencies. Of the examples given, dexamethasone is the most potent, with a dose of 750 micrograms being equivalent to prednisolone 5 mg and hydrocortisone 20 mg. Systemic corticosteroid treatment can be given orally or by IV or IM injection. In emergencies (e.g. treatment of the vasogenic oedema that may surround **brain tumours**), dexamethasone is prescribed at a high dose (e.g. 8 mg twice-daily orally or IV), then weaned slowly as symptoms improve. In acute asthma, prednisolone is usually prescribed at a dose of 40 mg orally daily. Where oral administration is inappropriate (e.g. **inflammatory bowel disease flares, anaphylaxis**), IV hydrocortisone may be used. In long-term treatment, e.g. for **inflammatory arthritis,** use the lowest dose of oral prednisolone that controls disease while limiting adverse effects. This may require co-prescription of steroid-sparing agents (e.g. azathioprine, methotrexate). In patients with relevant risk factors, consider the use of bisphosphonates and proton pump inhibitors to mitigate adverse effects.
Administration	Once-daily corticosteroid treatment should be taken in the morning, to mimic the natural circadian rhythm and reduce insomnia.
Communication	Explain to patients that treatment should suppress the underlying disease process and that they will usually **start to feel better within 1–2 days.** For patients who require prolonged treatment, warn them **not to stop treatment suddenly,** as this could make them very unwell. Give them a steroid card to carry with them at all times and show if they need treatment. Discuss the benefits and risks of steroids, including longer-term risks of osteoporosis, bone fractures and diabetes so that the patient can make an informed decision about taking treatment.
Monitoring	Monitoring of **efficacy** will depend on the condition treated, e.g. peak flow recordings for asthma, blood inflammatory markers for inflammatory arthritis. In prolonged treatment, monitor for **adverse effects** by, for example, measuring glucose and haemoglobin A_{1c} (HbA$_{1c}$) (to identify diabetes mellitus) or performing a dual-energy X-ray absorptiometry (DEXA) scan (to measure bone density).
Cost	Prednisolone, hydrocortisone and dexamethasone are all available in non-proprietary form and are inexpensive.

Clinical tip—Patients on long-term corticosteroid therapy have atrophic adrenal glands and may be unable to increase cortisol secretion in response to stress. You may therefore need to provide this artificially by increasing the dose of exogenous corticosteroid. Common practice is to double the dose during acute illness, reducing back to the maintenance dose on recovery.

The top 100 drugs

Corticosteroids (glucocorticoids), topical

CLINICAL PHARMACOLOGY

Common indications	Inflammatory skin conditions, e.g. **eczema,** to treat disease flares or to control chronic disease where <u>emollients</u> alone are ineffective.
Mechanisms of action	Corticosteroids have **immunosuppressive, metabolic** and **mineralocorticoid** effects, as discussed in detail under <u>Corticosteroids (glucocorticoids), systemic</u>. Where corticosteroids are applied topically, effects are mostly limited to the site of application. With potent or prolonged use of topical corticosteroids, systemic absorption and effects can occur. Topical corticosteroids can be classified as being mild, moderately potent, potent and very potent, depending on the type and concentration of corticosteroid in the formulation. Of the examples given, hydrocortisone 0.1–2.5% is mild and betamethasone valerate 0.1% is potent.
Important adverse effects	Adverse effects are uncommon with mild or moderately potent topical corticosteroids. However, potent and very potent topical corticosteroids can cause **local adverse effects** such as skin thinning, striae, telangiectasia and contact dermatitis. When used on the face, they can cause perioral dermatitis and cause or exacerbate acne. Withdrawal of topical corticosteroids can cause a **rebound worsening** of the underlying skin condition. Rarely, **adrenal suppression** and **systemic adverse effects** occur (see <u>Corticosteroids (glucocorticoids), systemic</u>).
Warnings	You should not use topical corticosteroids where ▲**infection** is present as this can cause the infection to worsen or spread. Where ▲**facial lesions** are present, potent corticosteroids should be avoided and treatment courses should be short.
Important interactions	There are generally no significant drug interactions when corticosteroids are used topically. If several topical agents are being used on the same area of skin, applications should be spaced out to allow absorption of pharmacologically active agents; <u>emollients</u> should be applied last.

PRACTICAL PRESCRIBING

Prescription	General advice when prescribing topical corticosteroids is to use as mild a corticosteroid as possible for as short a time as possible, usually for no more than 2 weeks (1 week for facial lesions). When prescribing for **eczema,** choose mild corticosteroids for mild flares, moderately potent corticosteroids for moderate flares and potent corticosteroids for severe flares. Indicate the potency of the steroid alongside its name as part of the prescription. Your prescription should state the name and strength of the corticosteroid, the formulation required (e.g. lotion, cream, ointment [see Emollients]), and the amount to be supplied, e.g. *hydrocortisone 1% (mild) cream, supply 30 g*. Note that the strength of hydrocortisone is expressed as a percentage (1%), which indicates the number of grams of drug (1 g) in 100 g of cream. You also need to define the area of skin that the corticosteroid should be applied to and state that it should be applied one to two times daily. The amount to be supplied will depend on the area of skin to be covered. On average, 30–60 g of cream or ointment should cover both arms for a 2-week course.
Administration	Corticosteroids should be **applied very thinly** and **only to the area of skin where disease is active.** You may find that creams are easier to apply to moist lesions, while ointments are more suitable where skin has become thick and leathery (lichenified). Wash hands after application (unless they are being treated!).
Communication	Explain to patients that you are providing a therapy that will relieve inflammation and improve their skin problem, but that the full effect may take 1–2 weeks. Inform them how and when to apply the topical corticosteroid and that emollients should be applied 5 minutes after this**. Warn them of the risk of skin damage if the treatment is applied to the wrong areas or for too long.** The pharmacist should make sure that the instructions are stuck directly onto the tube of cream or ointment and not onto the outside packaging, which may be discarded.
Monitoring	Review the patient after 1–2 weeks of treatment to ensure that symptoms are improving and treatment instructions are being followed correctly.
Cost	All topical corticosteroids are relatively inexpensive. Mild topical corticosteroids can be purchased over the counter with advice from a pharmacist.

Clinical tip—Explaining how to apply the correct amount of topical corticosteroid can be tricky. The BNF advises that if a length of cream or ointment is squeezed from its tube to run from the fingertip to the first crease of an adult finger, this should provide enough cream or ointment to cover an area of skin approximately twice the size of the palm.

Digoxin

CLINICAL PHARMACOLOGY

Common indications	**❶** In **atrial fibrillation (AF)** and **atrial flutter,** digoxin is used to reduce the ventricular rate. However, a β-blocker or non-dihydropyridine calcium channel blocker is usually more effective. **❷** In **severe heart failure,** digoxin is an option in patients who are already taking an ACE inhibitor, β-blocker and either an aldosterone antagonist or angiotensin receptor blocker. It is used at an earlier stage in patients with co-existing AF.
Mechanisms of action	Digoxin is **negatively chronotropic** (it reduces the heart rate) and **positively inotropic** (it increases the force of contraction). In **AF and flutter** its therapeutic effect arises mainly via an indirect pathway involving increased vagal (parasympathetic) tone. This reduces conduction at the atrioventricular (AV) node, preventing some impulses from being transmitted to the ventricles, thereby reducing the ventricular rate. In **heart failure,** it has a direct effect on myocytes through inhibition of Na^+/K^+-ATPase pumps, causing Na^+ to accumulate in the cell. As cellular extrusion of Ca^{2+} requires low intracellular Na^+ concentrations, elevation of intracellular Na^+ causes Ca^{2+} to accumulate in the cell, increasing contractile force.
Important adverse effects	Adverse effects of digoxin include **bradycardia, gastrointestinal disturbance, rash, dizziness** and **visual disturbance** (blurred or yellow vision). Digoxin is proarrhythmic and has a low therapeutic index: that is, the safety margin between the therapeutic and toxic doses is narrow. A wide range of arrhythmias can occur in **digoxin toxicity** and these may be life threatening.
Warnings	Digoxin may worsen conduction abnormalities, so is contraindicated in ✖**second-degree heart block** and ✖**intermittent complete heart block.** It should not be used in patients with or at risk of ✖**ventricular arrhythmias.** The dose should be reduced in ▲**renal failure,** as digoxin is eliminated by the kidneys. Certain electrolyte abnormalities increase the risk of digoxin toxicity, including ▲**hypokalaemia,** ▲**hypomagnesaemia** and ▲**hypercalcaemia.** Potassium disturbance is probably the most important of these, as digoxin competes with potassium to bind the Na^+/K^+-ATPase pump. When serum potassium levels are low, competition is reduced and the effects of digoxin are enhanced.
Important interactions	Loop and thiazide diuretics can increase the risk of digoxin toxicity by causing hypokalaemia. Amiodarone, calcium channel blockers, spironolactone and quinine can all increase the plasma concentration of digoxin and therefore the risk of toxicity.

PRACTICAL PRESCRIBING

Prescription	Digoxin is available as an oral or IV preparation. The effect of IV digoxin is seen at about 30 minutes, compared with about 2 hours following an oral dose. Intravenous administration is therefore usually unnecessary. By either route, a **loading dose** is required if a rapid effect is needed. A common approach is to give 500 micrograms of digoxin, followed by 250–500 micrograms 6 hours later, depending on response. Thereafter, the usual maintenance dose is 125–250 micrograms daily. For hospital inpatients, the loading doses are prescribed in the once-only section of the drug chart, while the maintenance dose is prescribed in the regular section (starting on day 2). Be sure to write 'micrograms' in full.
Administration	Oral digoxin can be taken with or without food. Intravenous doses must be given slowly.
Communication	Explain to patients that you are offering a treatment which, as applicable, should slow down their abnormally fast heart rate and make their heart beat more strongly. You should warn your patient of common side effects such as sickness, diarrhoea and headache. Ask them to seek advice if side effects are particularly bad or seem to get progressively worse, as this may suggest the dose is too high.
Monitoring	The best guide to the effectiveness of digoxin is the patient's **symptoms** and **heart rate.** Check their ECG, electrolytes and renal function periodically, and particularly when these may change (e.g. during acute illnesses or after a change in medication). You should note that therapeutic doses of digoxin can cause ST-segment depression (the **'reverse tick'** sign) on the ECG. This is an expected effect and does not signify toxicity. In acute therapy, continuous cardiac monitoring is advisable. You do not need to monitor digoxin levels routinely, but it may be helpful to measure these if you suspect toxicity. High plasma concentrations of digoxin do not always indicate toxicity, but the likelihood of toxicity increases as digoxin plasma concentrations increase. Conversely, toxicity can occur even when digoxin concentration is within the 'therapeutic range'.
Cost	Digoxin is available in non-proprietary form at low cost.

Clinical tip—Because digoxin's effect on ventricular rate in AF relies on parasympathetic ('rest and digest') tone, it tends to be lost during stress and exercise. Digoxin is therefore now rarely used on its own for AF, although it may be an option in sedentary patients.

Dipeptidylpeptidase-4 inhibitors

CLINICAL PHARMACOLOGY

Common indications	**Type 2 diabetes:** In *combination* with metformin (and/or other hypoglycaemic agents) where blood glucose is not adequately controlled on a single agent. As a *single agent* to control blood glucose and reduce complications where <u>metformin</u> is contraindicated or not tolerated.
Mechanisms of action	The **incretins** (glucagon-like peptide-1 [GLP-1] and glucose-dependent insulinotropic peptide [GIP]) are released by the intestine throughout the day, but particularly in response to food. They promote insulin secretion and suppress glucagon release, lowering blood glucose. The incretins are rapidly inactivated by hydrolysis by the enzyme **dipeptidylpeptidase-4 (DPP-4)**. DPP-4 inhibitors ('gliptins') therefore lower blood glucose by preventing incretin degradation and increasing plasma concentrations of their active forms. The actions of the incretins are **glucose dependent**, occurring when blood glucose is elevated, so they do not stimulate insulin secretion at normal blood glucose concentrations or suppress glucagon release in response to hypoglycaemia. This means that DPP-4 inhibitors are less likely to cause hypoglycaemia than <u>sulphonylureas</u>, which stimulate insulin secretion irrespective of blood glucose.
Important adverse effects	DPP-4 inhibitors are generally well tolerated. Patients may experience GI upset, headache, nasopharyngitis or peripheral oedema. **Hypoglycaemia** can occur, particularly where DPP-4 inhibitors are prescribed in combination with other drugs that cause hypoglycaemia such as <u>sulphonylureas</u> or <u>insulin</u>. All the DPP-4 inhibitors are associated with a small risk of **acute pancreatitis**, affecting 0.1–1% people taking the drugs. This should be suspected in patients experiencing persistent abdominal pain and usually resolves on stopping the drug.
Warnings	DPP-4 inhibitors are contraindicated in people with a history of ✖**hypersensitivity** to the drug class and should not be used in the treatment of ✖**type 1 diabetes** or ✖**ketoacidosis**. As there is animal evidence of reproductive toxicity and insufficient human data to ascertain safety, they should not be used during ✖**pregnancy** or ✖**breastfeeding**. They should be used with caution in the ▲**elderly (>80 years)** and people with a ▲**history of pancreatitis**. Many of the DPP-4 inhibitors are renally excreted, so a dose reduction may be required for patients with ▲**moderate-to-severe renal impairment**.
Important interactions	Risk of hypoglycaemia is increased by co-prescription of other antidiabetic drugs, including <u>sulphonylureas</u> and <u>insulin</u>, and by alcohol. β-<u>blockers</u> may mask symptoms of hypoglycaemia. The efficacy of DPP-4 inhibitors is reduced by drugs that elevate blood glucose, e.g. <u>prednisolone</u>, <u>thiazide</u> and <u>loop diuretics</u>.

PRACTICAL PRESCRIBING

Prescription	DPP-4 inhibitors are prescribed **to be taken orally**, usually once daily: e.g. sitagliptin 100 mg daily, linagliptin 5 mg daily, saxagliptin 5 mg daily. They are also formulated in **fixed-dose combinations** with metformin. As metformin needs to be taken 2–3 times daily, these fixed-dose combinations contain half the daily dose of the DPP-4 inhibitor (e.g. sitagliptin 50 mg with metformin 1 g) and are prescribed twice daily. Advantages of combined preparations include reduced tablet burden and improved treatment adherence. Disadvantages include limited dosage options, which can make it difficult to customise the dose for individuals. Also, the culprit drug can be more difficult to identify where adverse effects occur.
Administration	DPP-4 inhibitors are formulated as tablets. They may be taken with or without food.
Communication	Advise patients that a 'gliptin' has been prescribed to help control their blood sugar level and reduce the risk of diabetic complications, such as kidney disease. Explain that tablets are not a replacement for **lifestyle measures** and should be taken in addition to a healthy, balanced diet and regular exercise. Advise them to stop taking the drug and seek urgent medical attention if they develop symptoms that could indicate **acute pancreatitis** (e.g. severe and persistent stomach pain radiating to the back) or **allergy** (e.g. rash, swelling of face, lips, tongue or throat).
Monitoring	Assess blood glucose control by measuring **HbA$_{1c}$.** When a DPP-4 inhibitor is used as monotherapy, the **target HbA$_{1c}$** is <48 mmol/mol; when used as part of combination therapy the target is <53 mmol/mol. An HbA$_{1c}$ >58 mmol/mol is generally a **trigger to intensify therapy** with another agent. Home capillary blood glucose monitoring is not routinely required. Measurement of renal function before treatment can determine need for dose adjustment for sitagliptin and saxagliptin.
Cost	Monotherapy with a DPP-4 inhibitor is around 10-fold more expensive than monotherapy with metformin. The cost of a DPP-4 inhibitor alone is the same as its cost in a fixed-dose combination with metformin. However, in the long term, as generic products emerge and their cost falls, using fixed-dose combinations (which are less amenable to generic substitution) generally costs more.

Clinical tip—Although DPP-4 inhibitors improve glycaemic control, there is no evidence that they reduce the risk of vascular complications. This contrasts with metformin and a new class of antihyperglycaemic drugs, the **sodium–glucose co-transporter 2 (SGLT-2) inhibitors** (e.g. dapagliflozin, empagliflozin). SGLT-2 inhibitors interfere with reabsorption of glucose from the renal tubule, increasing urinary glucose losses. They lower blood glucose and improve vascular outcomes, without a significant risk of hypoglycaemia. Although SGLT-2 inhibitors do not currently feature in the 'Top 100', we anticipate they soon will.

Direct oral anticoagulants

CLINICAL PHARMACOLOGY

Common indications	❶ **Venous thromboembolism** (VTE, the collective term for deep vein thrombosis and pulmonary embolism): Direct oral anticoagulants (DOACs) are an option for treatment and prevention of recurrence (secondary prevention) of VTE. <u>Heparin</u> and <u>warfarin</u> are alternatives. DOACs are also indicated for primary prevention of VTE in patients undergoing elective hip or knee replacement surgery. ❷ **Atrial fibrillation (AF):** Anticoagulation with DOACs is indicated to prevent stroke and systemic embolism in patients with non-valvular AF who have at least one risk factor (including previous stroke, symptomatic heart failure, diabetes mellitus or hypertension). <u>Warfarin</u> is an alternative.
Mechanisms of action	The coagulation cascade is a series of reactions triggered by vascular injury that generates a fibrin clot. The DOACs act on the **final common pathway** of the coagulation cascade, comprising factor X, thrombin and fibrin. Api**xa**ban, edo**xa**ban and rivaro**xa**ban directly inhibit activated factor X (**Xa**), preventing conversion of prothrombin to thrombin. Dabigatran directly inhibits thrombin, preventing the conversion of fibrinogen to fibrin. All DOACs therefore inhibit fibrin formation, preventing clot formation or extension in the veins and heart. They are less effective in the arterial circulation where clots are largely platelet driven, and are better prevented by <u>antiplatelet</u> agents.
Important adverse effects	**Bleeding** is a common adverse effect, particularly epistaxis, GI and genitourinary haemorrhage. The risk of intracranial haemorrhage and major bleeding is less with DOACs than with <u>warfarin</u>. However, the risk of **GI bleeding** is greater, possibly due to intraluminal drug accumulation causing local anticoagulant effects. Other adverse effects include **anaemia**, **GI upset**, **dizziness** and **elevated liver enzymes**.
Warnings	DOACs should be avoided in people with ✖**active, clinically significant bleeding** and in those with ✖**risk factors for major bleeding**, such as peptic ulceration, cancer, and recent surgery or trauma, particularly of the brain, spine or eye. As DOACs are excreted by multiple routes, including cytochrome P450 (CYP) enzyme metabolism and elimination in faeces and urine, dose reduction or an alternative agent may be required in ▲**hepatic** or ▲**renal disease**. DOACs are contraindicated in ✖**pregnancy** and ✖**breastfeeding**, where the risk of harm to offspring is unknown.
Important interactions	Risk of bleeding with DOACs is increased by concurrent therapy with **other antithrombotic agents** (e.g. ▲<u>heparin</u>, ▲<u>antiplatelets</u> and ▲<u>NSAIDs</u>). Other interactions can arise with drugs that affect the **metabolism** of DOACs (e.g. CYP inducers/inhibitors) or their **excretion** (through induction/inhibition of transport proteins). For example, the anticoagulant effect can be *increased* by ▲<u>macrolides</u>, ▲protease inhibitors and ▲<u>fluconazole</u> and *decreased* by ✖rifampicin and ✖phenytoin.

apixaban, dabigatran, edoxaban, rivaroxaban

PRACTICAL PRESCRIBING

Prescription	The **dosage regimens** of DOACs vary by indication. For example, rivaroxaban is prescribed at 15 mg 12-hrly for VTE treatment, 20 mg daily for prevention of stroke in AF and 10 mg daily to prevent VTE following hip or knee replacement. **Duration of treatment** also varies by indication: e.g. 14 days following knee replacement; lifelong for AF. DOACs are usually started without need for initial heparin treatment, as onset of action is rapid. However, where dabigatran or edoxaban are used to treat VTE, 5 days of prior anticoagulation with heparin is recommended to align with the clinical trial evidence base.
Administration	DOACs are taken **orally**. This gives them an important advantage over heparin in the outpatient prevention or treatment of VTE, as patients can take them without the need for training in administering SC injections. Rivaroxaban, but not the other DOACs, must be taken with food as this affects its absorption.
Communication	You should advise patients that DOACs work by reducing the ability of the blood to clot and thus that the **main side effect is an increased risk of bleeding**. Patients should be provided with an **alert card** and advised to show this on all healthcare contacts, particularly if they have an accident, need surgery or start a new medication which may interact. They should contact a healthcare professional immediately if they develop prolonged or serious bleeding, or weakness, tiredness or breathlessness that could be signs of anaemia. Otherwise they should take their prescribed DOAC at the same time each day until told to stop.
Monitoring	**DOACs do not require routine monitoring**. Where knowledge of exposure to factor Xa inhibitors can inform clinical decisions (e.g. overdose, emergency surgery), a calibrated, quantitative factor Xa assay can be performed. This should be done with advice from a haematologist. **Reversal agents** for DOACs, to use if major bleeding occurs, are emerging but are not yet universally available. Idarucizumab is a humanised monoclonal antibody fragment that binds to dabigatran and its metabolites, reversing its effects. Ande**xa**net α is a potential reversal agent for factor **Xa** inhibitors, which is likely to be authorised soon.
Cost	In the UK, 1 month's supply of DOACs at a dose required to treat VTE costs around £50, whereas a similar supply of warfarin tablets costs <£1. However, this difference may be mitigated by lower monitoring costs with DOACs than warfarin.

Clinical tip—Even if you don't expect to initiate these drugs yourself, make sure you recognise the names of all the DOACs. This will help you to identify patients who are anticoagulated (which may not be evident from their laboratory clotting profile) and minimise the risk of, for example, an erroneous 'knee jerk' prescription of VTE prophylaxis when they are admitted to hospital.

Diuretics, loop

CLINICAL PHARMACOLOGY

Common indications	❶ For relief of breathlessness in **acute pulmonary oedema** in conjunction with <u>oxygen</u> and <u>nitrates</u>. ❷ For symptomatic treatment of fluid overload in **chronic heart failure.** ❸ For symptomatic treatment of fluid overload in **other oedematous states,** e.g. due to renal disease or liver failure, where they may be given in combination with other diuretics.
Mechanisms of action	As their name suggests, loop diuretics act principally on the ascending limb of the **loop of Henle,** where they **inhibit the Na⁺/K⁺/2Cl⁻ co-transporter.** This protein is responsible for transporting sodium, potassium and chloride ions from the tubular lumen into the epithelial cell. Water then follows by osmosis. Inhibiting this process has a potent diuretic effect. In addition, loop diuretics have a direct effect on blood vessels, causing **dilatation of capacitance veins.** In acute heart failure, this reduces preload and improves contractile function of the 'overstretched' heart muscle. Indeed, this is probably the main benefit of loop diuretics in acute heart failure, as illustrated by the fact that a clinical response usually occurs before diuresis is evident.
Important adverse effects	Water losses due to diuresis can lead to **dehydration** and **hypotension.** Inhibiting the Na⁺/K⁺/2Cl⁻ co-transporter increases urinary losses of sodium, potassium and chloride ions. Indirectly, this also increases excretion of magnesium, calcium and hydrogen ions. You can therefore associate loop diuretics with almost any **low electrolyte state** (i.e. hyponatraemia, hypokalaemia, hypochloraemia, hypocalcaemia, hypomagnesaemia and metabolic alkalosis). A similar Na⁺/K⁺/2Cl⁻ co-transporter is responsible for regulating endolymph composition in the inner ear. At high doses, loop diuretics can affect this too, leading to **hearing loss** and **tinnitus.**
Warnings	Loop diuretics are contraindicated in patients with severe ✖**hypovolemia** or ✖**dehydration**. They should be used with caution in patients at risk of ▲**hepatic encephalopathy** (where hypokalaemia can cause or worsen coma) and in patients with severe ▲**hypokalaemia** and/or ▲**hyponatraemia.** Taken chronically, loop diuretics inhibit uric acid excretion and this can worsen ▲**gout.**
Important interactions	Loop diuretics have the potential to affect **drugs that are excreted by the kidneys.** For example, ▲lithium levels are increased due to reduced excretion. The risk of ▲<u>digoxin</u> toxicity may also be increased, because of diuretic-associated hypokalaemia. Loop diuretics can increase the ototoxicity and nephrotoxicity of ▲<u>aminoglycosides</u>.

PRACTICAL PRESCRIBING

Prescription	Loop diuretics are available in oral and IV preparations. In the management of acute pulmonary oedema, you usually prescribe the initial dose of the loop diuretic intravenously, due to its more rapid and reliable effect. A typical choice is furosemide 40 mg IV, prescribed in the once-only section. Then, depending on your patient's response (see Monitoring), you may need to prescribe additional IV bolus doses, regular oral maintenance doses or, in resistant cases, an IV infusion.
Administration	Intravenous doses of furosemide should be administered slowly, at a rate no greater than 4 mg/min. Oral maintenance doses should be taken in the morning (with a second dose in the early afternoon in the case of twice-daily administration) to avoid causing nocturia.
Communication	Explain to your patients that their body is overloaded with water. You are therefore offering a treatment to increase urine flow, which will hopefully improve this. The medicine will inevitably cause them to need to **pass water more often.** Provided they do not take doses late in the day it should not affect them at night.
Monitoring	For **efficacy** in the acute management of pulmonary oedema, evidence for a good response will include improvements in the patient's symptoms, tachycardia, hypertension and oxygen requirement. Increased urine output typically occurs later and indicates onset of the diuretic effect. In longer-term therapy, you should monitor your patient's symptoms, signs and body weight (aiming for losses of no more than 1 kg/day). For **safety,** periodic monitoring of serum sodium, potassium and renal function is also advisable, particularly in the first few weeks of therapy.
Cost	Tablet and injectable forms of furosemide and bumetanide are cheap. Oral solutions are considerably more expensive (about 20 times more in the case of furosemide; over 100 times for bumetanide).

Clinical tip—The proportion of furosemide absorbed from the gut (its *bioavailability*) is highly variable, both between and within individuals. It tends to be particularly low in the context of severe fluid overload, presumably due to gut wall oedema. This problem can be circumvented by administering furosemide IV, but this will not always be possible or desirable. In such cases, bumetanide may be a better choice, as there is some evidence that its bioavailability is more predictable. Bumetanide 1 mg is equivalent to about 40 mg of furosemide.

Diuretics, thiazide and thiazide-like

CLINICAL PHARMACOLOGY

Common indications	❶ As an **alternative first-line treatment for hypertension** where a <u>calcium channel blocker</u> would otherwise be used, but is either unsuitable (e.g. due to oedema) or there are features of heart failure. ❷ **Add-on treatment for hypertension** in patients whose BP is not adequately controlled by a <u>calcium channel blocker</u> plus an <u>ACE inhibitor</u> or <u>angiotensin receptor blocker (ARB)</u>.
Mechanisms of action	Thiazide diuretics (e.g. bendroflumethiazide) and thiazide-like diuretics (e.g. indapamide, chlortalidone) differ chemically but have similar effects and clinical uses; we refer to them collectively as 'thiazides.' **Thiazides inhibit the Na⁺/Cl⁻ co-transporter in the distal convoluted tubule of the nephron.** This prevents reabsorption of sodium and its osmotically associated water. The resulting diuresis causes an initial fall in extracellular fluid volume. Over time, compensatory changes (e.g. activation of the renin–angiotensin system) tend to reverse this, at least in part. The longer-term antihypertensive effect may be mediated by **vasodilatation,** the mechanism of which is incompletely understood.
Important adverse effects	Preventing sodium ion reabsorption from the nephron can cause **hyponatraemia,** although this is not usually problematic. The increased delivery of sodium to the distal tubule, where it can be exchanged for potassium, increases urinary potassium losses and may therefore cause **hypokalaemia.** This, in turn, may cause **cardiac arrhythmias.** Thiazides may increase plasma concentrations of glucose (which may unmask type 2 diabetes), low density lipoprotein (LDL)-cholesterol and triglycerides. However, their net effect on cardiovascular risk is protective. They may cause **impotence** in men.
Warnings	Thiazides should be avoided in patients with ✖**hypokalaemia** and ▲**hyponatraemia.** As they reduce uric acid excretion, they may precipitate acute attacks in patients with ▲**gout.**
Important interactions	The effectiveness of thiazides may be reduced by <u>NSAIDs</u> (although low-dose <u>aspirin</u> is not a concern). The combination of thiazides with other drugs that lower the serum potassium concentration (e.g. ▲<u>loop diuretics</u>) is best avoided. If combination is essential, it should prompt more intensive electrolyte monitoring.

PRACTICAL PRESCRIBING

Prescription	Thiazides are taken orally as part of the patient's regular medication. Indapamide (e.g. 2.5 mg daily) and chlortalidone (12.5–25 mg daily) are recommended for hypertension. Historically in UK practice, bendroflumethiazide 2.5 mg daily has been widely used, but this is not recommended because there is limited evidence to support it. There is little to be gained from higher-dose treatment, as this tends just to increase side effects without significantly improving the antihypertensive effect.
Administration	It is generally best to take the tablet in the morning, so that the diuretic effect is maximal during the day rather than at night and does not therefore interfere with sleep.
Communication	Explain to patients that you are offering treatment with a 'water tablet' for their high blood pressure. If they have leg swelling, it may also help with this. Enquire whether they have any difficulty getting to the toilet in time (either because of mobility issues or sensations of urgency), since the water tablet is likely to make them pass water more often. Advise patients that antiinflammatory drugs like ibuprofen, which can be bought without prescription, may reduce the effectiveness of diuretics. At review, ask men directly about the possible side effect of impotence, as this may not be volunteered without prompting.
Monitoring	The best measure of efficacy is the patient's BP and, if applicable, the severity of the patient's oedema. Measure the patient's serum electrolyte concentrations before starting the drug, at 2–4 weeks into therapy, and after any change in therapy that might alter electrolyte balance.
Cost	Indapamide, chlortalidone and bendroflumethiazide are available in non-proprietary forms and are inexpensive. Indapamide is also available in branded MR forms. These are more expensive but there is no convincing evidence that they are clinically superior.

Clinical tip—One of the main adverse effects of thiazides is *hypokalaemia*, while one of the main adverse effects of ACE inhibitors and ARBs is *hyperkalaemia*. Moreover, these drug classes have a synergistic BP lowering effect: thiazides tend to activate the renin–angiotensin system, while ACE inhibitors/ARBs block it. Consequently, the combination of a thiazide and an ACE inhibitor/ARB is very useful in practice, both to improve BP control and to maintain neutral potassium balance.

Dopaminergic drugs for Parkinson's disease

CLINICAL PHARMACOLOGY

Common indications	❶ Dopaminergic drugs are used in **early Parkinson's disease,** when dopamine agonists (e.g. ropinirole, pramipexol) may be preferred over levodopa. ❷ In **later Parkinson's disease,** levodopa is an integral part of management, while dopamine agonists are an option for add-on therapy. ❸ Levodopa and dopamine agonists may be options for **secondary parkinsonism** (parkinsonian symptoms due to a cause other than idiopathic Parkinson's disease), but addressing the underlying cause (e.g. discontinuation of an offending drug) generally takes precedence.
Mechanisms of action	In Parkinson's disease, there is a **deficiency of dopamine in the nigrostriatal pathway** that links the substantia nigra in the midbrain to the corpus striatum in the basal ganglia. Via direct and indirect circuits, this causes the basal ganglia to exert greater inhibitory effects on the thalamus which, in turn, reduces excitatory input to the motor cortex. This generates the features of Parkinson's disease, such as bradykinesia and rigidity. Treatment seeks to increase dopaminergic stimulation to the striatum. It is not possible to give dopamine itself because it does not cross the blood–brain barrier. By contrast, levodopa (L-dopa) is a **precursor of dopamine** that can enter the brain via a membrane transporter. Ropinirole and pramipexol are relatively selective **agonists for the D_2 receptor,** which predominates in the striatum.
Important adverse effects	All dopaminergic drugs can cause **nausea, drowsiness, confusion, hallucinations** and **hypotension.** A major problem with levodopa is the **wearing-off effect,** where the patient's symptoms worsen towards the end of the dosage interval. This seems to get worse as duration of therapy increases. It can be partially overcome by increasing the dose and/or frequency, but this can generate the opposite effect: excessive and involuntary movements **(dyskinesias)** at the beginning of the dosage interval. When these occur together, this is called the **on–off effect.**
Warnings	Dopaminergic drugs should be used cautiously in the ▲**elderly** and in those with existing ▲**cognitive or psychiatric disease,** due to the risk of causing confusion and hallucinations. Caution is also required in ▲**cardiovascular disease,** because of the risk of hypotension.
Important interactions	Levodopa is always given with a peripheral dopa-decarboxylase inhibitor (e.g. carbidopa) to reduce its conversion to dopamine outside the brain. This desirable interaction reduces nausea and lowers the dose needed for therapeutic effect. Dopaminergic agents should not usually be combined with ▲first-generation antipsychotics (and, to a lesser extent, second-generation) or ▲metoclopramide because of their opposing effects on dopamine receptors.

levodopa (as co-careldopa, co-beneldopa), ropinirole, pramipexol

PRACTICAL PRESCRIBING

Prescription	Treatment decisions in **Parkinson's disease** should be made by a specialist. Dopamine agonists are often preferred over levodopa in early, non-severe disease, whereas levodopa is the more effective option when symptoms are disabling. By deferring initiation of levodopa until as late as possible, the emergence of problematic on–off effects may also be delayed, since these increase in proportion to duration of levodopa therapy. Levodpa is always formulated as a combined preparation with a peripheral dopa-decarboxylase inhibitor: with benserazide (co-beneldopa) or carbidopa (co-careldopa).
Administration	It is very important with levodopa that doses are taken at times that produce the best symptom control for the patient. This is especially important if the patient is admitted to hospital (see Clinical tip).
Communication	Close communication is essential between the patient and specialists in Parkinson's disease. Often a clinical nurse specialist will form the vital link in this partnership. You should engage with the specialist team to support this.
Monitoring	The best form of monitoring for clinical efficacy and side effects is an assessment by a specialist multidisciplinary team. BP should be monitored in all patients receiving dopaminergic therapy, particularly those with existing cardiovascular disease.
Cost	The dopaminergic drugs mentioned here are available in non-proprietary forms. There may be good reasons to use a more expensive branded product in some cases (e.g. when the on–off effect is prominent, switching to an MR form may mitigate this). A gel formulation, administered continuously via a percutaneous jejunostomy tube, is substantially more expensive. It is initiated in specialist practice only.

Clinical tip—As a foundation doctor you are unlikely to play a major role in active prescribing decisions regarding antiparkinsonian therapy. However, you may be integral in *ensuring that the patient's therapy is maintained* if they are admitted to hospital. Adhering to the correct timing of doses is essential: ask the patient exactly what time they take each dose and prescribe accordingly. Discuss the importance of this with nursing staff and, where appropriate, consider implementing a self-medication approach. Avoid switching brands if possible. You should also know that dopaminergic therapy should never be stopped abruptly. As well as causing an inevitable deterioration in symptom control, there is a risk that this may precipitate neuroleptic malignant syndrome. In patients who become unable to take tablets, a transdermal dopamine-agonist preparation may be useful.

Emollients

CLINICAL PHARMACOLOGY

Common indications	As a topical treatment for all **dry** or **scaling skin disorders.** Specifically, emollients are used alone or in combination with <u>topical corticosteroids</u> in the treatment of **eczema.** They can reduce skin dryness and cracking in **psoriasis,** where, depending on severity, they are used alone or in combination with other therapies.
Mechanisms of action	Emollients help to **replace water** content in dry skin. They contain oils or paraffin-based products that help to soften the skin and can **reduce water loss** by protecting against evaporation from the skin surface. Many preparations can be used as a soap substitute (as soap is drying to the skin) and there are also specific bath or shower emollient preparations available.
Important adverse effects	Emollients have few adverse effects. The main tolerability issue is that they cause **greasiness** of the skin, but this is integral to their therapeutic effect. Emollient ointments can **exacerbate acne vulgaris** and **folliculitis** by blocking pores and hair follicles.
Warnings	While these drugs are usually very safe to use, paraffin-based emollients are a significant **fire hazard** when the oil content is high (>50%).
Important interactions	There are no significant interactions with other medications. However, when using more than one topical product, applications should be spaced out. This ensures that small volumes of topical drugs (e.g. topical corticosteroids) are not prevented from reaching the affected skin by large quantities of emollient.

PRACTICAL PRESCRIBING

Prescription	Emollients are emulsions of oil and water formulated as semi-solid **creams** (50% oil, 50% water), semi-liquid **lotions** (less oil, more water) or **ointments** (80% oil, 20% water). The choice of preparation will depend on the amount of skin to cover (lotions and creams spread further) and the severity of the condition (ointments are more occlusive and potent and last longer), as well as patient preference. You should prescribe emollients to be applied at least two or three times a day in active disease as their effect is quite short lasting. **You should prescribe a sufficiently large amount,** e.g. 500 g, to ensure adequate supply for frequent and widespread application. Treatment should continue after improvement of symptoms to prevent recurrence.
Administration	Apply emollients in the direction of hair growth to reduce the risk of folliculitis.
Communication	Explain to patients that you are offering a therapy that should improve skin dryness, but that it may take several days or weeks of treatment for the full effect to be seen. Encourage patients to apply emollients as often as possible. Advise them to use emollients instead of soap for hand-washing as well as when washing in a bath or shower. Warn them that **emollients can make bathroom fittings slippery.** When treating **eczema,** advise the patient to apply emollient to the whole body, rather than just the affected skin, and to keep using emollients even when the disease is controlled, to stop it returning. If patients are using other topical agents, advise them to apply these first and leave 5 minutes before applying an emollient.
Monitoring	When treating conditions like **eczema** or **psoriasis** you should review the patient to determine whether therapy has been effective. If emollients are ineffective, you may need to prescribe a second agent, such as a topical corticosteroid.
Cost	Non-proprietary emollients are cheap, around £2–£5 for 500 g. Proprietary preparations are often double this.

Clinical tip—Most people who find emollients ineffective are not applying them frequently enough. Sometimes this is because they find them greasy and unpleasant. In this case encourage them to try a cream or a lotion instead of an ointment and apply the treatment more often.

Fibrinolytic drugs

CLINICAL PHARMACOLOGY

Common indications	**1** In **acute ischaemic stroke,** alteplase increases the chance of living independently if it is given within 4.5 hours of the onset of the stroke. **2** In **acute ST elevation myocardial infarction,** alteplase and streptokinase can reduce mortality when they are given within 12 hours of the onset of symptoms in combination with antiplatelet agents and anticoagulants. However, primary percutaneous coronary intervention (where available) has largely superseded fibrinolytics in this context. **3** For **massive pulmonary embolism (PE) with haemodynamic instability** fibrinolytic drugs reduce clot size and pulmonary artery pressures, but there is no clear evidence that they improve mortality.
Mechanisms of action	Fibrinolytic drugs, also known as thrombolytic drugs, catalyse the conversion of plasminogen to plasmin, which acts to **dissolve fibrinous clots** and **re-canalise occluded vessels.** This allows reperfusion of affected tissue, preventing or limiting tissue infarction and cell death and improving patient outcomes.
Important adverse effects	Common adverse effects include **nausea** and **vomiting, bruising** around the injection site and **hypotension.** Adverse effects that require treatment to be stopped include **serious bleeding, allergic reaction, cardiogenic shock** and **cardiac arrest.** Serious bleeding may require treatment with coagulation factors and antifibrinolytic drugs, e.g. tranexamic acid, but this is usually avoidable as fibrinolytic agents have a very short half-life. Reperfusion of infarcted brain or heart tissue can lead to **cerebral oedema** and **arrhythmias,** respectively.
Warnings	There are many contraindications to thrombolysis, which are mostly factors that predispose to ✖**bleeding,** including: recent haemorrhage; recent trauma or surgery; bleeding disorders; severe hypertension; and peptic ulcers. In acute stroke, ✖**intracranial haemorrhage** must be excluded with a computed tomography (CT) scan before treatment. ✖**Previous streptokinase treatment** is a contraindication to repeat dosing (although other fibrinolytics can be used), as development of antistreptokinase antibodies can block its effect.
Important interactions	The risk of haemorrhage is increased in patients taking <u>anticoagulants</u> and <u>antiplatelet</u> agents. <u>ACE inhibitors</u> appear to increase the risk of anaphylactoid reactions.

PRACTICAL PRESCRIBING

Prescription	Fibrinolytic drugs should be prescribed only by clinicians with expertise in their use. The dose varies depending on the indication, timing from the onset of symptoms and the patient's weight. They are available as injectable preparations only. A bolus dose is usually given first, followed by an IV infusion.
Administration	Fibrinolytic drugs should be administered in a high dependency area such as the emergency department, hyperacute stroke unit or coronary care unit, by staff with expertise in their use. Alteplase comes as a powder, which is reconstituted with sterile water (also provided in the package), and then either given directly as an IV bolus injection or diluted further in 0.9% <u>sodium chloride</u> and given as an IV infusion.
Communication	The decision to 'thrombolyse' (prescribe fibrinolytic therapy) should be made by an expert clinician, and the risks and benefits discussed with the patient and next of kin. For example, in acute stroke, explain that part of the brain is being starved of blood and oxygen due to a blocked artery, which will cause long-term damage. Giving a 'clot-busting drug' can reduce damage to the brain by dissolving the blood clot and restoring blood flow. However, it works only if given soon after the onset of the stroke. With or without treatment people may show some improvement, but symptoms may also get worse and one in three strokes is fatal. Although the chance of death is increased initially after receiving a clot-busting drug (due to bleeding), after the first week the chances of living independently are increased. For licensed indications, written consent is not essential but verbal consent should be obtained. If neurological impairment prevents consent, treatment can still be given if judged to be in the patient's best interests.
Monitoring	Patients should be monitored in a high dependency area, with vital signs checked every 15 minutes for the first 2 hours. This should include observation for signs of bleeding, anaphylaxis and, particularly in the case of acute stroke, neurological deterioration.
Cost	Fibrinolytic agents are currently available as branded products only. Treatment with alteplase costs around £300–£600 and with streptokinase costs around £80.

Clinical tip—In patients with acute ischaemic stroke, likely benefits of thrombolysis diminish rapidly with time. Compared with untreated patients, the chance of being alive and independent at 6 months is increased by 10% for patients who receive thrombolysis within 3 hours of symptom onset, but by 2% if thrombolysis is performed between 3 and 6 hours. Campaigns that encourage patients to present early, rapid triage and CT scanning, and good organisation of thrombolysis services are essential for treatment to be effective.

Gabapentin and pregabalin

CLINICAL PHARMACOLOGY

Common indications	❶ Both drugs are options for **add-on treatment of focal epilepsies** (with or without secondary generalisation) when other antiepileptic drugs (e.g. <u>carbamazepine</u>, <u>lamotrigine</u>, <u>valproate</u>) provide inadequate control. They are *not* recommended in absence and myoclonic seizures. ❷ Both drugs are first-line options for **neuropathic pain,** including painful diabetic neuropathy (<u>carbamazepine</u> is preferred in trigeminal neuralgia). ❸ Pregabalin is an option in **generalised anxiety disorder.**
Mechanisms of action	From a structural point of view, gabapentin and pregabalin are related to γ-aminobutyric acid (GABA), the major inhibitory neurotransmitter in the brain. However, they do not bind with GABA receptors and their mechanism of action, although not completely understood, seems to be mediated through binding with pre-synaptic **voltage-sensitive calcium (Ca^{2+}) channels.** This inhibits release of excitatory neurotransmitters, interfering with neurotransmitter release. The resulting **reduction of neuronal excitability** in the brain probably explains the drugs' anticonvulsant effects. These central effects, along with similar effects in peripheral nerves, may also explain the mechanism by which they reduce neuropathic pain.
Important adverse effects	Gabapentin and pregabalin are generally better tolerated than older antiepileptic drugs. Their main side effects are **drowsiness, dizziness** and **ataxia,** which usually improve over the first few weeks of treatment.
Warnings	Both drugs depend on the kidneys for their elimination, so their doses should be reduced in ▲**renal impairment.**
Important interactions	The sedative effects of gabapentin and pregabalin may be enhanced when combined with other ▲**sedating drugs** (e.g. <u>benzodiazepines</u>). Other than this, gabapentin and pregabalin are notable in having relatively few drug interactions – in contrast to many other antiepileptic drugs, including <u>carbamazepine</u>, <u>lamotrigine</u> and <u>valproate</u>. This makes them particularly useful where combination regimens are necessary.

gabapentin, pregabalin

PRACTICAL PRESCRIBING

Prescription	Gabapentin and pregabalin are taken orally. To improve tolerability, they should be started at a low dose. The dose is then increased over subsequent days and weeks to reach a dose that strikes the optimal balance between benefits and side effects. Appropriate escalating-dose regimens are listed in the BNF.
Administration	There are no special considerations with regard to the oral administration of gabapentin and pregabalin.
Communication	Explain to patients that you are offering a medicine which you anticipate will reduce the severity of their symptoms (e.g. seizure frequency or pain severity, as applicable). Explain that the medicine commonly causes some drowsiness or dizziness. For this reason, you will prescribe a low dose initially, then increase this gradually (make sure they are clear on the dosing instructions). Explain that these side effects should improve over the first few weeks. They should avoid driving or operating machines until they are confident that the symptoms have settled. For patients with epilepsy, advise that driving is prohibited unless they have been seizure-free for 12 months, and for 6 months after changing or stopping treatment.
Monitoring	The best guide to clinical effectiveness is to enquire about symptoms (e.g. seizure frequency) and side effects. Plasma concentration measurement is not required.
Cost	Gabapentin and pregabalin are available in both branded and non-proprietary forms. The brand name products are more expensive; there is no reason to prefer them. At the time of writing, pregabalin was more expensive than gabapentin. Due to its cost and prescribing volume, pregabalin represents a significant drug cost for the NHS.

Clinical tip—Gabapentin may cause false-positive results for detection of protein on urine dipstick testing. In this case, a sample should be sent to the laboratory for quantitative analysis (e.g. a spot sample for protein:creatinine ratio), which is not affected by gabapentin.

H₂-receptor antagonists

CLINICAL PHARMACOLOGY

Common indications	❶ **Peptic ulcer disease:** for treatment and prevention of gastric and duodenal ulcers and <u>NSAID</u>-associated ulcers, although <u>proton pump inhibitors</u> (PPIs) are more effective and therefore usually preferred. ❷ **Gastro-oesophageal reflux disease (GORD)** and **dyspepsia:** for relief of symptoms. <u>PPIs</u> are the main alternative, and preferred in more severe cases.
Mechanisms of action	Histamine H_2-receptor antagonists ('H_2-blockers') **reduce gastric acid secretion.** Acid is normally produced by the proton pump of the gastric parietal cell, which secretes H^+ into the stomach lumen in exchange for drawing K^+ into the cell. The proton pump is regulated, among other things, by histamine. Histamine is released by local paracrine cells and binds to H_2-receptors on the gastric parietal cell. Via a second-messenger system, this activates the proton pump. Blocking H_2-receptors therefore reduces acid secretion. However, as the proton pump can also be stimulated by other pathways, H_2-blockers cannot completely suppress gastric acid production. In this respect they differ from <u>PPIs</u>, which tend to have a more complete suppressive effect.
Important adverse effects	H_2-blockers are generally well tolerated with **few side effects.** Most common among these are bowel disturbance (diarrhoea or, less often, constipation), headache and dizziness.
Warnings	H_2-blockers are excreted by the kidneys, so their dose should be reduced in patients with renal impairment. Like <u>PPIs</u>, they can **disguise the symptoms of gastro-oesophageal cancer,** so it is important not just to treat symptoms without considering and, if appropriate, investigating their cause.
Important interactions	Ranitidine has **no major drug interactions**.

PRACTICAL PRESCRIBING

Prescription	Ranitidine can be purchased over the counter, but only for short-term use. You will need to write a prescription if you intend for the patient to take it for more than 2 weeks. The dose varies according to the indication, but 150 mg 12-hrly is typical. Likewise, the duration of therapy varies according to the indication.
Administration	Oral preparations can be taken before, with or after food.
Communication	Explain to patients that you are offering treatment to reduce stomach acid. This will hopefully improve their symptoms and, if applicable, allow their ulcer to heal. It is reasonable to say that side effects are pretty uncommon with this medicine. Ensure that both you and the patient are clear on the intended duration of therapy and the need to report any 'alarm' symptoms (e.g. weight loss, swallowing difficulty), should they arise.
Monitoring	For treatment of peptic ulcer disease, repeat endoscopy may be necessary in some cases to confirm healing. For symptomatic treatment of dyspepsia and GORD, the patient's symptoms are the best guide to the effect of therapy.
Cost	Standard ranitidine tablets are inexpensive; effervescent tablets and oral solution are about 10 times more expensive.

Clinical tip—H$_2$-blockers have been superseded by PPIs for most indications, due to their more complete acid suppressing effect. One advantage that H$_2$-blockers retain, however, is a more rapid onset of effect. This probably makes them a better choice for suppressing gastric acid production pre-operatively. In a patient with significant GORD due to undergo general anaesthesia, there is a risk that gastric acid may reflux and then be aspirated, causing pneumonitis. The anaesthetist may prescribe a dose of ranitidine to mitigate this. You may score 'brownie points' if you identify such patients and prescribe ranitidine yourself. You are looking for patients with active reflux symptoms—the sensation of acid coming up the gullet—who are due to undergo a procedure involving sedation or general anaesthesia. Offer ranitidine 300 mg orally, to be taken with a sip of water at least 2 hours before the start of the surgical list.

Heparins and fondaparinux

CLINICAL PHARMACOLOGY

Common indications	❶ Heparin, usually low molecular weight heparin (LMWH), is used for primary prevention of **deep vein thrombosis** and **pulmonary embolism** (collectively **venous thromboembolism, VTE**) in hospital inpatients. It is also an option for initial treatment of VTE, until oral anticoagulation (e.g. with warfarin, dabigatran) is established. Fondaparinux and DOACs (e.g. rivaroxaban) are alternatives. ❷ **Acute coronary syndrome (ACS):** Heparin (usually LMWH) or fondaparinux is used with antiplatelet agents to reduce clot progression or maintain revascularisation.
Mechanisms of action	In simplistic terms, venous and intracardiac clot formation is driven largely by the coagulation cascade, while arterial thrombosis is more a phenomenon of platelet activation. The coagulation cascade is an amplification reaction between clotting factors that generates a fibrin clot. **Antithrombin** (AT) inactivates clotting factors, particularly factors IIa (thrombin) and Xa, providing a natural break to the clotting process. Heparins and fondaparinux act by **enhancing the anticoagulant effect of AT.** The size of heparin molecules determines their molecular specificity: *unfractionated heparin (UFH)* (large and small molecules) promotes inactivation of both factors IIa and Xa, whereas *LMWH* (smaller molecules) is more specific for factor Xa. Fondaparinux is a synthetic pentasaccharide that mimics the sequence of the binding site of heparin to AT and is very specific for factor Xa.
Important adverse effects	The main adverse effect is **haemorrhage.** This risk may be lower with fondaparinux than with LMWH or UFH. Bruising or other reactions may occur at the **injection site. Hyperkalaemia** occurs occasionally due to an effect on adrenal aldosterone secretion. Rarely, patients may experience a dangerous immune reaction to heparin, characterised by low platelet count and thrombosis **(heparin-induced thrombocytopenia, HIT).** This is less likely with LMWH than UFH, and does not occur with fondaparinux.
Warnings	Anticoagulants should be used with caution in patients at increased risk of bleeding, including: ▲**clotting disorders;** ▲**severe uncontrolled hypertension;** and ▲**recent surgery or trauma.** They should be withheld immediately before and after ▲**invasive procedures,** particularly lumbar puncture and spinal anaesthesia. In ▲**renal impairment,** LMWH and fondaparinux accumulate, so a lower dose or UFH should be used instead.
Important interactions	Combining heparins with other antithrombotic drugs (e.g. antiplatelets, warfarin) has an additive effect. This is sometimes desirable (e.g. in treating ACS), but it is associated with an increased risk of bleeding, so should otherwise be avoided. In major bleeding, protamine is an option to reverse heparin anticoagulation. This is effective for UFH but much less so for LMWH, and ineffective against fondaparinux. Andexanet α is in development and appears to be an effective reversal agent.

enoxaparin, dalteparin, fondaparinux, unfractionated heparin

PRACTICAL PRESCRIBING

Prescription	LMWH, given SC, is preferred in most indications. Dosage is specified in units (*never* abbreviate this to 'U', which can easily be misread as '0'), and varies with indication and body weight. A typical VTE prophylaxis regimen is dalteparin 5000 units SC daily, but you should refer to local protocols. UFH may be preferred in renal impairment (e.g. heparin 5000 units SC 12-hrly for VTE prophylaxis) or when rapid onset and offset of anticoagulation is required (when it is given as a variable-rate IV infusion).
Administration	SC injections of these drugs should be given into the SC tissue of the abdominal wall. The arm should not be used because this can cause uncomfortable and disabling bruising.
Communication	In the context of VTE prophylaxis, explain to patients that you are offering a daily injection to reduce the risk of blood clots. In longer-term therapy (e.g. for the treatment of VTE in cancer, when LMWH may be preferred over warfarin), discuss the risks and benefits of anticoagulation. Advise patients to avoid activities that may increase their risk of bleeding and to inform healthcare professionals they encounter that they are taking anticoagulants. The patient (or their carer) will need to be trained in SC injection technique. If this is not possible, administration by a district nurse may be arranged.
Monitoring	A major advantage of LMWH and fondaparinux over UFH is that their anticoagulant effect is sufficiently predictable to obviate the need for routine laboratory monitoring. Where required in selected cases (e.g. renal impairment, pregnancy), plasma **antifactor Xa activity** is measured. UFH has a less predictable effect and, when used to achieve full ('therapeutic' as opposed to 'prophylactic') anticoagulation, the dosage is titrated against the activated partial thromboplastin ratio (APTR) (usual target 1.5–2.5). Full blood count, baseline clotting and renal profiles should be checked before starting treatment. In prolonged therapy (>4 days), **platelet count** and **serum potassium concentration** should be monitored, as the risk of thrombocytopenia and hyperkalaemia increases with duration of therapy. Seek immediate specialist advice if the platelet count drops significantly, as this may signify HIT, which requires urgent management.
Cost	When used for VTE prophylaxis, LMWH costs approximately £3 per day, whereas fondaparinux and UFH cost ~£6 per day. For UFH infusion, consumables and monitoring increase the costs. Cost is not generally a driver of drug choice for heparins and fondaparinux.

Clinical tip—When warfarin is to be used for VTE treatment, another anticoagulant (often LMWH) may be given alongside it initially. In this context, LMWH provides **'bridging anticoagulation'** during the period in which warfarin may be briefly pro-thrombotic (due to its initial inhibition of natural anticoagulants [proteins C and S], before its effect on other clotting factors [II, VII, IX, X] is established). LMWH should be continued for 5 days or until the INR (see Warfarin) is in the therapeutic range, whichever is longer.

Insulin

CLINICAL PHARMACOLOGY

Common indications	❶ For insulin replacement in people with **type 1 diabetes** and control of blood glucose in people with **type 2 diabetes** where oral hypoglycaemic treatment is inadequate or poorly tolerated. ❷ Given intravenously, in the treatment of **diabetic emergencies** such as diabetic ketoacidosis and hyperglycaemic hyperosmolar syndrome, and for **perioperative glycaemic control** in *selected* diabetic patients. ❸ Alongside <u>glucose</u> to treat **hyperkalaemia**, while other measures (such as treatment of the underlying cause) are initiated.
Mechanisms of action	In **diabetes mellitus,** exogenous insulin **functions similarly to endogenous insulin.** It stimulates glucose uptake from the circulation into tissues, including skeletal muscle and fat, and increases the use of glucose as an energy source. Insulin stimulates glycogen, lipid and protein synthesis and inhibits gluconeogenesis and ketogenesis. For the treatment of **hyperkalaemia, insulin drives K⁺ into cells,** reducing serum K⁺ concentrations. However, once insulin treatment is stopped, K⁺ leaks back out of the cells into the circulation, so this is a short-term measure while other treatment is commenced. The wide choice of insulin preparations for treatment of diabetes mellitus can be classified as: **rapid acting** (immediate onset, short duration) – e.g. NovoRapid® (insulin aspart); **short acting** (early onset, short duration) – e.g. Actrapid® (soluble insulin); **intermediate acting** (intermediate onset and duration) – e.g. Humulin I® (isophane or NPH insulin); and **long acting** (flat profile with regular administration) – e.g. Lantus® (insulin glargine), Levemir® (insulin detemir). **Biphasic insulin** preparations contain a mixture of rapid- and intermediate-acting insulins, e.g. NovoMix® 30 (30% insulin aspart, 70% insulin aspart protamine). Where IV insulin is required (hyperkalaemia, diabetic emergencies, peri-operative glucose control), soluble insulin (Actrapid®) is used.
Important adverse effects	The main adverse effect of insulin is **hypoglycaemia,** which can be severe enough to lead to coma and death. When administered by repeated SC injection at the same site, insulin can cause fat overgrowth (lipohypertrophy), which may be unsightly or uncomfortable.
Warnings	In patients with ▲**renal impairment,** insulin clearance is reduced, so there is an increased risk of hypoglycaemia.
Important interactions	Although often necessary, combining insulin with other hypoglycaemic agents increases the risk of hypoglycaemia. Concurrent therapy with <u>systemic corticosteroids</u> increases insulin requirements.

insulin aspart, insulin glargine, biphasic insulin, soluble insulin

PRACTICAL PRESCRIBING

Prescription	In **diabetes mellitus,** the goal of treatment is to attain good blood glucose control without problematic hypoglycaemia. Patients usually self-administer insulin by SC injection, and may adjust their own doses. Insulin doses are specified in 'units'. Typical daily insulin requirements are ~30–50 units, although this varies widely, depending on weight, diet, activity and insulin resistance. Insulin regimens need to provide 'peaks' of insulin to deal with the glucose absorbed at mealtimes, and lower 'basal' levels in between. Examples include *'basal–bolus' regimens,* e.g. Lantus® (glargine; long acting) taken once daily and NovoRapid® (insulin aspart; rapid acting) with meals and snacks; and *twice-daily regimens,* e.g. NovoMix® 30 (biphasic insulin). SC insulin is best prescribed by brand name. In **diabetic emergencies** and **peri-operative glycaemic control,** a 1-unit/mL IV solution is made by diluting Actrapid® 50 units in 0.9% sodium chloride 50 mL. The infusion rate is adjusted as necessary; consult a local protocol for details. Glucose and potassium are usually also infused. In **hyperkalaemia,** it is essential that glucose is given with insulin to avoid hypoglycaemia. A reasonable option is Actrapid® 10 units in 20% glucose 100 mL, infused over 15 minutes.
Administration	SC insulin is often administered using 'pens' containing insulin in solution (100 units/mL). These allow a patient to 'dial up' the number of units required and administer insulin discreetly, e.g. through clothes.
Communication	When starting patients with diabetes mellitus on insulin, explain that insulin will help to control blood sugar levels and prevent complications. Advise them that **lifestyle measures,** including a healthy, balanced diet and regular exercise, are needed as well as insulin to improve health. Warn them of the risk of **hypoglycaemia,** advising them of symptoms to watch out for (e.g. dizziness, agitation, nausea, sweating and confusion). Explain to patients that, if hypoglycaemia develops, they should take something sugary (e.g. glucose tablets or a sugary drink) then something starchy, e.g. a sandwich.
Monitoring	Patients should measure capillary blood glucose regularly and adjust insulin dose based on results. **Haemoglobin A$_{1c}$** should be measured at least annually to assess long-term glycaemic control. Where insulin is given as a continuous IV infusion, serum K$^+$ should be measured at least every 4 hours to guide need for replacement.
Cost	Insulin costs the NHS >£300 million/year (the fourth biggest drug cost).

Clinical tip—Try to avoid giving 'correction' doses of insulin to treat hyperglycaemia in inpatients. It is generally better to tolerate transient, mild hyperglycaemia and instead adjust the patient's scheduled insulin doses to avoid recurrence the next day. Correction doses add instability and can make titration of scheduled insulin more difficult. If, however, a correction dose is necessary, use a rapid-acting insulin (e.g. NovoRapid®). Short-acting insulin (e.g. Actrapid®) is best avoided, due to the 2–3-hr delay to its peak effect.

Iron

CLINICAL PHARMACOLOGY

Common indications	❶ **Treatment of iron-deficiency anaemia.** ❷ **Prophylaxis of iron-deficiency anaemia** in patients with risk factors such as poor diet, malabsorption, menorrhagia, gastrectomy, haemodialysis and infants with low birth weight.
Mechanisms of action	The aim of iron therapy is to replenish iron stores. Iron is essential for erythropoiesis (the formation of new red blood cells). It is required for the synthesis of the haem component of haemoglobin, which gives red blood cells the ability to carry oxygen. Iron is best absorbed in its ferrous state (Fe^{2+}) in the duodenum and jejunum. Its absorption is increased by stomach acid and dietary acids such as ascorbic acid (vitamin C). Once absorbed into the blood stream, iron is bound by transferrin. Transferrin transports it either to be used in the bone marrow for erythropoiesis, or to be stored as ferritin in the liver, reticuloendothelial system, bone marrow, spleen and skeletal muscle.
Important adverse effects	The most common adverse effect of oral iron salts is **gastrointestinal upset,** including nausea, epigastric pain, constipation and diarrhoea. Patients may notice that their bowel motions turn black on treatment. Intravenous iron administration can cause injection site irritation and hypersensitivity reactions, including anaphylaxis.
Warnings	*Oral iron* therapy may exacerbate bowel symptoms in patients with ▲**intestinal disease,** including inflammatory bowel disease, diverticular disease and intestinal strictures. *Intravenous iron* should be used with caution in people with an ▲**atopic predisposition** due to the risk of anaphylactic reaction.
Important interactions	Oral iron salts can reduce the absorption of other drugs, including <u>levothyroxine</u> and <u>bisphosphonates</u>. These medications should therefore be taken at least 2 hours before oral iron.

ferrous fumarate, ferrous sulfate

PRACTICAL PRESCRIBING

Prescription	Iron is available for oral or IV administration. Intravenous iron should be reserved for patients unable to tolerate sufficient oral iron to correct or prevent deficiency. It is also used for patients with end-stage renal disease, in whom it may be given with erythropoietin. Intravenous iron replacement does not lead to a more rapid increase in haemoglobin than oral iron. For **treatment of iron-deficiency anaemia,** you need to prescribe 100–200 mg of elemental iron per day. Different oral iron preparations contain different amounts of elemental iron. For example, ferrous sulfate 200 mg contains 65 mg elemental iron. A prescription for ferrous sulfate 200 mg two to three times daily will therefore provide 130–195 mg elemental iron a day. Once the haemoglobin has returned to normal, continue the prescription for a further 3 months to replenish iron stores fully. For **prophylaxis of iron-deficiency anaemia,** ferrous sulfate 200 mg daily should be sufficient. Gastrointestinal adverse effects may prevent patients from taking iron. Reducing the dose or switching to an alternative iron salt may improve tolerability.
Administration	Although oral iron salts are better absorbed on an empty stomach, they can be taken with food to reduce gastrointestinal side effects. Intravenous iron can be given as an injection over 10 minutes or as an infusion. Facilities for the management of anaphylaxis should be available.
Communication	Explain to patients that treatment should top up their iron stores and improve symptoms of anaemia, but that it may take a few months before the full benefit is felt. Warn them that iron may turn their stools black. Advise them to come back if the iron upsets their stomach, as treatment can be changed to reduce side effects.
Monitoring	Monitor full blood count until the haemoglobin has returned to normal. You should expect to see the haemoglobin rise by around 20 g/L per month.
Cost	Ferrous sulfate and ferrous fumarate are both available in non-proprietary forms, are equally efficacious and are cheap. Brand name compound preparations with ascorbic acid and modified-release preparations have minimal additional clinical benefit for a considerable increase in cost.

Clinical tip—People with iron deficiency often require colonoscopy to investigate the cause of their anaemia. However, oral iron can turn stools black and sticky. This is problematic for visualising the bowel during lower gastrointestinal endoscopy as the sticky black stool coats the colon and obscures the endoscopist's view. Iron treatment should therefore be stopped for 7 days before the procedure.

Lamotrigine

CLINICAL PHARMACOLOGY

Common indications	❶ Seizure prophylaxis in **epilepsy.** Epilepsy is classified by seizure type which, in turn, guides antiepileptic drug choice. Lamotrigine is an option for first-line monotherapy or add-on therapy in **focal seizures** (with or without secondary generalisation), **generalised tonic–clonic seizures** and **absence seizures.** ❷ **Bipolar depression**, but not mania or hypomania.
Mechanisms of action	The mechanism of action of lamotrigine is incompletely understood. Like <u>carbamazepine</u> and phenytoin, it binds to voltage-sensitive neuronal Na⁺ channels, interfering with Na⁺ influx into the neuron. This impedes repetitive neuronal firing, which is a characteristic of seizure activity. Additionally, it appears to have effects on synaptic function, including inhibition of a post-synaptic glutamate receptor (the α-amino-3-hydroxy-5-methyl-4-isoxazolepropionic acid [AMPA] receptor). These effects, and others, may contribute to its antiepileptic action. The mechanism by which it reduces depressive symptoms in bipolar disorder is uncertain.
Important adverse effects	The most common adverse effects are **headache, drowsiness, irritability, blurred vision, dizziness** and **gastrointestinal symptoms**. A minority of patients develop a **skin rash** within a few weeks of starting lamotrigine. This is usually mild, but requires urgent review and possibly discontinuation of the drug. This is because it may be the first sign of a **severe hypersensitivity reaction;** although rare, this may be life threatening, and early discontinuation of the drug is of paramount importance (see <u>Carbamazepine</u>).
Warnings	Lamotrigine should be avoided if possible in patients who have a prior history of ▲**hypersensitivity to other antiepileptic drugs**, due to the risk of cross-reactivity. Lamotrigine is metabolised by hepatic glucuronidation, so dosage reduction may be necessary in patients with moderate or severe ▲**hepatic impairment**. In general, there is no evidence that lamotrigine exposure in **pregnancy** increases the overall risk of congenital malformations, so it is a reasonable choice in women of child-bearing age. During pregnancy, due to changes in lamotrigine metabolism, plasma concentration measurement should be considered to guide dosage adjustment.
Important interactions	Lamotrigine has many interactions arising from its **metabolism by glucuronidation.** These are of sufficient importance to necessitate pre-emptive dosage modification (see Prescription). Drugs that **induce** glucuronidation include ▲<u>carbamazepine</u>, ▲phenytoin, ▲<u>oestrogens</u>, ▲rifampicin and ▲protease inhibitors. These can cause the lamotrigine concentration to fall, potentially leading to treatment failure. Glucuronidation is **inhibited** by ▲<u>valproate</u>, causing the lamotrigine concentration to rise, increasing the risk of toxicity. Severe hypersensitivity reactions are also more common when lamotrigine is co-administered with valproate.

PRACTICAL PRESCRIBING

Prescription	The dosage of lamotrigine depends on the patient's concomitant drug treatment. When used as monotherapy with no concomitant interacting drugs, the starting dosage in adults is 25 mg daily, increased at 2-weekly intervals to a usual maintenance dosage of 200 mg daily. If it is taken with <u>valproate</u>, the dosage should be halved (start at 25 mg on alternate days). If it is taken with a drug that induces glucuronidation (see Important interactions), the dosage is doubled (start at 50 mg daily).
Administration	Standard lamotrigine tablets should be swallowed whole with water. Chewable/dispersible tablets can be taken whole, chewed with a little water, or dispersed with water.
Communication	Explain to patients that the aim of treatment is to reduce seizure frequency, not to 'cure' epilepsy. Finding the right dosage may take a few weeks, so its effects may not be evident immediately. It is important for good seizure control to avoid missing doses. If patients miss a dose, they should take it as soon as they remember (unless the next dose is imminent, in which case they should just take that one). They should not stop treatment abruptly, as this can cause rebound seizures. Most patients tolerate lamotrigine well, but side effects such as headache, drowsiness and irritability can occur. In the first few months of treatment there is a risk of rare but serious allergic reactions. During this time particularly, patients should seek immediate medical attention if they develop a rash, ulcers, fever, swollen glands, bleeding/bruising or a sore throat. Advise patients that driving is prohibited unless they have been seizure-free for 12 months, and for 6 months after changing or stopping treatment.
Monitoring	Treatment **efficacy** is monitored by comparing seizure frequency before and after starting treatment or dose adjustment. **Safety** and **tolerability** are monitored by enquiring about adverse effects. This is particularly important in the initial few months of treatment, when patients should be advised to seek immediate medical attention for any symptoms that could suggest a hypersensitivity reaction (see Communication). Plasma lamotrigine concentration can be measured but it is not routinely required. It may be useful if there is an unexplained lack of efficacy, suspected poor adherence, or when altered pharmacokinetics are anticipated due to changes in concomitant therapy or pregnancy.
Cost	Lamotrigine is available in generic forms which are relatively inexpensive. The tablet formulations are generally cheaper than the dispersible formulations.

Clinical tip—Lamotrigine appears to be unique among agents used in bipolar disorder, in that it effectively treats depressive symptoms but does not increase the risk of a switch to mania.

Laxatives, osmotic

CLINICAL PHARMACOLOGY

Common indications	❶ **Constipation** and **faecal impaction.** ❷ **Bowel preparation** prior to surgery or endoscopy. ❸ **Hepatic encephalopathy.**
Mechanisms of action	These medicines are based on **osmotically active substances** (sugars or alcohols) that are not digested or absorbed, and which therefore remain in the gut lumen. **They hold water in the stool,** maintaining its volume and **stimulating peristalsis.** Lactulose, in particular, also reduces ammonia absorption. It does this by increasing gut transit rate and acidifying the stool, which inhibits the proliferation of ammonia-producing bacteria. This is helpful in patients with liver failure, in whom ammonia plays a major role in the pathogenesis of hepatic encephalopathy.
Important adverse effects	**Flatulence, abdominal cramps** and **nausea** are common adverse effects, although they may decrease with time. As with other laxatives, **diarrhoea** is a possible complication. Phosphate enemas can cause **local irritation** and **electrolyte disturbances.**
Warnings	Osmotic laxatives are contraindicated in ✖**intestinal obstruction** as there is a risk of perforation. Phosphate enemas can cause significant fluid shifts, so should be used with caution in ▲**heart failure,** ▲**ascites** and when ▲**electrolyte disturbances** are present.
Important interactions	There are no significant adverse drug interactions with osmotic laxatives, although the effects of ▲<u>warfarin</u> may be slightly increased.

lactulose, macrogol, phosphate enema

lactulose, macrogol, phosphate enema

The top 100 drugs

PRACTICAL PRESCRIBING

Prescription — Orally administered osmotic laxatives should generally be prescribed in the regular section of the drug chart. For example, when treating **constipation** or **faecal impaction** you might prescribe lactulose 15 mL 12-hrly, titrating this to response. Be aware that it may take a few days for an effect to be seen, as the drug needs to pass through the small intestine to the colon. When using a phosphate enema to treat **faecal impaction,** prescribe it in the once-only or as-required section for rectal administration. The dose should not usually exceed one enema in 24 hours. For **bowel preparation,** you should refer to a local protocol for prescribing advice. When using lactulose to treat or prevent **hepatic encephalopathy,** you might start with 30–50 mL (doubled in constipation) three times daily, aiming for the patient to produce three soft/loose stools daily.

Administration — Osmotic laxatives may be taken with or without food. Oral solutions can be taken as they are or diluted in another liquid; powdered forms are dissolved in water. Enemas are administered with the patient lying on their side, as for a rectal examination. They should stay in this position for a few minutes or until they need to open their bowels.

Communication — Explain to patients that you are offering treatment with a laxative that will hopefully make their stool softer and easier to pass. To work, it requires them to drink plenty of water: they should aim to have at least 6–8 glasses of liquid per day. Mention that side effects such as abdominal cramps and flatulence can occur, but these may get better over time. Advise that the dose should be adjusted to maintain comfort. If they are regularly passing more than two or three soft stools per day, the dose should be reduced or the laxative stopped (unless it is being used for hepatic encephalopathy).

Monitoring — When treating inpatients, a stool chart is useful to monitor the effects of treatment. This is particularly important when treating hepatic encephalopathy, where you should also monitor electrolytes.

Cost — Osmotic laxatives are cheap. Patients who pay for their prescriptions may save money if they buy them over the counter.

Clinical tip—When treating faecal impaction with rectally administered laxatives, try a glycerol suppository (stimulant laxative) before using a phosphate enema. Glycerol suppositories are less likely to cause electrolyte disturbance. Phosphate enemas are irritant and are contained in a significant volume of fluid (>100 mL), which can be quite uncomfortable. Reserve them for a second-line therapy.

Laxatives, stimulant

CLINICAL PHARMACOLOGY

Common indications	❶ **Constipation.** ❷ As suppositories for **faecal impaction.**
Mechanisms of action	Stimulant (also known as irritant or contact) laxatives **increase water and electrolyte secretion** from the colonic mucosa, thereby **increasing the volume of colonic content and stimulating peristalsis.** They also have a direct pro-peristaltic action, although the exact mechanism differs between agents. For example, bacterial metabolism of senna in the intestine produces metabolites that have a direct action on the enteric nervous system, stimulating peristalsis. Rectal administration of stimulant laxatives, such as glycerol suppositories, provokes a similar but more localised effect and can be useful to treat faecal impaction. Docusate sodium has both stimulant and faecal softening actions.
Important adverse effects	Abdominal pain or cramping may occur with stimulant laxative use and diarrhoea is an obvious potential adverse effect. With prolonged use, some stimulant laxatives cause melanosis coli (reversible pigmentation of the intestinal wall).
Warnings	Stimulant laxatives should not be used in patients in whom ✖**intestinal obstruction** is suspected as there is a risk that this could induce **perforation.** Rectal preparations are usually avoided if ▲**haemorrhoids** or ▲**anal fissures** are present.
Important interactions	There are no clinically significant adverse drug interactions with stimulant laxatives.

senna, bisacodyl, glycerol suppositories, docusate sodium

PRACTICAL PRESCRIBING

Prescription	For **constipation,** you should generally prescribe stimulant laxatives for regular administration. They are usually taken once or twice a day and the dose titrated to effect (e.g. 1–2 tablets of senna once or twice daily). When treating **faecal impaction,** rectal stimulant laxatives should usually be prescribed once only or as required with a maximum dose frequency of once in a 24-hour period.
Administration	Stimulant laxatives are usually administered orally, unless treating faecal impaction when glycerol suppositories may be administered rectally.
Communication	Explain to patients that you are offering treatment with a laxative that will help stool to pass. As with other laxatives, ensuring good oral fluid intake will also help. Aim for 6–8 glasses of liquid per day. Advise your patient that stimulant laxatives do not work immediately and they may need a few doses before a sustained effect is noticed. Explain that the dose can be adjusted if necessary to maintain comfort. If they are regularly passing more than two or three soft stools per day, the dose should be reduced or the laxative stopped. Mention that side effects such as abdominal cramps and flatulence can occur, but these may get better over time.
Monitoring	When treating inpatients, a stool chart is useful to monitor the effects of treatment.
Cost	Stimulant laxatives are cheap, around 10p a dose. Patients who pay for their prescriptions may save money if they buy them over the counter.

Clinical tip—When prescribing opioid analgesics to be taken regularly, consider co-prescribing a laxative to prevent constipation. A stimulant is a reasonable choice. Patients find constipation uncomfortable and it can contribute to confusion in the elderly, so prevention can increase adherence to opioid treatment and control of symptoms.

Leukotriene receptor antagonists

CLINICAL PHARMACOLOGY

Common indications	❶ **Adults:** leukotriene receptor antagonists may be considered as an add-on therapy for **asthma**, where symptoms are not adequately controlled by inhaled <u>corticosteroids</u> and <u>long acting β_2 agonists (LABAs)</u>. ❷ **Children aged 5–12 years:** as an alternative to <u>LABAs</u> as an add-on therapy where inhaled <u>corticosteroids</u> are insufficient to control **asthma** symptoms. ❸ **Children aged under 5 years:** as a first-line preventative therapy in young children with **asthma** who are unable to take an inhaled <u>corticosteroid</u>.
Mechanisms of action	In asthma, leukotrienes produced by mast cells and eosinophils (amongst other sources) activate the **G protein-coupled leukotriene receptor CysLT1.** This activates a cascade of pathways that result in the **inflammation and bronchoconstriction** that contribute to the pathophysiology of asthma. Leukotriene receptor agonists reduce inflammation and bronchoconstriction in asthma by blocking the CysLT1 receptor and damping down the inflammatory cascade.
Important adverse effects	Leukotriene receptor antagonists are generally well tolerated. **Headache** and **abdominal pain** are the most common adverse effects; they are usually mild. There is also an increased rate of upper respiratory tract infections in patients taking the drug. Uncommonly, **hyperactivity** and a **reduced ability to concentrate** may occur. **Churg–Strauss syndrome**, an eosinophilic autoimmune disorder, has been seen in association with leukotriene receptor antagonists; however, there is no conclusive evidence that it is an adverse effect of the drug.
Warnings	In general, leukotriene receptor antagonists should not be prescribed for asthma unless asthma is incompletely controlled with inhaled <u>corticosteroids</u> and long-acting <u>β_2-agonists</u>, except in the specific cases listed above. The safety of these drugs in pregnancy is uncertain because of a lack of evidence, although no harmful effects have been demonstrated. It is felt reasonable to continue treatment in pregnancy where leukotriene receptor antagonists are felt to have led to an improvement in asthma symptoms not achieved with other therapies.
Important interactions	There are no important drug interactions between leukotriene receptor antagonists (i.e. montelukast) and other commonly used drugs.

montelukast

PRACTICAL PRESCRIBING

Prescription	As leukotriene receptor antagonists are a third-line therapy for asthma, they should only be initiated by prescribers with appropriate knowledge and experience of managing complicated disease. Montelukast is prescribed at a dosage of 10 mg once daily.
Administration	Montelukast is taken orally and is available in tablet, chewable tablet and granule form. Young children may find it difficult to swallow or chew the tablet forms available. Granules can be dissolved in flavoured liquid and prescribing these may improve adherence to treatment.
Communication	Explain to patients that this medicine will reduce inflammation and relax their airways and therefore will hopefully help to **improve their symptoms and control their disease**. Make sure that they understand it will not help in an acute attack of breathlessness: they should seek medical advice in the event of an exacerbation, as they do currently. Explain to patients that it is important to continue to take their inhalers as well as this new tablet, as the inhalers work in different ways to control asthma. Advise them to report any worsening of symptoms, rash or numbness or weakness if they develop, as these are signs of a very uncommon, but serious adverse effect.
Monitoring	**Efficacy** should be monitored by symptom diary and serial measurement of peak expiratory flow rate.
Cost	Generic preparations are available and cheap

Clinical tip—The place in asthma therapy for leukotriene receptor antagonists continues to evolve. It may be that some subgroups of patients are more likely to benefit (e.g. those with exercise-induced bronchoconstriction or rhinitis-associated asthma), and some are less likely to benefit (e.g. children with viral-induced wheeze).

Levetiracetam

CLINICAL PHARMACOLOGY

Common indications	❶ Seizure prophylaxis in **epilepsy.** Epilepsy is classified by seizure type which, in turn, guides antiepileptic drug choice. Levetiracetam is an option for monotherapy or add-on therapy of **focal seizures** (with or without secondary generalisation) if <u>carbamazepine</u> or <u>lamotrigine</u> are unsuitable or not tolerated. It may be used for add-on therapy for **myoclonic seizures** and **generalised tonic–clonic seizures** if the first agent is insufficient. ❷ Selected cases of **established convulsive status epilepticus** that have not responded to adequate treatment with a <u>benzodiazepine</u>.
Mechanisms of action	The molecular target of levetiracetam is **synaptic vesicle protein 2A (SV2A)**. SV2A is expressed throughout the brain, in both excitatory and inhibitory synapses, as a glycoprotein located within the membranes of synaptic vesicles. Synaptic vesicles are where neurotransmitters are stored in the presynaptic nerve terminal. During depolarisation, synaptic vesicles fuse with the pre-synaptic membrane to release neurotransmitters into the synaptic cleft. It is presumably through **interfering with synaptic vesicle function** that levetiracetam **modulates neuronal excitability** and reduces the risk of seizures. The intermediate steps in this mechanism are, however, poorly understood.
Important adverse effects	In comparison with many other antiepileptic drugs, levetiracetam is generally well tolerated. Most patients have only mild adverse effects, or none at all. Drowsiness (affecting about 10%), weakness, dizziness and headache are the most common adverse effects. Mood disturbance and psychiatric adverse effects are less common (about 5% and 2.5%, respectively), but more likely to cause discontinuation. Suicidal ideation and serious hypersensitivity reactions have been reported rarely.
Warnings	Levetiracetam is eliminated by the kidneys, so dosage reduction may be required in ▲**renal impairment**. There is no evidence that levetiracetam increases the overall risk of congenital malformation when taken during pregnancy, although it is difficult to exclude effects on specific congenital defects.
Important interactions	In contrast to many other antiepileptic drugs, levetiracetam has few clinically significant interactions, and this is one of its major advantages. In particular, it does not have important interactions with other antiepileptic drugs, hormonal contraception, or warfarin.

levetiracetam

PRACTICAL PRESCRIBING

Prescription	A typical starting dose for seizure prophylaxis in adults with established epilepsy is 500 mg orally 12-hrly. This would usually be increased to 1 g orally 12-hrly after 2 weeks, and may then be titrated further according to clinical response (efficacy and adverse effects; max 1.5 g orally 12-hrly). When used in convulsive status epilepticus refractory to <u>benzodiazepine</u> treatment, the initial loading dose (40 mg/kg) is given IV.
Administration	Tablets should ideally be swallowed whole. They should not be chewed. If necessary to facilitate administration (e.g. in children), they may be crushed and taken with food. Intravenous doses are given by infusion, typically over 15–30 minutes.
Communication	Explain to patients that the aim of treatment is to reduce seizure frequency, not to 'cure' epilepsy. Finding the right dosage may take a few weeks, so its effects may not be evident immediately. It is important for good seizure control to avoid missing doses. If patients miss a dose, they should take it as soon as they remember (unless the next dose is imminent, in which case they should just take that one). They should not stop treatment abruptly, as this can cause rebound seizures. Side effects, such as drowsiness and headache, are infrequent and usually mild. A small minority of patients experience mood changes, and they should seek attention if they develop any symptoms of depression. Advise patients that driving is prohibited unless they have been seizure-free for 12 months, and for 6 months after changing or stopping treatment.
Monitoring	Treatment **efficacy** is monitored by comparing seizure frequency before and after starting treatment or dose adjustment. **Safety** and **tolerability** are monitored by enquiring about adverse effects, particularly in relation to mood disturbance and suicidal thoughts. There are no specific laboratory monitoring requirements, and measurement of plasma levetiracetam concentration is not required.
Cost	Due to the volume of prescribing and its unit cost, levetiracetam represents a significant drug cost for the NHS. It should be prescribed generically to allow the cheapest product to be dispensed. The IV formulation is considerably more expensive, so should be used only when oral administration is impossible (see Clinical tip).

Clinical tip—The bioavailability of levetiracetam is reliably high, so there is no need for dose modification when switching between oral and IV administration. For the same reason, IV administration should be stopped in favour of oral administration as early as possible, not least because the IV formulation is substantially more expensive.

Lidocaine

CLINICAL PHARMACOLOGY

Common indications	❶ Very commonly, as a first-choice **local anaesthetic** in, for example, **urinary catheterisation** and **minor procedures** (e.g. suturing). ❷ Uncommonly, as an antiarrhythmic drug in **ventricular tachycardia (VT)** and **ventricular fibrillation (VF) refractory to electrical cardioversion** (although <u>amiodarone</u> is preferred for the latter indication).
Mechanisms of action	Lidocaine (formerly known as lignocaine) enters cells in its uncharged form, then accepts a proton to become positively charged. From inside the cell, it enters and then **blocks voltage-gated sodium channels** on the surface membrane. This prevents initiation and propagation of action potentials in nerves and muscle, inducing local anaesthesia in the area supplied by blocked nerve fibres. In the heart, it reduces the duration of the action potential, slows conduction velocity and increases the refractory period. These effects may terminate VT and improve the chances of successfully treating VF.
Important adverse effects	The most common side effect is an initial **stinging** sensation during local administration. Systemic adverse effects are, predictably, more likely after systemic administration, whether intentional (in its use as an antiarrhythmic) or inadvertent (due to accidental intravascular injection during local administration). Its effects on the neurological system include **drowsiness, restlessness, tremor** and **fits.** It generally causes relatively little cardiovascular toxicity, but in overdose it may cause **hypotension** and **arrhythmias.**
Warnings	Used appropriately as a local anaesthetic, lidocaine is generally very safe. It depends heavily on hepatic blood flow for its elimination. Therefore, a lower dose should be used in states of ▲**reduced cardiac output.**
Important interactions	As the duration of action of local anaesthetics depends on how long they stay in contact with the neurons, co-administration with a vasoconstrictor (e.g. <u>adrenaline [epinephrine]</u>) produces a desirable interaction that may prolong the local anaesthetic effect.

PRACTICAL PRESCRIBING

Prescription	For **urinary catheterisation,** lidocaine is formulated as a gel, together with the antiseptic agent chlorhexidine, as a proprietary product (Instillagel®). This is provided in pre-filled syringes. The dose is 6–11 mL. It *should* be prescribed in the once-only section, although in practice this is often omitted. For **minor procedures,** you usually use a 1% (10 mg/mL) solution of lidocaine hydrochloride. The maximum dose is 200 mg or 3 mg/kg, whichever is lower (7 mg/kg, or up to 500 mg, is permitted when it is combined with adrenaline). This should be calculated using *ideal body weight.* In practice, you draw up the dose you think you will need (ensuring this does not exceed the maximum), then administer enough to produce adequate anaesthesia. It is therefore acceptable to write the prescription and sign for its administration after completing the procedure. Foundation doctors should not prescribe lidocaine for systemic administration.
Administration	In **urinary catheterisation,** you open the packaging and allow the Instillagel® syringe to drop into your sterile field, ensuring asepsis is maintained. To administer it, you remove the cap, press the plunger gently to free it and expel any air, and then slowly inject the gel into the urethra. In **minor procedures,** you initially infiltrate the skin and superficial layers using a fine (orange [25G]) needle, then step up to a larger needle (blue [23G] or green [21G]) as necessary for deeper layers. Briefly retract the plunger before each injection to ensure the tip has not entered a vessel; this is signified by blood appearing in the syringe.
Communication	Explain to patients that you are offering treatment with a local anaesthetic to numb the area before the procedure. Warn them that it will sting initially, but this will quickly disappear. They will still feel pushing and pulling sensations (from movement of surrounding non-anaesthetised tissues), but they should not feel pain. If they do, they should tell you.
Monitoring	Quality of anaesthesia is monitored clinically.
Cost	Lidocaine solution is cheap. Instillagel® costs about 10–20p per tube.

Clinical tip—A common mistake is not to wait long enough for lidocaine to reach maximal effect. There is no point infiltrating the area and then, 20 seconds later, repeatedly pricking the skin while saying 'Can you feel this?' to the patient. They will feel it, and they will then lose confidence in your ability to deliver adequate anaesthesia. *Be patient.* Administer the local anaesthetic early, then turn back to your trolley and complete any necessary preparatory work. Try to wait several minutes before testing its effect.

Macrolides

CLINICAL PHARMACOLOGY

Common indications	❶ Treatment of **respiratory, skin and soft tissue infections** as an alternative to a <u>penicillin</u> when use is contraindicated, e.g. by allergy. ❷ In **severe pneumonia** added to a penicillin to cover atypical organisms including *Legionella pneumophila* and *Mycoplasma pneumoniae*. ❸ Eradication of *Helicobacter pylori* (for example, causing **peptic ulcer disease**) in combination with a <u>proton pump inhibitor</u> and either <u>amoxicillin</u> or <u>metronidazole</u>.
Spectrum of activity	Erythromycin was isolated from *Streptomyces erythraeus* in the 1950s. It has a relatively **broad spectrum** of activity against Gram-positive and some Gram-negative organisms. Synthetic macrolides (e.g. clarithromycin and azithromycin) have increased activity against Gram-negative bacteria, particularly *Haemophilus influenzae*.
Mechanisms of action	Macrolides **inhibit bacterial protein synthesis.** They bind to the 50S subunit of the bacterial ribosome and block translocation, a process required for elongation of the polypeptide chain. Inhibition of protein synthesis is **bacteriostatic** (stops bacterial growth), which assists the immune system in killing and removing bacteria from the body. Bacterial resistance to macrolides is common, mainly due to ribosomal mutations preventing macrolide binding.
Important adverse effects	Adverse effects are most common and severe with erythromycin, but can occur with any macrolide. Macrolides are **irritant,** causing nausea, vomiting, abdominal pain and diarrhoea when taken orally and thrombophlebitis when given IV. Other important side effects include **allergy, antibiotic-associated colitis** (see <u>Penicillins, broad-spectrum</u>), liver abnormalities including **cholestatic jaundice, prolongation of the QT interval** (predisposing to **arrhythmias**) and **ototoxicity** at high doses.
Warnings	Macrolides should not be prescribed if there is a history of ✘**macrolide hypersensitivity,** although they are a useful option where penicillin is contraindicated by allergy as there is no cross-sensitivity between these drug classes. Macrolide elimination from the body is mostly hepatic with a small renal contribution, such that caution is required in ▲**severe hepatic impairment** and dose reduction in ▲**severe renal impairment.**
Important interactions	Erythromycin and clarithromycin (but not azithromycin) inhibit cytochrome P450 (CYP) enzymes. This increases plasma concentrations and the risk of adverse effects with ▲**drugs metabolised by CYP enzymes.** For example, with <u>warfarin</u> there is an increased risk of bleeding and with <u>statins</u> an increased risk of myopathy. Macrolides should be prescribed with caution in patients taking other ▲**drugs that prolong the QT interval** or cause arrhythmias, such as <u>amiodarone</u>, <u>antipsychotics</u>, <u>quinine</u>, <u>quinolone antibiotics</u> and <u>SSRIs</u>.

PRACTICAL PRESCRIBING

Prescription	**Erythromycin** has a short plasma half-life of around 2 hours and is usually prescribed at a dosage of 250–500 mg 6-hrly for the treatment of susceptible infections. **Clarithromycin** is concentrated in tissues and has a longer elimination half-life, and so is prescribed at a dosage of 250–500 mg 12-hrly. A modified-release preparation is also available that allows once-daily dosing. **Azithromycin**, which is highly concentrated in tissues and has a long half-life, is prescribed at a dosage of 250–500 mg daily. Higher doses and longer courses of treatment are used in more severe infections. All macrolides are also available for **IV prescription** where patients are unable to take or absorb drugs through the gut (e.g. due to vomiting). The indication, review date and duration of treatment should be documented on all inpatient antibiotic prescriptions to aid antibiotic stewardship.
Administration	Oral macrolides can be taken as tablets or oral suspension with or without food (although food may improve GI tolerability). Intravenous macrolides should be diluted **in a large volume**, e.g. 500 mg in 250 mL <u>sodium chloride</u> 0.9%, before infusion into a large proximal vein (to reduce the risk of thrombophlebitis) over at least 60 minutes (to reduce the risk of arrhythmias). They must not be given as a bolus IV or an IM injection.
Communication	Explain to patients that the aim of treatment is to get rid of infection and improve symptoms. Before prescribing, always check with your patient personally or get collateral history to ensure that they are not allergic to macrolides. Warn patients to seek medical advice if a rash or other unexpected symptoms develop. If an allergy develops during treatment, give patients written and verbal advice not to take this antibiotic in the future and make sure that the allergy is clearly documented in their medical records.
Monitoring	Check that infection resolves by patient report (e.g. resolution of symptoms), examination (e.g. resolution of pyrexia, lung crackles) and blood tests (e.g. falling C-reactive protein and white cell count), as appropriate.
Cost	Where IV macrolides are prescribed, switch to oral as soon as tolerated. Intravenous-to-oral switch is good practice as it reduces the cost of the drug (**oral macrolides cost around 50 times less than IV macrolides**), as well as reducing administration costs, treatment complications and duration of inpatient stay.

Clinical tip—In patients with lower respiratory tract infections (LRTIs), macrolides should generally only be added to penicillin treatment if there is **evidence of pneumonia** (e.g. consolidation on the chest X-ray). Macrolides are required to cover penicillin-resistant atypical organisms, e.g. *Legionella pneumophila* and *Mycoplasma pneumoniae*, which cause pneumonia but do not cause other LRTIs, e.g. COPD exacerbations.

Metformin

CLINICAL PHARMACOLOGY

Common indications	**Type 2 diabetes,** as the first-choice medication for control of blood glucose, used alone or in combination with other oral hypoglycaemic drugs (e.g. <u>sulphonylureas</u>, <u>DPP-4 inhibitors</u>) or <u>insulin</u>.
Mechanisms of action	Metformin (a biguanide) lowers blood glucose primarily by **reducing hepatic glucose output** (glycogenolysis and gluconeogenesis) and, to a lesser extent, increasing glucose uptake and utilisation by skeletal muscle. It does not stimulate insulin secretion and therefore does not cause hypoglycaemia. The cellular mechanisms are complex, involving **activation of adenosine monophosphate-activated protein kinase (AMP kinase).** This is a cellular metabolic sensor, activation of which has diverse effects on cell functions. Its effects on glucose metabolism can be accompanied by other metabolic changes, notably modest **weight loss**, which can be a desirable side effect (see Clinical tip).
Important adverse effects	Metformin commonly causes **GI upset,** including nausea, vomiting, taste disturbance, anorexia and diarrhoea. **Lactic acidosis** has been associated very rarely with metformin use, although the evidence for this is largely derived from case reports. There is no strong evidence of an increased risk in stable patients, but metformin may be a contributory factor among patients who develop an intercurrent illness that causes metformin accumulation (e.g. renal impairment), increased lactate production (e.g. sepsis, hypoxia) or reduced lactate metabolism (e.g. liver failure).
Warnings	Metformin is excreted unchanged by the kidney. It must therefore be used cautiously in ▲**renal impairment**, with dosage reduction required if the estimated glomerular filtration rate (eGFR) is <45 mL/min per 1.73 m^2 and the drug stopped if eGFR falls below 30 mL/min per 1.73 m^2. Metformin should be withheld acutely where there is ✖**acute kidney injury** or ✖**severe tissue hypoxia,** e.g. in sepsis, cardiac or respiratory failure, or myocardial infarction. Caution is required in ▲**hepatic impairment** as clearance of excess lactate may be impaired. Metformin should be withheld during ▲**acute alcohol intoxication**, and be used with caution in ▲**chronic alcohol abuse,** where there is a risk of hypoglycaemia.
Important interactions	Metformin must be withheld before and for 48 hours after injection of ▲**IV contrast media** (e.g. for CT scans, coronary angiography) when there is an increased risk of renal impairment, metformin accumulation and lactic acidosis. Other drugs (e.g. <u>ACE inhibitors</u>, <u>NSAIDs</u>, <u>diuretics</u>) with potential to impair renal function should also be used with caution (e.g. with renal function monitoring) in combination with metformin. <u>Prednisolone</u>, <u>thiazide</u> and <u>loop diuretics</u> elevate blood glucose, hence oppose the actions and reduce efficacy of metformin.

PRACTICAL PRESCRIBING

Prescription	Metformin is given orally. GI adverse effects of metformin are usually transient and are best tolerated if metformin is started at a **low dose** and **increased gradually.** A common regimen is to start metformin 500 mg once daily with breakfast, increasing the dose by 500 mg weekly to 500–850 mg three times daily with meals.
Administration	Patients should be started on a standard-release preparation of metformin and advised to swallow tablets whole with a glass of water **with or after food** to minimise GI side effects.
Communication	Advise patients that metformin has been prescribed as a **long-term treatment** to help control blood sugar and reduce the risk of diabetic complications, such as heart attacks. Explain that tablets are not a replacement for **lifestyle measures** and should be taken in addition to a healthy, balanced diet and regular exercise. Warn patients to seek **urgent medical advice** if they develop any significant illness (e.g. involving breathlessness, fever, chest pain) as, in addition to investigating and treating the illness, metformin may need to be stopped or withheld (due to the possibility of a rare but serious side effect called **lactic acidosis**). Advise them always to tell a doctor that they are taking metformin before having an **X-ray or operation,** as metformin may need to be stopped before the procedure.
Monitoring	Assess blood glucose control by measuring **haemoglobin A$_{1c}$ (HbA$_{1c}$)**. In treating type 2 diabetes with a single agent, the **target** HbA$_{1c}$ is usually <48 mmol/mol. Treatment is **intensified** by adding a second agent if the HbA$_{1c}$ is >58 mmol/mol, and a new target of <53 mmol/mol is then set (balancing the risks of hyperglycaemia against the risks of treatment, particularly hypoglycaemia). Home capillary blood glucose monitoring is not routinely required for patients with type 2 diabetes taking metformin. For **safety,** measure renal function before starting treatment, then at least annually during therapy. Renal function should be measured more frequently (at least twice per year) in people with deteriorating renal function or at increased risk of renal impairment.
Cost	Non-proprietary metformin 500 mg tablets cost around 3p each. More complicated formulations (e.g. oral solution, modified release, combinations with other oral hypoglycaemics) are more expensive.

Clinical tip—Increasing body weight increases insulin resistance, which can cause or worsen type 2 diabetes. Initial treatment for type 2 diabetes is therefore a healthy diet with increased physical activity, promoting weight loss if applicable, and this should be tried for at least 3 months before commencing drug therapy (started if HbA$_{1c}$ is >48 mmol/mol). As an anabolic hormone, insulin, and drugs which increase insulin secretion (e.g. sulphonylureas) cause weight gain, which can worsen diabetes mellitus over the long term. Metformin, which does not cause weight gain, is therefore usually the first-choice treatment unless contraindicated.

Methotrexate

CLINICAL PHARMACOLOGY

Common indications	❶ As a disease-modifying treatment for **rheumatoid arthritis.** ❷ As part of **chemotherapy** regimens for cancers, including **leukaemia**, **lymphoma** and some **solid tumours.** ❸ To treat severe **psoriasis** (including **psoriatic arthritis)** that is resistant to other therapies.
Mechanisms of action	Methotrexate **inhibits dihydrofolate reductase,** which converts dietary folic acid to tetrahydrofolate (FH4). FH4 is required for DNA and protein synthesis, so lack of FH4 **prevents cellular replication.** Actively dividing cells are particularly sensitive to the effects of methotrexate, accounting for its efficacy in **cancer.** Methotrexate also has antiinflammatory and immunosuppressive effects. These are mediated in part by inhibition of inflammatory mediators such as interleukin (IL)-6, IL-8 and tumour necrosis factor (TNF)-α, although the underlying mechanisms are not fully understood.
Important adverse effects	Dose-related adverse effects of methotrexate include **mucosal damage** (e.g. sore mouth, GI upset) and **bone marrow suppression** (resulting most significantly in neutropenia and an increased risk of infection). Rarely, **hypersensitivity reactions,** including cutaneous reactions, hepatitis or pneumonitis, may occur. Long-term use can cause **hepatic cirrhosis** or **pulmonary fibrosis.** As methotrexate is usually administered once weekly (see Prescription), there is a risk of accidental **overdose** if patients take treatment daily. Overdose causes severe dose-related adverse effects with renal impairment and hepatotoxicity. Neurological effects such as headache, seizures and coma may also occur. Treatment is with folinic acid, which 'rescues' normal cells from methotrexate effects, and with hydration and urinary alkalinisation to enhance methotrexate excretion.
Warnings	Methotrexate is **teratogenic** and must be avoided in ✖**pregnancy.** Both men and women taking the drug should use effective contraception during and for 3 months after stopping treatment. As methotrexate is renally excreted, it is contraindicated in ✖**severe renal impairment.** As it can cause hepatotoxicity, methotrexate should be avoided in patients with ▲**abnormal liver function.**
Important interactions	Methotrexate toxicity is more likely if it is prescribed with drugs that inhibit its renal excretion, e.g. ▲NSAIDs, ▲penicillins. Co-prescription with **other folate antagonists,** e.g. ▲trimethoprim and phenytoin, increases the risk of haematological abnormalities. The risk of neutropenia is increased if methotrexate is combined with ▲clozapine.

methotrexate

PRACTICAL PRESCRIBING

Prescription	Methotrexate should be prescribed only by specialists. For **autoimmune disease,** methotrexate is prescribed for oral administration. A typical dose would be 7.5–20 mg once weekly, adjusted according to response and adverse effects (which are more common at higher doses). **It is crucial to emphasise the once-weekly nature of this prescription.** Folic acid 5 mg weekly (taken on a different day to methotrexate) can be prescribed to limit adverse effects. For **cancer,** methotrexate may be given by IV, IM or intrathecal routes to induce remission, then orally for maintenance treatment.
Administration	**Intravenous** and **intrathecal administration** of methotrexate should be done only by healthcare practitioners who have appropriate training and expertise, and only in carefully regulated circumstances.
Communication	Explain to patients that methotrexate treatment should cause improvement in, for example, swollen painful joints, but that this may take some time to reach maximal effect. Emphasise that methotrexate should be **taken once a week** (not every day) by prompting patients to consider on what day they will take the drug. Warn patients to seek urgent medical advice if they develop sore throat or fever (infection), bruising or bleeding (low platelet count), nausea, abdominal pain or dark urine (liver poisoning) or breathlessness (lung toxicity). Give advice regarding contraception (see Warnings) to all patients (men and women) who have the potential to have a child. Patients should receive a **methotrexate treatment booklet** and **warning card.**
Monitoring	**Efficacy** should be monitored by symptoms, examination (e.g. of inflamed joints) and blood tests (e.g. inflammatory markers). **Safety** monitoring is essential as adverse effects can be life threatening, but may be reversible if detected early and treatment is stopped. Patients should be advised to report unexpected symptoms (see above). Measure FBC, liver and renal function before starting treatment, then 1–2 times weekly until treatment is established and 2–3 times monthly thereafter. Treatment should be stopped immediately if abnormalities develop or if the patient becomes breathless.
Cost	Non-proprietary oral methotrexate is available and is inexpensive.

Clinical tip—There are significant restrictions associated with the prescription of methotrexate in order to reduce medication errors and the risk of toxicity. Foundation year 1 doctors **should not** initiate a methotrexate prescription. They may have an important role in reviewing or continuing prescriptions: for example, at the time of hospital admission. If in any doubt about the appropriateness of a methotrexate prescription, always seek senior, expert advice.

Metronidazole

CLINICAL PHARMACOLOGY

Common indications	❶ **Antibiotic-associated colitis** caused by the Gram-positive anaerobe *Clostridium difficile*. ❷ **Oral infections** (such as dental abscess) or **aspiration pneumonia** caused by Gram-negative anaerobes from the mouth. ❸ **Surgical and gynaecological infections** caused by Gram-negative anaerobes from the colon, for example *Bacteroides fragilis.* ❹ **Protozoal infections** including trichomonal vaginal infection, amoebic dysentery and giardiasis.
Spectrum of activity	Anaerobic bacteria and protozoa.
Mechanisms of action	Metronidazole enters bacterial cells by passive diffusion. In **anaerobic bacteria,** reduction of metronidazole generates a nitroso free radical. This binds to DNA, reducing synthesis and causing widespread damage, **DNA degradation** and **cell death (bactericidal).** As aerobic bacteria are not able to reduce metronidazole in this manner, the spectrum of action of metronidazole is restricted to anaerobic bacteria (and protozoa). Bacterial resistance to metronidazole is generally low but is increasing in prevalence. Mechanisms include reduced uptake of metronidazole and reduced generation of nitroso free radicals.
Important adverse effects	As with many antibiotics, metronidazole can cause **GI upset** (such as nausea and vomiting) and immediate and delayed **hypersensitivity** reactions (see Penicillins, broad-spectrum). When used at high doses or for a prolonged course, metronidazole can cause neurological adverse effects, including **peripheral** and **optic neuropathy, seizures** and **encephalopathy.**
Warnings	Metronidazole is metabolised by hepatic cytochrome P450 (CYP) enzymes, so the dose should be reduced in people with ▲**severe liver disease.** Metronidazole inhibits the enzyme acetaldehyde dehydrogenase, which is responsible for clearing the intermediate alcohol metabolite acetaldehyde from the body. ✖**Alcohol** should not be drunk while taking metronidazole as the combination can cause a 'disulfiram-like' reaction, including flushing, headache, nausea and vomiting.
Important interactions	Metronidazole has some inhibitory effect on **CYP enzymes,** reducing metabolism of warfarin (increasing the risk of bleeding) and phenytoin (increasing the risk of toxicity, including impaired cerebellar function). The reverse interaction can occur with **CYP inducers** (e.g. phenytoin, rifampicin), resulting in reduced plasma concentrations and impaired antimicrobial efficacy. Metronidazole also increases the risk of toxicity with lithium.

PRACTICAL PRESCRIBING

Prescription	Metronidazole is available in a variety of formulations. The oral route is used for GI infection or where the patient is not systemically unwell. A typical starting dose would be 400 mg orally 8-hrly. The IV route, usually at a dose of 500 mg IV 8-hrly, is used for severe infection or where patients cannot take treatment by mouth. Rectal metronidazole is an alternative for patients who are nil by mouth. Metronidazole can be prescribed as a gel for topical administration to treat vaginal infection such as bacterial vaginosis or to reduce the odour from an infected skin ulcer.
Administration	Oral metronidazole may be taken as tablets or in an oral suspension. Intravenous metronidazole is given as an infusion over 20 minutes.
Communication	Explain to patients that the aim of treatment is to get rid of infection and improve symptoms. Before prescribing, always check with your patients personally or get collateral history to ensure that they have no **allergy** to metronidazole. If an allergy develops during treatment, give the patient written and verbal advice not to take this antibiotic in the future and make sure that the reaction (including its nature) is clearly documented in the patient's medical records. Warn patients not to take **alcohol** during or for 48 hours after treatment, explaining that if they do they may feel very unwell with nausea, vomiting, flushing and headache.
Monitoring	Check that infection resolves by review of symptoms, signs and blood tests (improvement in inflammatory markers) if appropriate. For treatment exceeding 10 days, measure full blood count and perform liver function tests to monitor for adverse effects.
Cost	A 7-day course of non-proprietary oral metronidazole tablets (one taken every 8 hours) currently costs around £4.50 if 400 mg tablets are prescribed, but around £38 if 500 mg tablets are prescribed. You should therefore select the lower dose unless there are overwhelming clinical reasons for the higher dose.

Clinical tip—Patients often ask if they can drink alcohol while they are taking a course of antibiotics. While it is sensible to moderate alcohol consumption when feeling unwell, **most antibiotics do not interact with alcohol** and do not preclude alcohol intake. **Metronidazole is a clear exception** to this as patients may feel extremely unwell (the disulfiram-like effect) if they take alcohol during, or for up to 48 hours after, metronidazole treatment. Co-trimoxazole rarely causes a similar reaction to metronidazole. Alcohol consumption can reduce or delay the effectiveness of doxycycline and erythromycin.

Naloxone

CLINICAL PHARMACOLOGY

Common indications	❶ Acute treatment of **opioid toxicity** associated with respiratory and/or neurological depression. ❷ A pre-filled syringe formulation, suitable for administration in the community by bystanders, may be indicated for individuals at high risk of recurrent opioid toxicity due to drug misuse. It is intended for administration (after appropriate training) by someone close to that person as a life-saving intervention.
Mechanisms of action	Naloxone binds to opioid receptors (particularly the pharmacologically important opioid μ-receptors), where it acts as a **competitive antagonist.** It has little or no effect in the absence of an exogenous opioid (e.g. morphine). However, if an opioid is present, naloxone displaces it from its receptors and, in so doing, it reverses its effects. In opioid toxicity, this is used to restore an adequate level of consciousness and respiratory rate.
Important adverse effects	Naloxone has few intrinsic adverse effects. However, the effect of opioid reversal in an opioid-dependent individual may be a significant **opioid withdrawal reaction**. This presents with pain (if the opioid was being taken for its analgesic effect), restlessness, nausea and vomiting, dilated pupils, and cold, dry skin with piloerection ('cold turkey').
Warnings	There are no specific contraindications to the use of naloxone. However, caution should be exercised in patients who may have developed ▲**opioid dependence** (whether from therapeutic or recreational use) because of the risk of precipitating opioid withdrawal. Lower doses should be used in the ▲**palliative care** setting to reduce the risk of complete reversal of analgesia.
Important interactions	Naloxone has no clinically important drug interactions other than its interaction with opioids, which is central to its pharmacological and therapeutic effects.

PRACTICAL PRESCRIBING

Prescription	Acute opioid toxicity can usually be adequately reversed with naloxone 400–1200 micrograms IV, titrated to effect (see Administration). If IV access is impractical, it can be given IM, SC, or intranasally. It should be prescribed in the once-only section of the drug chart, although in an emergency it is reasonable to treat first and prescribe later. The pre-filled syringe formulation (Prenoxad®), for individuals at high risk of opioid overdose, should be prescribed only after careful assessment and training. The practicalities of this will depend on local pathways; ideally, it should be co-ordinated by a specialist drugs misuse service.
Administration	In hospital, naloxone is usually administered by the prescriber or under their direct supervision. It is given in incremental doses (e.g. 200–400 micrograms IV) every 2–3 minutes until satisfactory reversal is achieved (patient rousable with adequate respiration). In patients who develop opioid toxicity in the context of chronic use (especially in palliative care), smaller incremental doses (e.g. 40–100 micrograms) should be used. The form of naloxone intended for non-medical use is given by IM injection in doses of 400 micrograms (0.4 mL of the 1 mg/mL solution) every 2–3 minutes until professional help arrives.
Communication	Once the patient is conscious, you can, as appropriate for the situation, explain that they required life-saving treatment for the overdose. Depending on the clinical context, you may need to discuss how this situation arose and how to avoid it in future. For individuals at high risk of recurrent overdose due to opioid misuse, it may be appropriate to discuss supplying naloxone for them to keep on their person, for emergency life-saving use by someone close to them.
Monitoring	Patients should be **closely monitored** during naloxone administration, as the dose is titrated to effect. Once adequate reversal is achieved, it is essential to continue monitoring for at least an hour. This is because the duration of action of naloxone (about 20–60 minutes, depending on route of administration) is shorter than that of most opioids. Consequently, **opioid toxicity can recur** when the effect of naloxone has dissipated, necessitating repeated doses or, occasionally, an infusion.
Cost	Naloxone is available in non-proprietary form and is inexpensive.

Clinical tip—When giving very small doses of naloxone (e.g. 40 micrograms), it is impractical to use the 400 microgram/mL solution that is usually available on the wards. Therefore take 1 mL (400 micrograms) of this solution in a 10-mL syringe and add 9 mL of 0.9% sodium chloride. Label the syringe immediately. The resulting 40-microgram/mL solution can then be administered in more practical 1-mL increments.

Nicotine replacement and related drugs

CLINICAL PHARMACOLOGY

Common indications	In **smoking cessation,** drug therapy to control physical symptoms of nicotine withdrawal is used alongside non-pharmacological measures to address the psychological and behavioural aspects of dependence.
Mechanisms of action	Nicotine obtained from tobacco use has complex actions. In the central nervous system, it **activates nicotinic acetylcholine receptors,** increasing neurotransmitter levels and causing euphoria and relaxation. Nicotine withdrawal causes intense craving, anxiety, depression and irritability with increased appetite and weight gain. During abstinence from tobacco, *nicotine replacement therapy* **prevents withdrawal symptoms** by maintaining receptor activation. *Varenicline,* a partial agonist of the nicotinic receptor, reduces both withdrawal symptoms and the rewarding effects of smoking by preventing binding of tobacco-derived nicotine to receptors. *Bupropion* increases concentrations of noradrenaline and dopamine in the synaptic cleft by inhibiting reuptake. The mechanism underlying its benefits in smoking cessation are not fully understood.
Important adverse effects	It is generally considered safer for smokers to take nicotine replacement therapy than to continue smoking. Adverse effects include **local irritation** (for example, from patches, lozenges, nasal spray) or **GI upset** with oral nicotine. Palpitations and abnormal dreams may occur. Common side effects of *varenicline* include nausea, headache, insomnia and abnormal dreams. Rarely, patients may develop **suicidal ideation.** *Bupropion* commonly causes **dry mouth, GI upset, neurological** (e.g. headache, impaired concentration, dizziness) and **psychiatric** (e.g. insomnia, depression, agitation) adverse effects. Hypersensitivity is common and more often manifests as a skin rash (for example, urticaria) than a severe reaction (such as anaphylaxis).
Warnings	*Nicotine replacement therapy* should be used with caution in people who are ▲**haemodynamically unstable:** for example, following myocardial infarction. *Bupropion* and *varenicline* should be used with caution in people ▲**at risk of seizures** as they can precipitate convulsions. This includes people with prior seizures or head injury and those who abuse alcohol or who take other drugs that lower the seizure threshold. They should be used with care in people with ▲**psychiatric disease** due to risk of suicidal ideation. All these drugs should be used with caution in people with ▲**hepatic** or ▲**renal impairment.**
Important interactions	*Nicotine replacement* and *varenicline* have no clinically significant drug interactions. *Bupropion* is metabolised by cytochrome P450 (CYP) enzymes, so its plasma levels are increased by **CYP inhibitors,** e.g. valproate, and reduced by **inducers,** e.g. phenytoin, carbamazepine. Use of bupropion with monoamine oxidase inhibitors or tricyclic antidepressants increases stimulation of catecholaminergic pathways and risk of adverse effects.

PRACTICAL PRESCRIBING

Prescription	*Nicotine replacement therapy* is prescribed as a **continuous-release patch** to reduce or prevent cravings and/or an **immediate-release preparation** (for example, sublingual (SL) tablets, sprays, gum) to control the acute urge to smoke. Treatment should start either before a cessation attempt to reduce the number of cigarettes smoked or when the patient stops smoking. For people smoking >10 cigarettes/day, start treatment with a high-dose nicotine patch for 6–8 weeks, then wean to a medium- then low-dose patch for 2 weeks each before stopping. Treatment with *varenicline* or *bupropion* should start 1–2 weeks before the target quit date. A low starting dose is titrated over the first week to the optimal treatment dose and continued for 9–12 weeks. The drug is stopped if the smoking cessation attempt fails.
Administration	**Nicotine patches** should be applied in the morning to an area of dry hairless skin and taken off at night to prevent insomnia. They should be applied to a different site each day to reduce skin irritation. **Immediate-release nicotine** in any formulation should be taken as soon as the urge to smoke strikes.
Communication	Explain to patients that the medicine offered can help to **reduce the craving** for a cigarette and the feeling of irritability that can occur when stopping smoking. Advise them that treatment works best if they have a plan as to how and when they will stop and have thought about how they might change their habits to stay off cigarettes. Offer **support and counselling,** for example through a smoking cessation clinic, as this increases the chance of a successful quit attempt.
Monitoring	Monitoring the success of a quit attempt and side effects of treatment is usually by **patient report,** but a salivary cotinine test (a marker of tobacco exposure) may be helpful to confirm abstinence. Patients should be reviewed monthly, for example, as part of a smoking cessation clinic.
Cost	Drugs to help with smoking cessation can be **prescribed on the NHS,** but only for patients who have a clear idea of how and when they will quit. A course of any treatment to support smoking cessation (10–12 weeks) costs approximately £150. Treatment should therefore be stopped if the attempt fails and should not usually be repeated within 6 months, unless exceptional circumstances have interrupted the attempt.

Clinical tip—Acute hospital admission causes anxiety and immobility, both of which can encourage people to stop smoking. Nicotine withdrawal can add to symptoms and precipitate patients to discharge themselves before medical treatment is complete. Ask all inpatients about smoking and offer nicotine replacement as patches and/or immediate-release preparations to current smokers. Refer those interested to smoking cessation services for ongoing support on discharge.

Nitrates

CLINICAL PHARMACOLOGY

Common indications	❶ Short-acting nitrates (glyceryl trinitrate) are used in the treatment of **acute angina** and chest pain associated with **acute coronary syndrome (ACS).** ❷ Long-acting nitrates (e.g. isosorbide mononitrate) are used for **prophylaxis of angina** where a β-blocker and/or a calcium channel blocker are insufficient or not tolerated. ❸ Intravenous nitrates are used in the treatment of **pulmonary oedema,** usually in combination with furosemide and oxygen.
Mechanisms of action	Nitrates are converted to nitric oxide (NO). NO increases cyclic guanosine monophosphate (cGMP) synthesis and reduces intracellular Ca^{2+} in vascular smooth muscle cells, causing them to relax. This results in venous and, to a lesser extent, arterial vasodilatation. **Relaxation of the venous capacitance vessels** reduces cardiac preload and left ventricular filling. These effects **reduce cardiac work and myocardial oxygen demand,** relieving angina and cardiac failure. Nitrates can relieve coronary vasospasm and dilate collateral vessels, improving coronary perfusion. They also relax the systemic arteries, reducing peripheral resistance and afterload. However, most of the antianginal effects are mediated by reduction of preload.
Important adverse effects	As vasodilators, nitrates commonly cause **flushing, headaches, light-headedness** and **hypotension.** Sustained use of nitrates can lead to **tolerance,** with reduced symptom relief despite continued use. This can be minimised by careful timing of doses to avoid significant nitrate exposure overnight, when it tends not to be needed.
Warnings	Nitrates are contraindicated in patients with ✖**severe aortic stenosis,** in whom they may cause cardiovascular collapse. This is because the heart is unable to increase cardiac output sufficiently through the narrowed valve area to maintain pressure in the now dilated vasculature. Nitrates should also be avoided in patients with ✖**haemodynamic instability,** particularly ✖**hypotension.**
Important interactions	Nitrates must not be used with ✖phosphodiesterase (PDE) inhibitors (e.g. sildenafil) because these enhance and prolong the hypotensive effect of nitrates. Nitrates should also be used with caution in patients taking antihypertensive medication, in whom they may precipitate hypotension.

PRACTICAL PRESCRIBING

Prescription	In patients with **stable angina,** glyceryl trinitrate (GTN) is prescribed to be taken **sublingually** as tablets or spray for immediate relief of chest pain. GTN has a plasma half-life of <5 minutes, so has a very quick onset and offset of action. In patients with **ACS** or **heart failure,** GTN is prescribed as a **continuous IV infusion.** Isosorbide mononitrate (ISMN) has a plasma half-life of 4–5 hours and is prescribed two to three times daily as immediate-release **tablets** for the prevention of recurrent angina. ISMN is also available as modified-release (MR) tablets or transdermal **patches,** which are prescribed once daily. When prescribing MR preparations, prescribe by the brand name, since there are important differences between preparations.
Administration	Intravenous GTN is usually administered as a solution containing GTN 50 mg in 50 mL (1 mg/mL). You should give nursing staff clear instructions on the starting dose, normally expressed as an infusion rate, e.g. 1 mL/hr. You should provide instructions on how to increase the dose to relieve symptoms (e.g. 'Increase GTN infusion rate by 0.5 mL/hr every 15–30 minutes until chest pain is relieved') while avoiding hypotension (e.g. 'Keep systolic blood pressure >90 mmHg').
Communication	Explain to patients that you are prescribing a nitrate to relieve chest pain and/or breathlessness. Advise patients that they may develop a headache when starting nitrates, but that this is normally short-lived. As nitrates are probably more effective at preventing than terminating angina, patients should be advised to use sublingual GTN *before* tasks that normally bring on their angina. Due to the risks of postural hypotension, it is a good idea to advise them to sit down and rest before and for 5 minutes after taking GTN. For regularly administered nitrates, advise on the times that doses should be taken (see Clinical tip).
Monitoring	The best indicators of efficacy are the patient's **symptoms** (e.g. chest pain, breathlessness). When administering nitrates by IV infusion, **blood pressure** should be monitored frequently, and the infusion rate adjusted to ensure the systolic blood pressure does not drop below 90 mmHg.
Cost	Non-proprietary GTN and ISMN are inexpensive. GTN tablets must be discarded after 8 weeks, so a spray may be a better choice for patients with infrequent symptoms.

Clinical tip—Where nitrates are taken regularly, there is a risk of tolerance (tachyphylaxis), which can reduce efficacy. To prevent this, time doses to ensure there is a 'nitrate-free period' every day during a time of inactivity, usually overnight. For example, patients should be advised to take twice-daily ISMN morning and mid-afternoon (rather than evening) to provide a longer (about 18-hour) gap between doses in the afternoon and the following morning. Transdermal patches should be applied in the morning and removed at bedtime.

Nitrofurantoin

CLINICAL PHARMACOLOGY

Common indications	❶ Nitrofurantoin is a first-choice treatment **for acute, uncomplicated lower urinary tract infection (UTI)** (alternatives are <u>trimethoprim</u>, <u>amoxicillin</u> and <u>cefalexin</u>). ❷ It can also be used for **prophylaxis** of UTI in patients with recurrent infections. As nitrofurantoin requires concentration in the urine by renal excretion for therapeutic effect, it is not effective against clinical infections elsewhere in the body.
Spectrum of activity	Nitrofurantoin is active against most organisms that cause uncomplicated UTIs, including *Escherichia coli* (Gram negative) and *Staphylococcus saprophyticus* (Gram-positive).
Mechanisms of action	Nitrofurantoin is metabolised (reduced) in bacterial cells by nitrofuran reductase. Its **active metabolite damages bacterial DNA** and causes cell death (bactericidal). Bacteria with lower nitrofuran reductase activity are resistant to nitrofurantoin. Some organisms that are less common causes of UTI (such as *Klebsiella* and *Proteus* species) have intrinsic resistance to nitrofurantoin. It is relatively rare for *E. coli* to acquire nitrofurantoin resistance.
Important adverse effects	As with many antibiotics, nitrofurantoin can cause **GI upset** (including nausea and diarrhoea) and immediate and delayed **hypersensitivity** reactions (see <u>Penicillins, broad-spectrum</u>). Nitrofurantoin, specifically, can turn urine dark yellow or brown. Less commonly, it may cause **chronic pulmonary reactions** (including inflammation [pneumonitis] and fibrosis), **hepatitis** and **peripheral neuropathy,** which all are more likely with prolonged administration. In neonates, **haemolytic anaemia** may occur because immature red blood cells are unable to mop up nitrofurantoin-stimulated superoxides, which damage red blood cells.
Warnings	Nitrofurantoin should not be prescribed for ✖**pregnant women towards term** or for ✖**babies in the first 3 months of life.** It is contraindicated in patients with ✖**renal impairment**, as impaired excretion increases toxicity and reduces efficacy due to lower urinary drug concentrations. Caution is required when using nitrofurantoin for ▲**long-term prevention** of UTIs, as chronic use increases the risk of adverse effects, particularly in elderly patients.
Important interactions	There are no significant interactions between nitrofurantoin and other commonly prescribed drugs.

PRACTICAL PRESCRIBING

Prescription	Nitrofurantoin is only available for oral administration. Maximum urinary concentrations are usually achieved 2–4 hours after dosing. For treatment of acute UTI, a typical dosage regimen is 50–100 mg 6-hrly. Treatment duration depends on nature and severity of infection, with a 3-day course being sufficient for uncomplicated UTIs in women and 7 days of treatment being required for men or for people with more complicated infection. For **prevention of recurrent UTI,** a single nightly dose of 50–100 mg is prescribed. Treatment duration should only be longer than 6 months if strongly indicated, and this requires monitoring (see below).
Administration	Oral nitrofurantoin is available as tablets, capsules and in suspension. It should be **taken with food or milk** to minimise GI effects.
Communication	Explain to patients that the aim of treatment is to get rid of infection and improve symptoms. Where antibiotics are for **prophylaxis,** emphasise that this is a long-term medication that should be renewed, rather than a course that should stop. Before prescribing, always check with patients personally or get collateral history to ensure that they do not have an **allergy** to nitrofurantoin. Advise them that their **urine colour** may change to dark yellow or brown during treatment; this is harmless and temporary. For long-term treatment, warn patients to report any unexplained symptoms, particularly **pins and needles** or **breathlessness,** which could indicate development of serious side effects.
Monitoring	Efficacy of **treatment for acute UTI** is determined by resolution of symptoms and, less commonly, by ensuring sterility of urine on repeat culture. Success in **preventing recurrent UTI** is determined by comparing UTI frequency before and during prophylaxis. Safety of long-term treatment is a particular concern, and patients should be advised to report any symptoms (see Communication) that could indicate the onset of neuropathy or pulmonary adverse effects.
Cost	The drug tariff price (amount paid to pharmacy contractors for dispensing the drug) of a 7-day course of nitrofurantoin is £10–15 where capsules or tablets are prescribed. A similar course of nitrofurantoin as oral suspension is around 30 times more expensive. This preparation should be reserved for patients who truly are unable to take tablets or capsules.

Clinical tip—As tissue concentrations of nitrofurantoin are very low, you should not prescribe it for pyelonephritis or other complicated UTIs, which should be treated with an IV broad-spectrum antibiotic such as a broad-spectrum penicillin with β-lactamase inhibitor, a cephalosporin, or a quinolone, with or without an aminoglycoside.

Non-steroidal antiinflammatory drugs

CLINICAL PHARMACOLOGY

Common indications	❶ 'As needed' treatment of **mild-to-moderate pain** (e.g. dysmenorrhoea, dental pain) as an alternative to or in addition to paracetamol. Analgesia from a single dose of a non-steroidal anti-inflammatory drug (NSAID) is similar to that from paracetamol. Paracetamol is therefore preferred, particularly in those at risk of adverse effects. ❷ Regular treatment for **pain related to inflammation,** particularly of the musculoskeletal system, e.g. in rheumatoid arthritis, severe osteoarthritis and acute gout.
Mechanisms of action	NSAIDs inhibit prostaglandin synthesis from arachidonic acid by **inhibiting cyclo-oxygenase (COX)**. COX exists as two main isoforms. COX-1 is the *constitutive* form. It stimulates prostaglandin synthesis that is essential to preserve integrity of the gastric mucosa; maintains renal perfusion (by dilating afferent glomerular arterioles); and inhibits thrombus formation at the vascular endothelium. COX-2 is the *inducible* form, expressed in response to inflammatory stimuli. It stimulates production of prostaglandins that cause inflammation and pain. The therapeutic benefits of NSAIDs are principally mediated by COX-2 inhibition and adverse effects by COX-1 inhibition, although there is some overlap between the two. Selective COX-2 inhibitors (e.g. etoricoxib) were developed in an effort to reduce the adverse gastrointestinal effects of NSAIDs.
Important adverse effects	The main adverse effects of NSAIDs are **gastrointestinal (GI) toxicity, renal impairment** and increased risk of **cardiovascular events** (e.g. myocardial infarction and stroke). The likelihood of adverse effects differs between NSAIDs. Of all the non-selective NSAIDs (>20 are available), ibuprofen is associated with the lowest risk of GI effects. Naproxen and low-dose ibuprofen are associated with the lowest risk of cardiovascular events. COX-2 inhibitors cause fewer GI side effects than non-selective NSAIDs, but are associated with an increased risk of cardiovascular events. All NSAIDs, including COX-2 inhibitors, can cause renal impairment. Other adverse effects include **hypersensitivity reactions,** e.g. bronchospasm and angioedema, and **fluid retention,** which can worsen hypertension and heart failure.
Warnings	Avoid NSAIDs in ✖**severe renal impairment,** ✖**heart failure,** ✖**liver failure** and known ✖**NSAID hypersensitivity.** If NSAID use is unavoidable in patients at high risk of adverse effects (e.g. prior ▲**peptic ulcer disease** or ▲**GI bleeding,** ▲**cardiovascular disease,** ▲**renal impairment**), use the safest NSAID at the lowest effective dose for the shortest possible time.
Important interactions	Many drugs increase the risk of NSAID-related adverse effects, including *peptic ulceration* – low-dose ▲aspirin, corticosteroids; *GI bleeding* – ▲anticoagulants (e.g. warfarin, direct-oral anticoagulants), ▲SSRIs, ▲venlafaxine; and *renal impairment* – ▲ACE inhibitors, diuretics. NSAIDs also reduce the therapeutic effects of other antihypertensives.

PRACTICAL PRESCRIBING

Prescription	NSAIDs are generally taken orally, but are also available as topical gels, suppositories and injectable preparations. Most NSAIDs have similar antiinflammatory efficacy, but there may be considerable differences in individual patient response to and tolerance of individual drugs. The choice of drug and dosage will depend on the condition to be treated, as well as on safety considerations and patient choice. For example, in a patient with **rheumatoid arthritis,** naproxen 500 mg orally 12-hrly may be prescribed. Regular treatment for at least 3 weeks is required before full antiinflammatory effect is seen, when treatment may be continued or switched to an alternative NSAID if ineffective. By contrast, a patient with **acute pain** may be treated with naproxen 250 mg orally 6–8-hrly as needed, to be stopped as soon as pain has resolved.
Administration	Oral NSAIDs should be taken with food to minimise GI upset.
Communication	Explain to patients that you are recommending an antiinflammatory drug to help improve symptoms of pain, swelling and/or fever. Warn patients that the most common side effect is indigestion and advise them to stop treatment and seek medical advice if this occurs. For patients with acute pain, explain that long-term use, e.g. beyond 10 days, is not recommended due to the risk of side effects. Advise patients requiring long-term treatment (particularly if they have renal impairment) to stop NSAIDs if they become acutely unwell or dehydrated to reduce the risk of damage to the kidneys.
Monitoring	Control of pain and inflammation can be assessed by enquiry about symptoms, examination and by using scoring systems, e.g. a visual analogue scale for pain. Routine biochemical monitoring is not usually required but renal function should be monitored closely in patients with existing renal impairment. The NSAID should be stopped if there is significant deterioration.
Cost	NSAIDs are available in non-proprietary formulations, which are inexpensive. For patients who pay for their prescriptions, it may be cheaper for them to buy non-proprietary NSAIDs over the counter.

Clinical tip—Gastroprotection should be considered for all patients taking NSAIDs who are at increased risk of GI complications. Risk factors include age >65 years, previous peptic ulcer disease, co-morbidities (such as cardiovascular disease, diabetes), and concurrent therapy with other drugs with GI side effects, particularly low-dose aspirin and prednisolone. The preferred strategy in at-risk patients is to use low-dose ibuprofen (which has the lowest risk of gastric side effects) with a PPI (e.g. lansoprazole 15 mg daily). Although COX-2 inhibitors are an alternative, they confer a higher risk of adverse vascular events.

Ocular lubricants (artificial tears)

CLINICAL PHARMACOLOGY

Common indications	For first-line symptomatic treatment of **dry eye conditions,** including **keratoconjunctivitis sicca** and **Sjögren's syndrome,** alongside environmental coping strategies and avoiding precipitants.
Mechanisms of action	In dry eye conditions, ocular lubricants have a **soothing effect** and help **protect the eye surfaces from abrasive damage.** Lubricant *eye drops* typically consist of an electrolyte solution with a viscosity agent, such as a cellulose polymer (e.g. hypromellose). *Gels,* such as carbomer 980 (the active ingredient of Viscotears®), have greater viscosity and are retained in the eye for longer. *Ointments* such as white soft paraffin with liquid paraffin (e.g. Lacri-Lube®) are highly viscous and may provide greater protection, but at a cost of causing blurred vision.
Important adverse effects	Ocular lubricants have **few side effects** other than mild **stinging** on application and temporary **blurring of vision.** The risk of blurring increases with viscosity and is therefore greatest for ointments. Unless specified as 'preservative-free', it can be assumed that the preparation contains some form of preservative. This may incite a local **inflammatory (allergic) reaction** in some patients.
Warnings	As ocular lubricants are not absorbed, there are no major safety considerations from a systemic illness perspective.
Important interactions	No clinically important interactions arise from the pharmacological effects of ocular lubricants. If patients need to take more than one type of eye drop, they should separate them by about 5 minutes. Ocular lubricants should be taken last, otherwise they may be 'washed away' by the other eye drops.

hypromellose, carbomers, liquid and white soft paraffin

PRACTICAL PRESCRIBING

Prescription	Most ocular lubricants can be purchased from pharmacies without a prescription. In the absence of an underlying condition requiring medical supervision (such as Sjögren's syndrome), it is generally easier for the patient to purchase the product over the counter. Hypromellose 0.3% eye drops are usually tried first at a dose of 1–2 drops three times daily as required. They can be taken more often (up to hourly) if necessary, but if they are required more than four times daily on a regular basis, it may be worth trying a gel (e.g. Viscotears® 1 drop three times daily as required). In severe cases an ointment (e.g. Lacri-Lube®) may be added, although this is generally restricted to bedtime use due to its visual blurring effect.
Administration	Ocular lubricants are usually self-administered. After washing their hands, the patient tips the head back ('looks at the ceiling') and pulls down slightly on the lower eyelid. Then, with the bottle held upside-down just above the eye, they squeeze to release a drop. For drops, they should then close the eye and press gently on the corner nearest the nose for 1 minute. For gels, they should blink a few times to spread it over the eye. They should try not to let the tip of the dispenser touch the eye (or anything else), and should replace the cap directly after use to prevent infection.
Communication	Explain to patients that you are recommending 'artificial tears' in the hope of improving their dry eyes. Explain how to take them and warn that, like most eye drops, they can sting a little when applied. This wears away quickly and they should then experience some relief from their dry eye symptoms. With continued use over days and weeks their symptoms may improve further as previous abrasive damage is repaired. They will probably need to take the treatment indefinitely.
Monitoring	The best form of monitoring is by patients themselves. Ask them to return if their symptoms fail to improve or any problems develop.
Cost	Patients who pay for their prescriptions will generally save money if they purchase the product over the counter.

Clinical tip—Critically ill patients in intensive care units may suffer from corneal erosions and microbial keratitis, due to poor eyelid closure and suppression of protective reflexes in the context of impaired consciousness. Eye care should be a routine part of intensive care, but is sometimes neglected. Prescription of an ocular lubricant, e.g. hypromellose 0.3%, one drop per eye 4-hrly, should be considered for all critically ill patients.

Oestrogens and progestogens

CLINICAL PHARMACOLOGY

Common indications	❶ **Hormonal contraception** in women who require highly effective and reversible contraception, particularly if they may also benefit from its other effects, such as improved acne symptoms with oestrogens. ❷ **Hormone replacement therapy (HRT)** to delay **early menopause** in women <50 years old and treat distressing **menopausal symptoms** (any age).
Mechanisms of action	Luteinising hormone (LH) and follicle-stimulating hormone (FSH) control ovulation and ovarian production of oestrogen and progesterone. In turn, oestrogen and progesterone exert predominantly negative feedback on LH and FSH release. In hormonal contraception, oestrogens (e.g. ethinylestradiol) and/or progestogens (e.g. desogestrel) are given to **suppress LH/FSH release and hence ovulation.** Oestrogens and progestogens also have effects outside the ovary. Some, such as in the cervix and endometrium, may contribute to their contraceptive effect (most relevant in progestogen-only contraception). Others offer additional benefits, e.g. reduced menstrual pain and bleeding, and improvements in acne. At the menopause, a fall in oestrogen and progesterone levels may generate symptoms such as vaginal dryness and vasomotor instability ('hot flushes'). Oestrogen replacement (usually combined with a progestogen) alleviates these.
Important adverse effects	Hormonal contraception may cause **irregular bleeding** and **mood changes.** It does not appear to cause weight gain. The oestrogens in combined hormonal contraception (CHC) double the risk of venous thromboembolism (VTE), but the absolute risk is low. They also increase the risk of **cardiovascular disease** and **stroke,** but this is probably relevant only in women with other risk factors. They may be associated with increased risk of **breast and cervical cancer.** In both cases the effect is small, and for breast cancer, it gradually resolves after stopping the pill. Progestogen-only pills do not increase the risk of VTE or cardiovascular disease. The adverse effects of **HRT** are similar to those of CHC but, as baseline rates of disease are higher, the relative risks have more significant effects.
Warnings	All forms of oestrogens and progestogens are contraindicated in patients with ✖**breast cancer.** CHC should be avoided in patients at increased risk for **VTE** (✖personal or ▲family history; ✖known thrombogenic mutation) or ▲**cardiovascular disease** (age >35 years; risk factors; migraine with aura; heavy smoking history).
Important interactions	Non-enzyme–inducing antibiotics do not interact significantly with hormonal contraceptives. ▲**Cytochrome P450 inducers** (e.g. rifampicin, <u>carbamazepine</u>) may reduce contraceptive efficacy, particularly of progestogen-only forms. Absorption of ▲<u>lamotrigine</u> may be reduced, potentially impairing seizure control.

combined ethinylestradiol products, desogestrel

PRACTICAL PRESCRIBING

Prescription	Hormonal contraception should be prescribed by appropriately trained health professionals only. CHC is commonly taken as a combined oral contraceptive (COC) pill. A pill containing ethinylestradiol 30 or 35 micrograms is appropriate for most women. Refer to the **UK Medical Eligibility Criteria for Contraceptive Use** from the Faculty of Sexual and Reproductive Healthcare (FSRH) for guidance on cautions and contraindications. Where CHC is contraindicated, a progesterone-only pill (POP) may be suitable. For HRT, combined oestrogen–progestogen therapy is preferred, although women who have had a hysterectomy may receive oestrogen alone. For women with vaginal symptoms only, a vaginal oestrogen preparation is best.
Administration	If a COC pill is started within the first 6 days of the woman's cycle, no additional contraception is needed. If started from day 7 onwards, a barrier method should be used or sex avoided for the first 7 days. Most combined pills are designed to be taken for 21 days followed by a 7-day pill-free interval, during which a withdrawal bleed occurs. Some ('everyday') pills are taken throughout the cycle, but the tablets for days 22–28 are inactive. Detailed guidance on **how to deal with missed pills** is provided by the FSRH and summarised in the BNF. In general, missing 1 COC pill does not significantly reduce contraceptive efficacy, but missing two or more necessitates additional contraceptive precautions for 7 days.
Communication	Hormonal contraception should be offered only after a discussion of the risks and benefits of the various contraceptive methods available. Explain that the usual method of taking the pill (with either no pills or inactive pills in days 22–28) results in a withdrawal bleed each month, although irregular bleeding may occur initially. Explain how to deal with missed pills, and support this with written guidance.
Monitoring	Baseline assessment should include a relevant history, BP check and body mass index (BMI). A woman starting a COC pill should be seen again at 3 months for a BP check and to discuss any issues. She should then be seen yearly to discuss health changes and for BP and BMI checks.
Cost	Hormonal contraception accounts for significant health expenditure. You should generally follow local policies on which pill to use. These take cost into account.

Clinical tip—Continuous or extended use of the COC pill (without pill-free intervals) is unlicensed for most brands, but is safe and effective. It eliminates or reduces withdrawal bleeding, which some women may consider desirable.

Opioids, strong

CLINICAL PHARMACOLOGY

Common indications	❶ Rapid relief of **acute severe pain,** including post-operative pain and pain associated with acute myocardial infarction. ❷ Relief of **chronic pain,** when paracetamol, NSAIDs and weak/moderate opioids are insufficient ('rung 3' of the World Health Organization (WHO) pain ladder). ❸ Relief of breathlessness in the context of **end-of-life care**. ❹ Relief of breathlessness and anxiety in **acute pulmonary oedema,** alongside oxygen, furosemide and nitrates.
Mechanisms of action	The term *opioids* encompasses naturally occurring *opiates* (e.g. morphine) and *synthetic analogues* (e.g. oxycodone). Morphine and oxycodone are *strong opioids*. The therapeutic action of opioids arises from **activation of opioid μ receptors** in the central nervous system (CNS). Activation of these G protein-coupled receptors has several effects that, overall, reduce neuronal excitability and pain transmission. In the medulla, they blunt the response to hypoxia and hypercapnoea, reducing respiratory drive and breathlessness. By relieving pain, breathlessness and associated anxiety, opioids **reduce sympathetic nervous system (fight or flight) activity.** Thus in myocardial infarction and acute pulmonary oedema they may reduce cardiac work and oxygen demand, as well as relieving symptoms. That said, although commonly used, the efficacy and safety of morphine in acute pulmonary oedema is not firmly established.
Important adverse effects	Opioids cause **respiratory depression** by reducing respiratory drive. They may cause euphoria and detachment, and in higher doses, **neurological depression.** They can activate the chemoreceptor trigger zone, causing **nausea and vomiting,** although this tends to settle with continued use. **Pupillary constriction** occurs due to stimulation of the Edinger–Westphal nucleus. In the large intestine, activation of μ receptors increases smooth muscle tone and reduces motility, leading to **constipation.** In the skin, opioids may cause histamine release, leading to **itching,** urticaria, vasodilatation and sweating. Continued use can lead to **tolerance** (a state in which the dose required to produce the same effect increases over time) and **dependence.** Dependence becomes apparent on cessation of the opioid, when a **withdrawal reaction** occurs (see Clinical tip).
Warnings	Most opioids rely on the liver and the kidneys for elimination, so doses should be reduced in ▲**hepatic failure** and ▲ **renal impairment** and in the ▲**elderly.** Do not give opioids in ▲**respiratory failure** except under senior guidance (e.g. in palliative care). Avoid opioids in ▲**biliary colic,** as they may cause spasm of the sphincter of Oddi, which may worsen pain.
Important interactions	Opioids should ideally not be used with ▲**other sedating drugs** (e.g. antipsychotics, benzodiazepines and tricyclic antidepressants). Where their combination is unavoidable, close monitoring is necessary.

PRACTICAL PRESCRIBING

Prescription	When treating **acute severe pain** in high dependency areas, morphine is given IV for rapid effect (onset at about 5 minutes). An initial dose of 2–10 mg, tailored to pain, age and other individual factors, is prescribed in the once-only section. On a general ward, IM or SC administration is preferred. For **chronic pain,** the oral route is safest and usually most appropriate. Immediate-release oral morphine is preferred initially (e.g. Oramorph® 5 mg orally every 4 hours). Then, having found the optimum dose, this is converted to an modified-release (MR) form (e.g. MST Continus® 15 mg every 12 hours). Alongside regular treatment, 'breakthrough analgesia' should be prescribed. Prescribe immediate-release morphine at a dose of about one-sixth of the total daily regular dose (e.g. Oramorph® 5 mg 2-hrly) in the as-required section. For safety reasons, we favour **brand name prescribing** for strong oral opioids, although local practices may vary.
Administration	Intravenous morphine should be given only in high dependency areas as adverse effects may be more pronounced. It should be given incrementally (1–2 mg every few minutes) to achieve the desired response.
Communication	Patients may be reluctant to accept morphine, due to the stigma associated with abuse and dependence. Explain that it is a highly effective painkiller and that 'addiction' is not an issue when it is used for pain control. That said, you should warn patients that the dose may need to be increased over time as they become tolerant to its effects; this is normal and should not cause alarm. Explain how patients should take their morphine: e.g. to take 'slow-release' tablets every 12 hours for background pain and use a 'fast-acting' solution when required for breakthrough pain. Explain that nausea usually settles after a few days, but offer an antiemetic (e.g. metoclopramide). Constipation is very common; pre-emptive use of a laxative (e.g. senna), along with good hydration, is advisable. Advise patients not to drive or operate heavy machinery if they feel drowsy or confused.
Monitoring	For **acute pain,** review your patients' response to analgesia within an hour, as well as for adverse effects such as respiratory depression. For **chronic pain,** schedule a review after a couple of weeks to assess the need to step up or down the analgesic ladder and/or specialist referral.
Cost	Morphine is relatively inexpensive. Synthetic opioids may be more expensive.

Clinical tip—The features of opioid withdrawal are the opposite of the clinical effects of opioids: anxiety, pain and breathlessness increase; the pupils dilate; and the skin is cool and dry with piloerection ('cold turkey'). Opioid dependence is less problematic when opioids are taken therapeutically rather than recreationally; do not let this concern deter you from offering opioids for severe or chronic pain, especially in end-of-life care.

Opioids, weak/moderate

CLINICAL PHARMACOLOGY

Common indications	**Mild-to-moderate pain,** including post-operative pain, as second-line agents when simple analgesics, such as <u>paracetamol</u>, are insufficient. Weak opioids are on the second 'rung' of the World Health Organisation (WHO) pain ladder.
Mechanisms of action	In unmodified form, codeine and dihydrocodeine are very weak opioids. They are metabolised in the liver to produce relatively small amounts of morphine (from codeine) or dihydromorphine (from dihydrocodeine). These metabolites, which are stronger **agonists of opioid μ (mu) receptors** (see <u>Opioids, strong</u>), probably account for most of the analgesic effect. About 10% of Caucasians have a less active form of the key metabolising enzyme (CYP 2D6), and these people may find codeine and dihydrocodeine largely ineffective. Tramadol is a synthetic analogue of codeine; it is perhaps best classified as a 'moderate-strength' opioid. Like codeine, tramadol and its active metabolite are μ-receptor agonists. Unlike other opioids, tramadol also affects serotonergic and adrenergic pathways, where it is thought to act as a serotonin and noradrenaline reuptake inhibitor (SNRI). This probably contributes to its analgesic effect.
Important adverse effects	Common side effects of weak opioids include **nausea, constipation, dizziness** and **drowsiness.** All opioids can cause **neurological and respiratory depression** when taken in overdose. Tramadol may cause less constipation and respiratory depression than other opioids. **Codeine and dihydrocodeine must never be given intravenously,** as this can cause a severe reaction similar to anaphylaxis. This is mediated by histamine release, but does not have an 'allergic' basis.
Warnings	Caution must be exercised when prescribing an opioid in the context of ▲**significant respiratory disease.** Tramadol, codeine and dihydrocodeine rely on both the liver and the kidneys for their elimination. Doses should therefore be reduced in ▲**renal impairment,** ▲**hepatic impairment** and in the ▲**elderly.** Tramadol lowers the seizure threshold, so is best avoided in patients with ▲**epilepsy,** and certainly should not be used in those with ✖**uncontrolled epilepsy.**
Important interactions	Opioids should ideally not be used with ▲**other sedating drugs** (e.g. <u>antipsychotics</u>, <u>benzodiazepines</u> and <u>tricyclic antidepressants</u>). Where their combination is unavoidable, closer monitoring is necessary. Tramadol should not be used with other ▲**drugs that lower the seizure threshold,** such as <u>antipsychotics</u>. Due to its serotonin-modulating effects, tramadol may increase the risk of serotonin syndrome when taken with other ▲**serotonergic drugs** (e.g. monoamine oxidase inhibitors, <u>selective serotonin reuptake inhibitors</u>, <u>tricyclic antidepressants</u>, <u>tramadol</u>).

tramadol, codeine, dihydrocodeine

PRACTICAL PRESCRIBING

Prescription	Weak opioids are usually prescribed orally as a regular or as-required prescription. A common starting prescription might be for codeine or dihydrocodeine 30 mg orally 4-hrly, or tramadol 50 mg orally 4-hrly (to max 400 mg/day). Whenever an opioid is to be administered regularly, you should consider the need for a laxative (e.g. a <u>stimulant laxative</u> such as senna) to mitigate its constipating effects. Codeine and dihydrocodeine are available in combination with paracetamol as oral preparations in varying ratios. For example, 'co-codamol 8/500' tablets contain codeine 8 mg and paracetamol 500 mg; 'co-dydramol 10/500' contains dihydrocodeine 10 mg and paracetamol 500 mg.
Administration	Doses should be taken at regular intervals. They may be taken with or without food. If they are being administered IM, care must be taken to avoid inadvertent IV administration.
Communication	Explain to patients that you are offering a painkiller that is like a weaker version of morphine. It will work best if taken regularly at equal intervals. Discuss common side effects, and if appropriate, offer a laxative to prevent constipation. Advise patients to avoid driving or operating heavy machinery if they become drowsy or confused while taking the new painkiller. Mention that painkillers should be stored out of reach of children. When prescribing weak opioids as a compound preparation, advise patients not to take other medications that contain paracetamol to avoid accidental overdose.
Monitoring	**Efficacy** of analgesics is best established by symptom enquiry and/or with a pain score: e.g. a visual analogue scale. In acute pain, review the response to analgesia 1–2 hours after an oral dose. For chronic pain, schedule a review after 1–2 weeks to assess the need to step up or down the analgesic ladder, to assess side effects, and to consider the need for specialist referral.
Cost	Weak opioids are available in inexpensive non-proprietary forms, and some are available over the counter. Avoid using expensive branded products, such as modified-release tramadol, unless there is a clear reason to do so. For patients who pay for prescriptions it may be cheaper to buy them over the counter.

Clinical tip—Combining two analgesics with different mechanisms of action, such as paracetamol and codeine, may offer better pain control than can be achieved with either drug alone. Putting them together in a fixed-ratio compound product improves convenience for the patient, although at a cost of reduced flexibility in terms of dose titration. It is often preferable to use the drugs as separate products, at least initially. For example, you might prescribe codeine 15 mg tablets to be added to the patient's existing regimen of paracetamol 1 g 6-hrly. Under your guidance, the patient may then adjust the dose in the range 15–60 mg 6-hrly without having to obtain a new prescription each time. Having found the optimum balance between efficacy and side effects, it may *then* be appropriate to switch to the equivalent compound preparation.

Oxygen

CLINICAL PHARMACOLOGY

Common indications	❶ To increase tissue oxygen delivery in **acute hypoxaemia.** ❷ To accelerate reabsorption of pleural gas in **pneumothorax.** ❸ To reduce carboxyhaemoglobin half-life in **carbon monoxide (CO) poisoning.** *Long-term oxygen therapy* in patients with chronic hypoxaemia is outside the scope of this monograph.
Mechanisms of action	An abnormally low partial pressure of oxygen (PO_2) in arterial blood (PaO_2), termed *hypoxaemia*, may be a consequence of a wide range of disease processes. It reduces delivery of oxygen to tissues *(hypoxia)*, increasing their reliance on anaerobic metabolism for energy generation. Supplemental oxygen therapy increases the PO_2 in alveolar gas (P_AO_2), driving more rapid diffusion of oxygen into blood. The resultant increase in PaO_2 **increases delivery of oxygen to the tissues,** which in effect 'buys time' while the underlying disease is corrected. In *pneumothorax,* supplemental oxygen has an additional benefit of reducing the fraction of nitrogen in alveolar gas. This **accelerates the diffusion of nitrogen out of the body.** Since pleural air is composed mostly of nitrogen, this increases its rate of reabsorption. In *CO poisoning,* oxygen competes with CO to bind with haemoglobin and thereby **shortens the half-life of carboxyhaemoglobin,** returning haemoglobin to a form that can transport oxygen to tissues.
Important adverse effects	The most common adverse effects of oxygen are related to the delivery device (e.g. the **discomfort of a face mask**; nasal cannulae may be more comfortable) or its lack of water vapour (**dry throat**; humidification may improve this). Except in pneumothorax and CO poisoning, there is little to be gained from an *abnormally high* PaO_2 and, indeed, there is some evidence that **hyperoxaemia may be harmful**. For example, it has been observed that routine oxygen administration to *non-hypoxaemic* patients with stroke and myocardial infarction does not improve, and may worsen, outcomes. This may be because the vascular effects of hyperoxaemia.
Warnings	Patients with **chronic type 2 respiratory failure** (e.g. those with severe COPD) exhibit several adaptive changes in response to persistent hypoxaemia and hypercapnia. If exposed to high inspired oxygen concentrations, this finely balanced adaptive state may be disturbed, resulting in a rise in $PaCO_2$. This may lead to respiratory acidosis, depressed consciousness and worsened tissue hypoxia. This necessitates a different approach to oxygen therapy (see Prescription and Administration). Oxygen accelerates combustion and therefore presents a fire risk if exposed to a **heat source or naked flame,** including from smoking.
Important interactions	There are no clinically important interactions.

PRACTICAL PRESCRIBING

Prescription	Oxygen therapy should always be guided by a written prescription, except in emergencies when it may be administered first and prescribed later. The key feature of the oxygen prescription is the specification of a **target oxygen saturation range,** as measured by pulse oximetry (SpO_2). The target SpO_2 should be 94–98% in most patients and 88–92% in those with chronic type 2 respiratory failure. For the **initial delivery device,** in general, prescribe a reservoir ('non-rebreathing') mask in critical illness and patients with SpO_2 <85%; a Venturi mask (28%) for patients in chronic type 2 respiratory failure; and nasal cannulae for everyone else.
Administration	**Reservoir masks** have a bag (reservoir) that is continuously filled by the incoming oxygen supply. Inspired gas is drawn from the bag and so contains a high oxygen concentration (at least 60–80%). The oxygen flow rate should be 15 L/min. **Venturi masks** blend oxygen with air in a fixed ratio. The oxygen concentration is defined by the characteristics of the device. It is identified by a colour-coding system and written information on the device. This will also specify the oxygen flow rate that, with entrained air, produces a total gas flow rate sufficient to maintain a fixed inspired oxygen concentration. **Nasal cannulae** deliver a variable oxygen concentration (roughly 24–50% at flow rates of 2–6 L/min). **Simple face masks** are also variable-performance devices; they have few advantages over nasal cannulae and are less comfortable.
Communication	Explain to patients that the face mask or nasal cannulae should generally be kept in place continuously. Face masks may briefly be removed to allow eating and drinking. Ask patients to report any discomfort, as it may be possible to improve this with a different device or the addition of humidification.
Monitoring	**Frequent SpO_2 monitoring** is essential in all patients receiving oxygen for acute illness. The device and/or flow rate should be adjusted as necessary to keep the SpO_2 within the target range. In addition, **arterial blood gas measurement** is essential in patients with critical illness; those with chronic type 2 respiratory failure or those at risk of hypercapnoea; and those with hypoxaemia that is unexpected, progressive, or disproportionate to their illness.
Cost	Cost is not a consideration when using oxygen at the bedside.

Clinical tip—Remember that the PaO_2 is only one determinant of the amount of oxygen reaching the tissues. The other determinants are cardiac output and haemoglobin concentration. Neglecting to correct these, if they are significantly abnormal, may render oxygen therapy worthless.

Paracetamol

CLINICAL PHARMACOLOGY

Common indications	❶ Paracetamol is a first-line analgesic for most forms of **acute and chronic pain.** The World Health Organization (WHO) pain ladder (originally designed to guide the treatment of cancer pain) uses regular paracetamol as the basis of treatment, with <u>weak/moderate</u> then <u>strong opioids</u> added incrementally until pain is controlled. ❷ Paracetamol is an antipyretic that can reduce **fever** and its associated symptoms (e.g. shivering).
Mechanisms of action	The mechanisms of action of paracetamol are **poorly understood.** Paracetamol is a **weak inhibitor of cyclo-oxygenase (COX)**, the enzyme involved in prostaglandin metabolism. In the brain, COX inhibition appears to increase the pain threshold and reduce prostaglandin E_2 (PGE_2) concentrations in the thermoregulatory region of the hypothalamus, controlling fever. Paracetamol has specificity for COX-2 (the isoform induced in inflammation) rather than COX-1 (the isoform involved in protecting the gastric mucosa and regulating renal blood flow and clotting). However, despite its COX-2 selectivity, paracetamol is a weak antiinflammatory, as its actions are inhibited in inflammatory lesions by the presence of peroxides. It is likely that other mechanisms, which have not been fully elucidated, contribute to the effects of paracetamol.
Important adverse effects	At treatment doses, paracetamol is very safe with **few side effects.** Lack of COX-1 inhibition means that it does not cause peptic ulceration or renal impairment or increase the risk of cardiovascular events (unlike <u>NSAIDs</u>). Its safety makes it a popular choice as a first-line analgesic. In **overdose,** paracetamol causes **liver failure.** Paracetamol is, in part, metabolised by cytochrome P450 (CYP) enzymes to a toxic metabolite (N-acetyl-p-benzoquinone imine, NAPQI), which is conjugated with glutathione before elimination. After overdose, this elimination pathway is saturated, and NAPQI accumulation causes hepatocellular necrosis. Hepatotoxicity can be prevented by treatment with the glutathione precursor <u>acetylcysteine</u>.
Warnings	Paracetamol dose should be reduced in people at increased risk of liver toxicity, either because of *increased NAPQI production* (e.g. in ▲**chronic excessive alcohol use,** inducing metabolising enzymes) or *reduced glutathione stores* (e.g. in ▲**malnutrition,** ▲**low body weight** (<50 kg) and ▲**severe hepatic impairment**). This is particularly important where paracetamol is given by IV infusion.
Important interactions	There are few clinically significant interactions between paracetamol and other drugs. **CYP inducers,** e.g. phenytoin and <u>carbamazepine,</u> increase the rate of NAPQI production and risk of liver toxicity **after paracetamol overdose.**

paracetamol

PRACTICAL PRESCRIBING

Prescription

Oral paracetamol is on the 'general sales list', which means that it can be purchased from any retail outlet, although it is also available on prescription. For patients unable to take drugs by mouth, paracetamol can be prescribed for **IV infusion** or **rectal** administration. By all routes, the **usual adult dose** is 0.5–1 g every 4–6 hours, maximum 4 g daily (see Warnings). Paracetamol can be prescribed for **regular** administration or to be taken only **as required,** depending on the nature of the pain. When prescribed 'as required' the maximum daily dose must always be stated.

Administration

Oral paracetamol is available as tablets, caplets, capsules, soluble tablets and oral suspension. **Intravenous paracetamol** solution may be infused neat over 15 minutes or diluted in 0.9% sodium chloride or 5% glucose solution before administration, depending on the product.

Communication

Explain to patients that you are prescribing paracetamol with the aim of reducing or relieving pain. Effects should be felt around half an hour after taking it. Where regular paracetamol is prescribed, explain the importance of taking it every 6 hours. Warn them not to exceed the recommended **maximum daily dose** because of the potential risk of liver poisoning. Advise patients that many medicines purchased from the chemist (e.g. **cold and flu preparations**) contain paracetamol. Warn them to check the label or ask the pharmacist before taking these with paracetamol.

Monitoring

Efficacy of paracetamol in pain control can be established by enquiry about symptoms or by using a pain score, e.g. a visual analogue scale. For acute pain, review response to analgesia 1–2 hours after an oral dose. For chronic pain, schedule a review to assess the need to step up or down the analgesic ladder. After **overdose,** blood tests including international normalised ratio, serum alanine aminotransferase activity and creatinine concentration, are required to establish efficacy of acetylcysteine treatment and determine the need for further treatment.

Cost

A single dose of **oral paracetamol** 1 g can cost as little as 2p. Advise patients purchasing paracetamol from a shop or pharmacist to ask for the cheapest brand. As **IV paracetamol** is around 60 times more expensive (£1.25 for 1 g plus infusion costs) than oral formulations, it should be reserved for patients unable to take medicines by mouth and administration should be switched from IV to oral as soon as possible.

Clinical tip—If you are writing up paracetamol on an inpatient chart, always check that it has not already been prescribed. For example, if you are prescribing paracetamol regularly, cross it off the 'as required' side. Look out for 'co-' drugs such as co-codamol or co-dydramol with 'hidden' paracetamol.

Penicillins

CLINICAL PHARMACOLOGY

Common indications	❶ Streptococcal infection, including **tonsillitis, pneumonia** (with a <u>macrolide</u> or <u>tetracycline</u>), **endocarditis** (usually with <u>gentamicin</u>) and **skin and soft tissue infections** (with <u>flucloxacillin</u>). ❷ Meningococcal infection, for example **meningitis, septicaemia.** ❸ Clostridial infection, for example **gas gangrene** (clostridial myonecrosis).
Spectrum of activity	Benzylpenicillin and phenoxymethylpenicillin have a relatively **narrow** antimicrobial spectrum, with activity against some Gram-positive organisms (e.g. streptococci, bacillus and some anaerobes [clostridia]) and Gram-negative cocci (e.g. *Neisseria meningitidis* and *N. gonorrhoeae*). They are not active against Gram-negative bacilli (rods).
Mechanisms of action	Penicillins inhibit the enzymes responsible for cross-linking peptidoglycans in bacterial cell walls. This **weakens cell walls,** preventing them from maintaining an osmotic gradient. Uncontrolled entry of water into bacteria causes **cell swelling, lysis and death.** Penicillins contain a **β-lactam ring,** which is responsible for their **bactericidal** activity. **Side chains** attached to the β-lactam ring can be modified to make semi-synthetic penicillins. The nature of the side chain determines the antimicrobial spectrum and other properties of the drug. Bacteria **resist** the actions of penicillins by making **β-lactamases,** enzymes which break the β-lactam ring. Other resistance mechanisms include limiting the intracellular concentration of the drug (by reduced bacterial permeability or increased extrusion) and changes in the target enzyme to prevent penicillin binding. As the antimicrobial spectrum of benzylpenicillin and phenoxymethylpenicillin is relatively narrow, they are often combined with other antibiotics (see Common indications).
Important adverse effects	Penicillin **allergy** affects 1–10% of people exposed to the drug. This usually presents as a **skin rash** 7–10 days after first exposure or 1–2 days after repeat exposure (subacute [delayed] IgG-mediated reaction). Less commonly (0.05% of patients), an immediate (minutes to hours) life-threatening IgE-mediated **anaphylactic reaction** occurs, with some or all of hypotension, bronchospasm, and orofacial, pharyngeal and laryngeal oedema. **Neurological toxicity** (including convulsions and coma) can occur with very high-dose therapy or accumulation due to severe renal impairment.
Warnings	Penicillin can generally be used safely in most clinical situations, although a dose reduction is required for patients with ▲**renal impairment.** The main contraindication to penicillins is a history of ✖**penicillin allergy.** Note that allergy to one type of penicillin implies allergy to all types as it is due to a reaction to the basic penicillin structure. Patients with immediate hypersensitivity to penicillins may also react to <u>cephalosporins</u> and other β-lactam antibiotics.
Important interactions	All penicillins reduce renal excretion of ▲<u>methotrexate</u>, increasing the risk of toxicity.

benzylpenicillin, phenoxymethylpenicillin

PRACTICAL PRESCRIBING

Prescription	*Benzylpenicillin* can be administered by injection (IV or IM) only, as hydrolysis by gastric acid prevents GI absorption. It is prescribed for the treatment of severe infections, usually at a high dose (e.g. 1.2 g 4–6-hrly). *Phenoxymethylpenicillin* ('penicillin V') is stable in the presence of gastric acid and so can be taken orally as tablets or in solution. As absorption is unpredictable and phenoxymethylpenicillin is less active than benzylpenicillin, it is not used for severe infections. Benzylpenicillin and phenoxymethylpenicillin have a short plasma half-life of 30–60 minutes due to rapid renal excretion, so need to be administered 4–6-hrly. The indication, review date and duration of treatment should be documented on all inpatient antibiotic prescriptions to aid antibiotic stewardship.
Administration	Intravenous benzylpenicillin can be given either as a slow injection or by infusion.
Communication	Explain to patients that the aim of treatment is to get rid of infection and improve symptoms. Before prescribing, always check with your patient personally or get collateral history to ensure that they do not have an **allergy** to any form of penicillin, cephalosporin or other β-lactam antibiotic. Warn them to seek medical advice if rash or other unexpected symptoms develop. If an allergy develops during treatment, give the patient written and verbal advice not to take this antibiotic class in the future and make sure that the reaction (including its nature) is clearly documented in the patient's medical records.
Monitoring	Check that infection resolves by resolution of symptoms, signs (e.g. pyrexia, lung crackles) and blood markers (e.g. falling C-reactive protein and white cell count) as appropriate.
Cost	Both benzylpenicillin and phenoxymethylpenicillin are inexpensive. Cost is not the main consideration when choosing between these preparations.

Clinical tip—Where antibiotics are required to treat a young person with a sore throat caused by an unknown organism, make sure you choose phenoxymethylpenicillin, not amoxicillin. If the sore throat is due to Epstein–Barr virus (glandular fever), amoxicillin treatment commonly causes a rash. Although this is not truly an allergic reaction, it may lead erroneously to a lifetime label of 'penicillin allergy' for that patient.

Penicillins, antipseudomonal

CLINICAL PHARMACOLOGY

Common indications	Antipseudomonal penicillins are reserved for **severe infections,** particularly where there is a **broad spectrum of potential pathogens**; **antibiotic resistance** is likely (e.g. hospital-acquired infection); or patients are **immunocompromised** (e.g. neutropenia). Clinical infections treated with these drugs include: ❶ **Lower respiratory tract infections.** ❷ **Urinary tract infections.** ❸ **Intraabdominal sepsis.** ❹ **Skin and soft tissue infections.**
Spectrum of activity	Antipseudomonal penicillins (e.g. piperacillin) have a **broad spectrum** of activity against a wide range of Gram-positive and Gram-negative bacteria (notably including *Pseudomonas* spp.) and anaerobes. They are formulated with a β-lactamase inhibitor (e.g. tazobactam), which confers antimicrobial **activity against β-lactamase-producing bacteria** (e.g. *Staphylococcus aureus*, Gram-negative anaerobes).
Mechanisms of action	Penicillins inhibit the enzymes responsible for cross-linking peptidoglycans in bacterial cell walls. This **weakens cell walls,** preventing them from maintaining an osmotic gradient. Uncontrolled entry of water into bacteria causes **cell swelling, lysis and death.** Penicillins contain a **β-lactam ring,** which is responsible for their **bactericidal** activity. **Side chains** attached to the β-lactam ring can be modified to make semi-synthetic penicillins. For piperacillin, the side chain of broad-spectrum penicillins has been converted to a form of urea. This longer side chain may improve affinity to penicillin-binding proteins, increasing the spectrum of antimicrobial activity.
Important adverse effects	**Gastrointestinal (GI) upset,** including nausea and diarrhoea, is common. Less frequently, **antibiotic-associated colitis** occurs. Broad-spectrum antibiotics kill normal GI flora, allowing overgrowth of toxin-producing *Clostridium difficile*. This debilitating colitis can be complicated by colonic perforation and/or death. Delayed or immediate **hypersensitivity** may occur (see Penicillins).
Warnings	Antipseudomonal penicillins should be used with caution in people at risk of ▲*C. difficile* **infection,** particularly those in hospital and the elderly. The main contraindication is a history of ✖**penicillin allergy.** Note that allergy to one type of penicillin implies allergy to all types, as it is due to a reaction to the basic penicillin structure. Patients with immediate hypersensitivity to penicillins may also react to cephalosporins and other β-lactam antibiotics. The dose of antipseudomonal penicillins should be reduced in patients with ▲**moderate/severe renal impairment.**
Important interactions	All penicillins reduce renal excretion of ▲methotrexate, increasing the risk of toxicity. Antipseudomonal penicillins can enhance the anticoagulant effect of warfarin by killing normal GI flora that synthesise vitamin K.

piperacillin with tazobactam (e.g. Tazocin®)

PRACTICAL PRESCRIBING

Prescription	Piperacillin is always given with tazobactam. It can be prescribed using the drugs' generic names (piperacillin–tazobactam) or by brand name (e.g. Tazocin®, although note that non-proprietary compound preparations are now available). Piperacillin–tazobactam can only be given by IV infusion. Thus if it is the only effective agent, the whole course (usually 5–14 days) must be given IV as no oral switch is possible. The usual dose is 4.5 g, containing 4 g of piperacillin and 500 mg of tazobactam, given every 6–8 hours. The indication, review date and duration of treatment should be documented on all inpatient antibiotic prescriptions to aid antibiotic stewardship.
Administration	Piperacillin with tazobactam is formulated as a powder to be reconstituted in 10 mL sterile water or 0.9% sodium chloride. This is diluted further in 50–150 mL of 0.9% sodium chloride or 5% glucose for IV infusion. The duration of infusion varies according to local protocols.
Communication	Explain to patients that the aim of treatment is to get rid of infection and improve symptoms. Before prescribing, always check with your patients personally or get a collateral history to ensure that they do not have an **allergy** to any form of penicillin or other β-lactam antibiotics. Warn them to seek medical advice if a rash or other unexpected symptoms develop. If an allergy develops during treatment, give the patient written and verbal advice not to take this antibiotic class in the future and make sure that the reaction (including its nature) is clearly documented in the patient's medical records.
Monitoring	Check that infection resolves by resolution of symptoms, signs (e.g. pyrexia, lung crackles) and blood markers (e.g. falling C-reactive protein and white cell count) as appropriate.
Cost	The cost of a single 4.5-g dose of piperacillin–tazobactam is currently around £15. This, combined with the costs of administration and inpatient stay, makes IV antibiotic treatment expensive. Use of an outpatient parenteral antimicrobial therapy (OPAT) service to administer treatment can reduce duration and costs of inpatient stay.

Clinical tip—Each dose of piperacillin–tazobactam contains about 11 mmol Na$^+$ and is infused in 50–150 mL fluid (which may contain more sodium). Take this into account when determining the need for supplementary fluid and electrolyte therapy, particularly in patients with heart failure.

Penicillins, broad-spectrum

CLINICAL PHARMACOLOGY

Common indications	❶ Amoxicillin is used to treat a range of **susceptible infections,** including uncomplicated community-acquired pneumonia, otitis media, sinusitis and urinary tract infections. ❷ In the treatment of **_Helicobacter pylori_-associated peptic ulcers,** amoxicillin may be given in combination with <u>clarithromycin</u> or <u>metronidazole</u> and a <u>proton pump inhibitor</u>. ❸ Co-amoxiclav is a common choice for **severe, resistant** and **hospital-acquired infections,** including respiratory tract infection, genitourinary and abdominal infections, cellulitis, and bone and joint infections. Amoxicillin is not generally used empirically (without microbiological evidence of bacterial sensitivity) in this context, because of the risk of bacterial resistance.
Spectrum of activity	A **broad spectrum** of activity against a wide range of Gram-positive and Gram-negative cocci and bacilli (rods). However, they are inactivated by bacterial penicillinases, and resistance is increasingly prevalent. Addition of the β-lactamase inhibitor clavulanic acid restores activity of the combination (co-amoxiclav) against many amoxicillin-resistant strains.
Mechanisms of action	Penicillins inhibit the enzymes responsible for cross-linking peptidoglycans in bacterial cell walls. This **weakens cell walls,** preventing them from maintaining an osmotic gradient. Uncontrolled entry of water into bacteria causes **cell swelling, lysis** and **death.** Penicillins contain a **β-lactam ring,** which is responsible for their **bactericidal** activity. Broad-spectrum penicillins are synthesised by addition of an amino group to the β-lactam ring side chains, broadening activity against aerobic Gram-negative bacteria.
Important adverse effects	**Gastrointestinal (GI) upset** such as nausea and diarrhoea is common. Less frequently, **antibiotic-associated colitis** occurs. Broad-spectrum antibiotics kill normal gut flora, allowing overgrowth of toxin-producing _Clostridium difficile_. This debilitating colitis can be complicated by colonic perforation and/or death. Penicillin **allergy,** affecting 1–10% people exposed, usually presents as a **skin rash** 7–10 days after first, or 1–2 days after repeat exposure (delayed IgG-mediated reaction). In ~0.05% of treated patients, an immediate (minutes to hours) life-threatening IgE-mediated **anaphylactic reaction** occurs. **Acute liver injury** (cholestatic **jaundice** or hepatitis) may develop during or shortly after co-amoxiclav treatment and is generally self-limiting if treatment is stopped.
Warnings	The main contraindication is ✖**history of allergy** to any penicillin. Broad-spectrum penicillins should be used with caution in people at risk of ▲**_C. difficile_ infection,** particularly those in hospital and the elderly, or those with a history of ▲**penicillin-associated liver injury**. Dose should be reduced in ▲**severe renal impairment** (risk of crystalluria).
Important interactions	Broad-spectrum penicillins can enhance the anticoagulant effect of <u>warfarin</u> by killing normal gut flora that synthesise vitamin K.

PRACTICAL PRESCRIBING

Prescription	For **severe infection,** *amoxicillin* is prescribed at a high dose (e.g. 1 g 8-hrly) for IV administration. Intravenous antibiotics should be switched to oral administration after 48 hours if clinically indicated and the patient is improving (e.g. resolution of pyrexia, tachycardia) and able to take oral medication. **Prompt IV-to-oral switch** reduces complications and costs of antibiotic treatment and facilitates early discharge. For **mild-to-moderate infection** (e.g. without systemic features) oral amoxicillin should be prescribed at a lower dose (e.g. 250–500 mg 8-hrly). Where *co-amoxiclav* is prescribed, the strength (e.g. co-amoxiclav 500/125) indicates the relative amounts of amoxicillin (e.g. 500 mg) and clavulanic acid (e.g. 125 mg) in the preparation (in practice the dose prescribed is often these numbers combined, e.g. 625 mg). The **indication**, **review date** and **duration** of treatment should be documented on all inpatient antibiotic prescriptions to aid antibiotic stewardship.
Administration	Amoxicillin and co-amoxiclav are available as capsules/tablets and oral suspensions. Co-amoxiclav suspension may cause superficial staining of the teeth. Intravenous preparations may be given by slow injection or infusion.
Communication	Explain to patients that the aim of treatment is to get rid of infection and improve symptoms. Before prescribing, always check with patients personally or get a collateral history to ensure that they do not have an **allergy** to any form of penicillin, cephalosporin or other β-lactam antibiotic. Warn them to seek medical advice if a rash or other unexpected symptoms develop. If an allergy develops during treatment, give the patient written and verbal advice not to take this antibiotic class in the future and make sure that the reaction (including its nature) is clearly documented in the patient's medical records.
Monitoring	Check that infection resolves by resolution of symptoms, signs (e.g. pyrexia, lung crackles, dysuria) and blood markers (e.g. falling C-reactive protein and white cell count) as appropriate.
Cost	When prescribing *co-amoxiclav*, use this non-proprietary name rather than the brand name, allowing dispensing of the cheapest preparation. Generic prescribing also facilitates awareness of co-amoxiclav as a penicillin, reducing the risk of it being prescribed accidentally to a patient with penicillin allergy.

Clinical tip—Broad-spectrum antibiotics can usefully cover a wide range of organisms where the cause of infection is unknown. However, their disadvantages include generation of bacterial resistance and antibiotic-associated infections, such as *C. difficile* colitis. Avoiding unnecessary use of broad-spectrum antibiotics is a key aim of antimicrobial stewardship. You can contribute to this by following **local guidelines** to use the narrowest-spectrum antibiotic possible for the empirical treatment of infection and by using **microbiological test results** as soon as available to guide the change of antibiotics from a broader to a narrower spectrum.

Penicillins, penicillinase-resistant

CLINICAL PHARMACOLOGY

Common indications	Staphylococcal infection, usually as part of combination therapy, including: ❶ **Skin and soft tissue infections** such as cellulitis. ❷ **Osteomyelitis** and **septic arthritis.** ❸ Other infections, including **endocarditis.**
Spectrum of activity	Penicillinase-resistant penicillins have a **narrow spectrum** of activity against Gram-positive staphylococci.
Mechanisms of action	Penicillins inhibit the enzymes responsible for cross-linking peptidoglycans in bacterial cell walls. This **weakens cell walls,** preventing them from maintaining an osmotic gradient. Uncontrolled entry of water into bacteria causes **cell swelling, lysis** and **death.** Penicillins contain a **β-lactam ring,** which is responsible for their **bactericidal** activity. **Side chains** attached to the β-lactam ring can be modified to make semi-synthetic penicillins. The nature of the side chain determines the antimicrobial spectrum and other properties of the drug. For flucloxacillin, an acyl side chain protects the β-lactam ring from β-lactamases, which are enzymes made by bacteria to deactivate penicillin. This makes flucloxacillin **effective against β-lactamase-producing staphylococci.** Meticillin-resistant *Staphylococcus aureus* (MRSA) resists the actions of flucloxacillin by reducing penicillin-binding affinity. As penicillinase-resistant penicillins are active against staphylococci only, they are often combined with other antibiotics, particularly where the infecting organism has not been identified or infection is severe, e.g. with benzylpenicillin for severe cellulitis.
Important adverse effects	Minor **GI upset** is common. Penicillin **allergy** affects 1–10% of people exposed to the drug. This usually presents as a **skin rash** 7–10 days after first exposure or 1–2 days after repeat exposure (delayed IgG-mediated reaction). Less commonly (0.05% of patients), an immediate (minutes to hours) life-threatening IgE-mediated **anaphylactic reaction** occurs, with some or all of hypotension, bronchospasm, and orofacial, pharyngeal and laryngeal oedema. **Liver toxicity,** including cholestasis and hepatitis, is a rare but serious adverse effect which can occur even up to 2 months after treatment has been completed.
Warnings	Flucloxacillin can generally be used safely, although a dose reduction is required for patients with ▲**renal failure.** The main contraindication to flucloxacillin use is a ✖**history of penicillin allergy.** Note that allergy to one type of penicillin implies allergy to all types, as it is due to a reaction to the basic penicillin structure. Flucloxacillin is contraindicated in patients with ✖**prior flucloxacillin-related hepatotoxicity** and should be used with caution in patients with ▲**hepatic impairment.**
Important interactions	Penicillins reduce renal excretion of ▲methotrexate, increasing the risk of toxicity.

PRACTICAL PRESCRIBING

Prescription	Flucloxacillin is prescribed at high dose (e.g. 1–2 g 6-hrly) for IV administration for severe infection (e.g. where patients are systemically unwell). A prolonged course (e.g. 6 weeks) of high-dose IV flucloxacillin may be required for deep-seated infections such as osteomyelitis or endocarditis. Patients with less severe infection (such as cellulitis without systemic illness) can be treated with flucloxacillin orally at a lower dose, e.g. 250–500 mg. Flucloxacillin has a short plasma half-life of 45–60 minutes due to rapid renal excretion, so needs to be administered 6-hrly. The indication, review date and duration of treatment should be documented on all inpatient antibiotic prescriptions to aid antibiotic stewardship.
Administration	Intravenous flucloxacillin can be given either by slow injection or infusion. Oral flucloxacillin is available as capsules or as oral solutions (elixir or syrup) for infants and those with difficulty swallowing.
Communication	Explain to patients that the aim of treatment is to get rid of infection and improve symptoms. Before prescribing, always check with your patient personally or get collateral history to ensure that they do not have an **allergy** to any form of penicillin, cephalosporin or other β-lactam antibiotic. Warn them to seek medical advice if a rash or other unexpected symptoms develop. If an allergy develops during treatment, give the patient written and verbal advice not to take this antibiotic class in the future and make sure that the reaction (including its nature) is clearly documented in the patient's medical records.
Monitoring	Check that infection resolves by resolution of symptoms, signs (e.g. pyrexia, erythema of cellulitis) and blood markers (e.g. falling C-reactive protein and white cell count) as appropriate.
Cost	Flucloxacillin is inexpensive in oral and IV forms.

Clinical tip—Many patients will say they are 'allergic' to penicillin. Check this is a true hypersensitivity, with features of skin rash, bronchospasm or anaphylaxis, rather than a dose-related side effect such as severe vomiting. A ✖**prior anaphylactic reaction** to any penicillin is an **absolute contraindication** to prescription of any penicillin or other β-lactam antibiotic, whereas you can prescribe these antibiotics to intolerant patients (perhaps with an antiemetic) where there is a strong indication.

Phosphodiesterase (type 5) inhibitors

CLINICAL PHARMACOLOGY

Common indications	❶ Erectile dysfunction. ❷ Primary pulmonary hypertension.
Mechanisms of action	Sildenafil is a phosphodiesterase (PDE) inhibitor. It is **selective for PDE type 5 (PDE-5)** that is found predominantly in the smooth muscle of the corpus cavernosum of the penis and arteries of the lung. For an erection to occur, sexual stimulation is required. This releases nitric oxide (NO), which stimulates cyclic guanosine monophosphate (cGMP) production, causing arterial smooth muscle relaxation, vasodilatation and penile engorgement. As PDE-5 is responsible for the breakdown of cGMP, inhibition of this enzyme by **sildenafil increases cGMP concentrations, improving penile blood flow** and **erection quality.** Sildenafil does not cause an erection without sexual stimulation. In the pulmonary vasculature, sildenafil causes arterial vasodilatation by similar mechanisms and so is used to treat **primary pulmonary hypertension.**
Important adverse effects	Most of the adverse effects of sildenafil relate to its actions as a vasodilator. These include **flushing, headache, dizziness** and **nasal congestion.** More seriously, **hypotension, tachycardia** and **palpitations** can occur and there is a small associated risk of **vascular events** (e.g. myocardial infarction, stroke). If the erection fails to subside for a prolonged period despite absence of stimulation (**priapism**), urgent medical assistance is required to prevent penile damage. **Visual disorders** including colour distortion are due to inhibition of PDE-6 in the retina and should prompt urgent medical review.
Warnings	You should not prescribe sildenafil for patients in whom vasodilatation could be dangerous, including those with recent ✖**stroke** or ✖**acute coronary syndrome** or with a significant history of ✖**cardiovascular disease**. Sildenafil should be avoided or used at a lower dose in people with severe ▲**hepatic** or ▲**renal impairment** in whom sildenafil metabolism and excretion is reduced.
Important interactions	Do not prescribe sildenafil for people taking any drug that increases nitric oxide concentration, particularly ✖nitrates or ✖nicorandil, as their combined effects on cGMP (see Mechanisms of action) can cause marked arterial vasodilatation and cardiovascular collapse. Prescribe sildenafil with caution in patients taking other ▲**vasodilators,** including α-blockers (should not be taken within 4 hours of sildenafil) and calcium channel blockers, as there is an increased risk of hypotension. Plasma concentrations and adverse effects of sildenafil are increased by ▲**cytochrome P450 inhibitors,** e.g. amiodarone, diltiazem and fluconazole.

PRACTICAL PRESCRIBING

Prescription	**Erectile dysfunction**: the usual starting dose is 50 mg orally, taken as required before sex with a maximum of one dose per day. Non-proprietary (generic) preparations are available and should be prescribed in preference to branded products (e.g. Viagra®). **Pulmonary hypertension:** Treatment should only be started by a specialist. Non-proprietary sildenafil is used for this indication in doses from 25 to 100 mg three times daily, although this is an unlicensed use. **Revatio®** is the only licensed PDE-5 inhibitor for pulmonary hypertension, at a dose of 20 mg three times daily. The reason for this slight peculiarity in licensing arrangements is that the patent for Viagra®, the first PDE-5 inhibitor, has expired, whereas the patent for Revatio® has not. Viagra® was never licensed for the treatment of pulmonary hypertension. It is used for this indication because of the cost saving (see Cost).
Administration	Absorption of oral sildenafil and onset of effect will be delayed if it is taken with food.
Communication	For the treatment of erectile dysfunction, explain to men that you are prescribing a drug that will help them to have and maintain an erection, but that the **drug will not produce an erection without sexual stimulation.** Advise the patient that sildenafil should be **taken an hour before sex** to allow sufficient time for absorption. Warn them to seek medical advice if the erection does not subside within 2 hours after sexual activity has finished. They should also report any eyesight changes.
Monitoring	You should review the patient to enquire about therapeutic efficacy and side effects. Patients with pulmonary hypertension should have regular monitoring with a specialist.
Cost	Generic PDE-5 inhibitors have brought down the cost of treatment considerably. They can now be prescribed for any indication for erectile dysfunction (previously they could only be prescribed within the NHS where the problem was secondary to chronic disease or trauma). For pulmonary hypertension, the approximate annual cost of treatment with Revatio® is £5400, compared to £270 with generic sildenafil.

Clinical tip—Some people take the recreational drug amyl nitrate ('poppers') as an aphrodisiac. Warn them not to take this while they are on sildenafil as the combination may cause them to collapse.

Prostaglandin analogue eye drops

CLINICAL PHARMACOLOGY

Common indications	First-line agents to lower intraocular pressure in **open-angle glaucoma** and **ocular hypertension.** Prostaglandin analogues are generally preferred over topical β-blockers (the main alternative class) as they cause fewer systemic side effects.
Mechanisms of action	**Glaucoma** is characterised by progressive optic nerve damage associated with visual field loss and eventually blindness. It is usually associated with elevated intraocular pressure (**ocular hypertension**), and lowering intraocular pressure reduces glaucoma progression. Analogues of prostaglandin $F_{2\alpha}$ reduce intraocular pressure by increasing outflow of aqueous humour via the uveoscleral pathway. The exact mechanism for this is uncertain.
Important adverse effects	Prostaglandin analogue eye drops have few systemic side effects. Locally in the eye they may cause **blurred vision, conjunctival reddening (hyperaemia),** and **ocular irritation and pain.** They may also cause a **permanent change in eye colour** by increasing the amount of melanin in stromal melanocytes of the iris. This affects about one in three patients and is most noticeable when treatment is restricted to one eye.
Warnings	Caution is needed when contemplating prostaglandin analogue treatment in eyes in which the lens is absent (▲**aphakia**) or artificial (▲**pseudophakia**); and in patients with or at risk of ▲**iritis, uveitis or macular oedema.** In patients with **severe asthma** there is a theoretical risk of provoking bronchoconstriction, but in practice this does not seem to be a problem. It is certainly less of a concern than with topical β-blockers.
Important interactions	There are no clinically important adverse drug interactions with prostaglandin analogue eye drops.

latanoprost, bimatoprost

PRACTICAL PRESCRIBING

Prescription	The decision to offer pharmacological treatment in **ocular hypertension** is made by a specialist, taking into account the patient's age, intraocular pressure and central corneal thickness. All patients with confirmed **open-angle glaucoma** should be offered pharmacological treatment, again by a specialist. Usually this is with latanoprost 0.005% eye drop solution, 1 drop administered to the affected eye(s) once daily.
Administration	It is best to administer latanoprost eye drops in the evening. Contact lenses should be removed before instilling the drops. They may be reinserted 15 minutes later.
Communication	Explain to patients that the aim of treatment is to reduce the risk of sight loss. Advise patients how to administer the eye drops correctly. Warn them about the possibility of a change in eye colour. This advice may be tailored according to the patients' eye colour, since it is most likely in those with mixed-colour irides (i.e. brown plus another colour), and very rare in those with a homogenous eye colour ('pure' blue, grey, green, or brown). Explain that it is usually only slight and is not harmful, but if it occurs it is likely to be permanent.
Monitoring	Patients should be reviewed regularly by a clinician with expertise in glaucoma. The intensity of follow-up depends on intraocular pressure and risk of conversion to glaucoma.
Cost	The generic forms of latanoprost are substantially less expensive than the branded products.

Clinical tip—Advice that may be given for all eye drops is that the patient should gently compress the medial canthus (the nasal 'corner') of the eye for about 1 minute, immediately after instilling the drop. This reduces drainage through the lacrimal duct, lowering systemic absorption of the drug.

Proton pump inhibitors

CLINICAL PHARMACOLOGY

Common indications	❶ Prevention and treatment of peptic ulcer disease, including NSAID-associated ulcers. ❷ Symptomatic relief of dyspepsia and gastro-oesophageal reflux disease (GORD). ❸ Eradication of *Helicobacter pylori* infection, in which they are used in combination with antibiotic therapy.
Mechanisms of action	Proton pump inhibitors (PPIs) reduce gastric acid secretion. They act by **irreversibly inhibiting H^+/K^+-ATPase in gastric parietal cells.** This is the 'proton pump' responsible for secreting H^+ and generating gastric acid. An advantage of targeting the final stage of gastric acid production is that they suppress gastric acid production almost completely. In this respect they differ from H_2-receptor antagonists.
Important adverse effects	Common side effects of PPIs include **gastrointestinal disturbances** and **headache.** By increasing the gastric pH, PPIs may reduce the body's host defence against infection; there is some evidence of increased risk of *Clostridium difficile* infection in patients taking PPIs. Prolonged treatment with PPIs can cause **hypomagnesaemia,** which if severe can lead to tetany and ventricular arrhythmia.
Warnings	PPIs may **disguise symptoms of gastro-oesophageal cancer,** so prescribers should enquire about 'alarm symptoms' before and during treatment (see Communication). There is epidemiological evidence that PPIs, particularly when administered at high dose for prolonged courses in the elderly, can **increase the risk of fracture.** Patients at risk of ▲osteoporosis should therefore be identified and treated as appropriate.
Important interactions	There is some evidence that PPIs, particularly omeprazole, reduce the antiplatelet effect of ▲clopidogrel by decreasing its activation by cytochrome P450 enzymes. Understanding continues to evolve on this issue, but current evidence suggests that lansoprazole and pantoprazole have a lower propensity to interact with clopidogrel. As such, these are the preferred PPIs when prescribing alongside clopidogrel.

lansoprazole, omeprazole, pantoprazole

PRACTICAL PRESCRIBING

Prescription	Oral and injectable preparations are available. The dose of PPI depends on the drug and indication, and these are detailed in the BNF. Generally, the lowest effective dose should be used for the shortest period possible. The BNF provides a helpful table of recommended regimens for *H. pylori* eradication.
Administration	Oral preparations can be taken with food or on an empty stomach. They are best taken in the morning. Intravenous preparations should be given by slow injection or infusion.
Communication	Explain to patients that you are offering treatment to reduce stomach acid production. This will hopefully improve their symptoms and, if applicable, allow their ulcer to heal. Ensure that both you and the patient are clear on the intended duration of therapy (e.g. a 7-day course to eradicate *H. pylori,* or long-term therapy to protect against ulcers) and how success will be judged (e.g. evidence of healing on endoscopy, or simply by resolution of symptoms). Ask the patient to report any problems, particularly 'alarm' symptoms (e.g. weight loss, swallowing difficulty).
Monitoring	Response to treatment should be monitored in terms of symptomatic response and, in some cases (e.g. peptic ulcers), endoscopic appearance. In prolonged use (>1 year) you should check serum magnesium levels due to the risk of hypomagnesaemia.
Cost	Relatively inexpensive non-proprietary formulations are available and should be preferred in most cases.

Clinical tip—Patients undergoing investigation for *H. pylori* infection should ideally withhold their PPI for 2 weeks before testing. This is because it increases the chance of a false-negative result. This applies to all *H. pylori* tests.

Quinine

CLINICAL PHARMACOLOGY

Common indications	❶ Quinine is commonly used for the treatment and prevention of night-time **leg cramps,** but should really be reserved for cases when cramps regularly disrupt sleep and when non-pharmacological methods, such as passive stretching exercises, have failed. ❷ A first-line treatment option for ***Plasmodium falciparum* malaria.**
Mechanisms of action	**Leg cramps** are caused by sudden, painful involuntary contraction of skeletal muscle. Quinine is thought to act by reducing the excitability of the motor end plate in response to acetylcholine stimulation. This reduces the frequency of muscle contraction. In **malaria,** the mechanism of action of quinine is not well understood, but its overall effect leads to rapid killing of *Plasmodium falciparum* parasites in the schizont stage in the blood.
Important adverse effects	Although quinine is usually safe at recommended doses, it is potentially very toxic and can be fatal in overdose. It can cause **tinnitus, deafness** and **blindness** (which may be permanent), **gastrointestinal upset** and **hypersensitivity** reactions. Quinine **prolongs the QT interval,** and may therefore predispose to arrhythmias. **Hypoglycaemia** can occur and can be particularly problematic in patients with malaria, which also predisposes to hypoglycaemia.
Warnings	Quinine should be prescribed with caution in people with existing ▲**hearing or visual loss.** It is **teratogenic,** so should not be prescribed in the ▲**first trimester** of pregnancy, although in the case of malaria its benefit may outweigh this risk. Quinine should be avoided in people with ▲**glucose-6-phosphate dehydrogenase (G6PD) deficiency,** as it can precipitate haemolysis.
Important interactions	Quinine should be prescribed with caution in patients taking other ▲**drugs that prolong the QT interval** or cause arrhythmias such as amiodarone, antipsychotics, quinolones, macrolides and selective serotonin reuptake inhibitors.

PRACTICAL PRESCRIBING

Prescription	For nocturnal **leg cramps,** quinine should be prescribed for oral administration at a dose of 200–300 mg, to be taken at night. In the treatment of **malaria,** higher doses of quinine are required. It may be prescribed to be taken orally for uncomplicated cases (alongside another antimalarial medication such as <u>doxycycline</u>) or for IV administration in severe cases. Intravenous dosing should be based on the patient's weight.
Administration	Intravenous quinine should be given as a slow infusion.
Communication	For nocturnal **leg cramps,** explain to patients that you are recommending a 4-week trial of quinine in the hope of reducing the frequency of cramps. Explain that if there is no improvement after 4 weeks, they are unlikely to experience any benefit and should stop taking it. Ask the patient to report any adverse effects, such as hearing loss, visual disturbance and palpitations immediately, as quinine is potentially harmful to the ears, eyes and heart.
Monitoring	Review the patient's symptoms after 4 weeks and advise the patient to stop taking quinine if there has not been a significant improvement. If you decide to continue treatment, review the patient again at 3 months and consider a trial discontinuation at that stage. Aim to avoid long-term use due to the potential for serious adverse effects.
Cost	Quinine sulfate is available in non-proprietary formulations and is relatively inexpensive.

Clinical tip—Although quinine is commonly prescribed for people with nocturnal leg cramps, its benefit is relatively modest, reducing the frequency of cramps only by around 20%. Before starting treatment, you should first exclude reversible causes, such as electrolyte disturbances and drug causes (e.g. <u>statins</u>, β_2-<u>agonists</u>), and attempt non-pharmacological treatments such as passive stretching exercises. If you do decide to start treatment, review your patient after a month; if the patient has not experienced any significant benefit, discuss stopping treatment.

Quinolones

CLINICAL PHARMACOLOGY

Common indications	Quinolones are generally reserved as second or third-line treatment due to the potential for rapid emergence of resistance and an association with *Clostridium difficile* infection. With these caveats in mind, they are used in: ❶ **Urinary tract infection (UTI)** (mostly Gram-negative organisms). ❷ **Severe gastroenteritis** (e.g. due to *Shigella*, *Campylobacter*). ❸ **Lower respiratory tract infection (LRTI)** (Gram-positive and Gram-negative organisms; therefore moxifloxacin or levofloxacin preferred).
Spectrum of activity	Quinolones have a relatively **broad spectrum** of activity, particularly against Gram-negative bacteria. Ciprofloxacin is unusual among oral antibiotics in having significant activity against *Pseudomonas aeruginosa*. The newer quinolones, *moxifloxacin* and *levofloxacin*, have enhanced activity against Gram-positive organisms.
Mechanisms of action	Quinolones kill bacteria by **inhibiting DNA synthesis (bactericidal). Bacteria rapidly develop resistance** to quinolones. Some bacteria prevent intracellular accumulation of the drug by reducing permeability and/or increasing efflux. Others develop protective mutations in target enzymes. Quinolone resistance genes are spread horizontally between bacteria by plasmids, accelerating acquisition of resistance.
Important adverse effects	Quinolones are generally well tolerated although they can cause **GI upset** (including nausea and diarrhoea) and immediate and delayed **hypersensitivity** reactions (see Penicillins, broad spectrum). Class-specific adverse reactions include **neurological effects** (lowering of the seizure threshold and hallucinations), and inflammation and **rupture of muscle tendons.** Quinolones (particularly moxifloxacin) **prolong the QT interval** and therefore increase the risk of **arrhythmias.** Quinolones and cephalosporins are the broad-spectrum antibiotics most commonly associated with **C. difficile colitis**.
Warnings	Quinolones should be used with caution in people at heightened risk of adverse effects, including those with or at risk of ▲**seizures;** ▲**children** and young adults who are growing (potential risk of arthropathy); and with other risk factors for ▲**QT prolongation** (such as cardiac disease or electrolyte disturbance).
Important interactions	Drugs containing divalent cations (e.g. calcium, antacids) reduce absorption and efficacy of quinolones. Ciprofloxacin inhibits certain cytochrome P450 (CYP) enzymes, increasing risk of toxicity with some drugs, notably ▲**theophylline.** Co-prescription of ▲NSAIDs increases the risk of **seizures,** and of ▲prednisolone increases the risk of **tendon rupture.** Quinolones should be prescribed with caution in patients taking other ▲**drugs that prolong the QT interval** or cause arrhythmias, such as amiodarone, antipsychotics, quinine, macrolide antibiotics and SSRIs.

PRACTICAL PRESCRIBING

Prescription	Quinolones are rapidly and extensively absorbed in the intestine, so high plasma concentrations can be achieved by oral administration. Intravenous prescription should therefore usually be reserved for people unable to take drugs by mouth or absorb them in the intestine (also see Cost). They are eliminated by the kidney and have relatively long plasma half-lives, so are administered every 12–24 hours. Typical dosages are: *ciprofloxacin* 250–750 mg orally 12-hrly or 400 mg IV 12-hrly; *moxifloxacin* 400 mg oral/IV daily; and *levofloxacin* 500 mg oral/IV daily. Duration of therapy is determined by the type and severity of infection. The indication, review date and duration of treatment should be documented on all inpatient antibiotic prescriptions to aid antibiotic stewardship.
Administration	Oral quinolones are available as tablets, with ciprofloxacin also being formulated as a (more expensive) oral suspension. Intravenous quinolones come pre-prepared in solution for infusion over 60 minutes.
Communication	Explain to patients that the aim of treatment is to get rid of infection and improve symptoms. Before prescribing, always check with patients personally or get their collateral history to ensure they do not have an **allergy** to quinolones (any 'floxacin'). Warn them to seek medical advice if a rash or other unexpected symptoms develop. If an allergy develops during treatment, give the patient written and verbal advice not to take this antibiotic in the future and make sure that the allergy is clearly documented in the patient's medical records.
Monitoring	Check that infection resolves by resolution of symptoms, signs (e.g. pyrexia, lung crackles) and blood markers (e.g. falling C-reactive protein and white cell count) as appropriate.
Cost	Where IV quinolones are prescribed, switch to oral as soon as tolerated. Intravenous-to-oral switch is good practice as it reduces the cost of the drug (**oral quinolone preparations cost around 20 times less than IV quinolone preparations**), as well as reducing administration costs, treatment complications and duration of inpatient stay.

Clinical tip—Ciprofloxacin has good antibacterial activity against organisms causing severe traveller's diarrhoea, including *Shigella*, *Salmonella* and *Campylobacter*. You could ask your general practitioner for a pack to take on elective study trips to remote high-risk destinations! However, antibiotics should be reserved for severe infection (e.g. with systemic features), as use in milder infections will have little clinical benefit and may increase the risk of resistance.

Serotonin 5-HT₁-receptor agonists

CLINICAL PHARMACOLOGY

Common indications	In **acute migraine with or without aura,** serotonin 5-HT₁-receptor agonists, often referred to as 'triptans', are effective at reducing the duration and severity of headache symptoms.
Mechanisms of action	Serotonin 5-HT₁-receptor agonists relieve the symptoms of acute migraine. Although the exact mechanisms underlying migraines are not completely understood, dilatation of cranial blood vessels is thought to be important. Triptans **constrict cranial blood vessels** and **inhibit neurotransmission** in the peripheral trigeminal nerve and in the trigeminocervical complex.
Important adverse effects	Common adverse effects of triptans include **pain or discomfort in the chest and throat**, which can be intense but should resolve quickly. Rarely, **myocardial infarction** has been reported. Other common adverse effects include nausea and vomiting, tiredness, dizziness and transient high blood pressure.
Warnings	Due to their vasoconstrictor properties it is important that patients with ✖**coronary artery disease** (e.g. angina, myocardial infarction) and ✖**cerebrovascular disease** (e.g. stroke) do not take these drugs due to the risk of acute vascular events. Triptans should not be used in patients with ✖**hemiplegic or ✖basilar migraines**.
Important interactions	Triptans may increase the risk of **serotonin toxicity** and **serotonin syndrome** when given in combination with and other **serotonergic drugs**, such as ✖monoamine oxidase inhibitors, <u>tramadol</u>, <u>selective serotonin reuptake inhibitors</u> and <u>tricyclic antidepressants</u>.

PRACTICAL PRESCRIBING

Prescription	Serotonin 5-HT$_1$-receptor agonists are usually taken **orally**. The usual dose of sumatriptan for the treatment of migraine is 50–100 mg, repeated if the migraine recurs (but not if it failed to respond to the initial dose). **Intranasal** or **subcutaneous** formulations may be useful alternatives if vomiting precludes oral treatment.
Administration	Tablets should be swallowed whole with water. Patients using the nasal spray should be advised first to blow their nose if it is blocked. They should then insert the nozzle into a nostril, block the other nostril with their finger, then push the plunger as they breathe in through the nose.
Communication	Explain to patients that you are recommending a treatment they can use as needed to **reduce the severity** of their migraines. Explain that migraines can be caused by brief widening of blood vessels in the head and that the treatment acts to narrow the blood vessels and block the transmission of pain information to the brain. It should **shorten the duration and intensity** of the headache. Advise them to take the treatment **as soon as they feel the migraine coming on**, ideally within 6 hours of onset of a moderate-to-severe headache. Explain that it can be taken in combination with an antiinflammatory, like ibuprofen, and paracetamol. Explain the treatment only works when a migraine has started and **not to take it to prevent an attack**. Warn the patient of the **main side effects,** particularly that they may feel heaviness or pressure in the chest or throat but that this should pass quickly. However, if the pain does not pass quickly or is severe they should seek medical help as there is a **very small risk** they could have a **heart attack**. Encourage patients to return if they are having frequent migraines—4 or more attacks a month—as they may benefit from other treatments that prevent migraines from occurring in the first place.
Monitoring	Schedule a follow-up appointment for all patients taking triptans for the first time to check if the treatment is effective.
Cost	Triptans are available in non-proprietary form and are inexpensive. They can be issued by a qualified pharmacist without prescription.

Clinical tip—Triptans are an effective treatment in around two-thirds of patients, and if patients do not respond to one triptan they may still respond to another. However, if their headaches have not responded to several trials of different triptans, they are unlikely to be migrainous, and it is worth considering alternative diagnoses. Response to treatment with a triptan is supportive of the diagnosis of migraine, although it does not exclude other diagnoses.

Sex hormone antagonists for breast cancer

CLINICAL PHARMACOLOGY

Common indications	❶ **Early and locally advanced estrogen (oestrogen)-receptor positive (ER-positive) breast cancer,** as an adjuvant treatment option (e.g. after surgery) to reduce the risk of recurrent disease. ❷ **Advanced ER-positive positive breast cancer,** to slow disease progression. Hormonal therapy is given as a first-line treatment if the tumour does not express human epidermal growth factor receptor 2 (HER2-negative; because other options are available in HER2-positive disease). Aromatase inhibitors are used in post-menopausal women only. Tamoxifen is used in pre-menopausal women and in post-menopausal women who cannot take an aromatase inhibitor.
Mechanisms of action	Approximately two-thirds of breast cancers express oestrogen receptors (ER-positive). Oestrogen binds to these and stimulates cell proliferation. Sex hormone antagonists reduce tumour cell proliferation by **blocking the effects of oestrogen. Tamoxifen is a selective estrogen (oestrogen) receptor modulator** (SERM), which acts to prevent oestrogen binding to its receptor. **Aromatase inhibitors interfere with synthesis of oestrogens outside the ovary** (e.g. in fat and muscle) by inhibiting the enzyme (aromatase) that converts androgens to oestrogens. Aromatase inhibitors are superior to tamoxifen for ER-positive breast cancer in post-menopausal women, but ineffective in pre-menopausal women with functioning ovaries. This is because they have relatively **little effect on *ovarian* oestrogen synthesis**, which may even rise in response to aromatase inhibition. Antioestrogen therapies are ineffective if the tumour does not express oestrogen receptors.
Important adverse effects	The most common adverse effects of tamoxifen and aromatase inhibitors are symptoms of oestrogen depletion, including **vaginal dryness, hot flushes** and **loss of bone density**. Tamoxifen increases the risk of **venous thromboembolism** and **endometrial cancer**, so any unusual vaginal discharge or menstrual irregularity must be investigated. Other side effects include gastrointestinal upset and headache. Rarely, tamoxifen and aromatase inhibitors can cause **agranulocytosis** and **liver failure**.
Warnings	Tamoxifen may increase the risk of miscarriage and is contraindicated in **✖pregnancy,** and is secreted in breast milk so should be avoided in **✖lactation**. Aromatase inhibitors should not be used in **✖pre-menopausal women** unless ovarian function is suppressed or ablated (e.g. by oophorectomy).
Important interactions	Tamoxifen inhibits a cytochrome P450 enzyme (CYP2C9) responsible for metabolising **✖warfarin**, increasing the risk of bleeding. The SSRIs **✖fluoxetine** and **✖paroxetine** inhibit hepatic activation of tamoxifen. Aromatase inhibitors do not have clinically important drug interactions.

PRACTICAL PRESCRIBING

Prescription	Tamoxifen and aromatase inhibitors are taken orally. The usual dose for tamoxifen is 20 mg daily. The usual dose for anastrozole is 1 mg daily.
Administration	Tamoxifen and aromatase inhibitors are formulated as tablets to be taken with water. It does not matter if they are taken with or without food.
Communication	Explain to patients that hormone treatment is a **long-term treatment.** Depending on the clinical context, explain that it is intended to **reduce the risk of recurrence** or **slow the growth of the tumour**, and that most people take it for 5 years. Explain it works by blocking the effects of oestrogen (tamoxifen) or reducing the amount of oestrogen in the body (aromatase inhibitors). This prevents oestrogen from signalling the cancer cells to multiply. Warn patients that, because it blocks the effects of oestrogen, **side effects** include hot flushes, tiredness and vaginal symptoms (e.g. dryness, itching). For tamoxifen, explain that it can rarely cause **cancer of the lining of the womb** and they should report symptoms such as **vaginal bleeding** promptly. Explain that tamoxifen can also increase the **risk of blood clots** in the leg and lungs (deep vein thrombosis and pulmonary embolism) and advise them to contact their doctor immediately if they develop symptoms such as leg swelling or breathlessness. Patients should be advised that tamoxifen **can harm a baby in the womb**. Therefore women taking tamoxifen should **avoid becoming pregnant;** men with breast cancer should **avoid fathering a child** whilst taking tamoxifen. They should use barrier protection or non-hormonal contraceptives.
Monitoring	**Monitoring for disease recurrence or progression** should be guided by the multidisciplinary oncology team. Both tamoxifen and aromatase inhibitors can cause changes in liver enzymes and bone marrow suppression, so you should **check liver enzymes and obtain a full blood count** before starting treatment and repeat these if there is clinical suspicion of toxicity.
Cost	Tamoxifen and aromatase inhibitors are available in non-proprietary forms and are inexpensive.

Clinical tip—The combination of warfarin and tamoxifen should be avoided due to a significant drug interaction that increases the risk of bleeding. Interactions are common in cancer therapy, and this is one of the reasons that when anticoagulation is required in patients with cancer, a low molecular weight heparin is preferable, and perhaps superior, to warfarin.

Statins

CLINICAL PHARMACOLOGY

Common indications	❶ **Primary prevention of cardiovascular events:** to prevent cardiovascular events (e.g. myocardial infarction, stroke) in people over 40 years of age with a 10-year cardiovascular risk >10%, as assessed using the QRISK®2 tool. ❷ **Secondary prevention of cardiovascular events:** first line alongside lifestyle changes, to prevent events in patients with established cardiovascular disease. ❸ **Primary hyperlipidaemia:** first line, in conditions such as primary hypercholesterolaemia, mixed dyslipidaemia and familial hypercholesterolaemia.
Mechanisms of action	Statins reduce serum cholesterol levels. They **inhibit 3-hydroxy-3-methyl-glutaryl coenzyme A (HMG CoA) reductase,** an enzyme involved in making cholesterol. They decrease cholesterol production by the liver and increase clearance of low density lipoprotein (LDL)-cholesterol from the blood, reducing LDL-cholesterol levels. They also indirectly reduce triglycerides and slightly increase high density lipoprotein (HDL)-cholesterol levels. Through these effects they slow the atherosclerotic process and may even reverse it.
Important adverse effects	Statins are generally safe and well tolerated. The most common adverse effects are **headache** and **gastrointestinal disturbances.** Potentially more serious are their effects on muscle. These can range from simple **aches** to more serious **myopathy** or, rarely, **rhabdomyolysis.** They can also cause a **rise in liver enzymes** (e.g. alanine transaminase [ALT]); drug-induced hepatitis is a rare but serious adverse effect.
Warnings	Statins should be used with caution in patients with existing ▲**hepatic impairment.** They are excreted by the kidneys, so the dose should be reduced in people with ▲**renal impairment.** You should avoid prescribing statins to women who are ▲**pregnant** (cholesterol is essential for normal fetal development) or ▲**breastfeeding.**
Important interactions	The metabolism of statins is reduced by ▲**cytochrome P450 inhibitors,** such as <u>amiodarone</u>, <u>diltiazem</u>, <u>itraconazole</u>, <u>macrolides</u> and protease inhibitors. This leads to accumulation of the statin in the body, which may put patients at increased risk of adverse effects. ▲<u>Amlodipine</u> has a similar interaction, although the mechanism is less clear. To reduce this risk you may need to reduce the dose of the statin or, if the other drug is being used for a short period only (e.g. a course of clarithromycin therapy), withhold the statin.

simvastatin, atorvastatin, pravastatin, rosuvastatin

PRACTICAL PRESCRIBING

Prescription	Statins are prescribed for oral administration. A typical starting dose in primary prevention is simvastatin 40 mg daily or atorvastatin 20 mg daily. Higher doses may be used for secondary prevention.
Administration	Simvastatin, which has a short half-life, is traditionally taken in the **evening,** because cholesterol synthesis is greatest in the early-morning hours. This is not necessary for other statins that have a longer half-life.
Communication	Explain to patients that you are prescribing a medicine to lower cholesterol levels to reduce the risk of a heart attack or stroke in the future. Advise patients of common side effects, and to seek medical attention if they experience **muscle symptoms** (e.g. pain or weakness). Ask your patients to come back for **blood tests** in 3 and 12 months. Advise them to keep alcohol intake to a minimum. Those taking simvastatin or atorvastatin should **avoid grapefruit juice,** which reduces the body's ability breakdown the statin and may therefore increase the risk of side effects. This is not the case for pravastatin and rosuvastatin.
Monitoring	In **primary prevention** of cardiovascular disease, you should check a lipid profile before treatment and 3 months after initiating treatment, aiming for a 40% reduction in non-HDL cholesterol levels. In **secondary prevention,** a baseline lipid profile is informative but not essential if the patient has established cardiovascular disease, but **efficacy** should be monitored by checking target cholesterol levels are achieved, as specified in guidelines. If reductions in cholesterol are not achieved, you could consider increasing the dose, switching to an alternative statin or a different class of lipid-lowering agent. For **safety,** check liver enzymes (e.g. ALT) at baseline and again at 3 and 12 months. A rise in ALT up to three times the upper limit of normal may be acceptable but above this should lead to discontinuation. The statin can be restarted at a lower dose when liver enzymes have returned to normal. You do not need to check creatine kinase routinely, but you should ask patients to report muscle symptoms.
Cost	Statins that are available in non-proprietary form (e.g. simvastatin, atorvastatin) are inexpensive, and should be preferred over branded products.

Clinical tip—Do not forget to check the patient's thyroid status (by checking serum thyroid stimulating hormone [TSH] if there is any clinical uncertainty) before starting a statin. Hypothyroidism is a reversible cause of hyperlipidaemia, and should therefore be corrected before reassessing the need for lipid-lowering medications. Furthermore, hypothyroidism increases the risk of myositis with statins.

Sulphonylureas

CLINICAL PHARMACOLOGY

Common indications	In **type 2 diabetes:** ❶ In *combination* with metformin (and/or other hypoglycaemic agents) where blood glucose is not adequately controlled on a single agent. ❷ As a *single agent* to control blood glucose and reduce complications where <u>metformin</u> is contraindicated or not tolerated.
Mechanisms of action	Sulphonylureas lower blood glucose by **stimulating pancreatic insulin secretion.** They block ATP-dependent K^+ channels in pancreatic β-cell membranes, causing depolarisation of the cell membrane and opening of voltage-gated Ca^{2+} channels. This increases intracellular Ca^{2+} concentrations, stimulating insulin secretion. Sulphonylureas are effective only in patients with residual pancreatic function. As insulin is an anabolic hormone, stimulation of insulin secretion by sulphonylureas is associated with weight gain. Weight gain increases insulin resistance and can worsen diabetes mellitus in the long term.
Important adverse effects	Dose-related side effects such as **GI upset** (nausea, vomiting, diarrhoea, constipation) are usually mild and infrequent. **Hypoglycaemia** is a potentially serious adverse effect, which is more likely with high treatment doses, where drug metabolism is reduced (see Warnings) or where other hypoglycaemic medications are prescribed (see Important interactions). Sulphonylurea-induced hypoglycaemia may last for many hours and, if severe, should be managed in hospital. **Rare hypersensitivity reactions** include hepatic toxicity (e.g. cholestatic jaundice), drug hypersensitivity syndrome (rash, fever, internal organ involvement) and haematological abnormalities (e.g. agranulocytosis).
Warnings	Gliclazide is metabolised in the liver and has a plasma half-life of 10–12 hours. Unchanged drug and metabolites are excreted in the urine. A dose reduction may therefore be required in patients with ▲**hepatic impairment** and blood glucose should be monitored carefully in patients with ▲**renal impairment.** Sulphonylureas should be prescribed with caution for people at ▲**increased risk of hypoglycaemia,** including those with hepatic impairment (reduced gluconeogenesis), malnutrition, adrenal or pituitary insufficiency (lack of counter-regulatory hormones) and the elderly.
Important interactions	Risk of hypoglycaemia is increased by co-prescription of other antidiabetic drugs, including <u>metformin</u>, <u>DPP-4 inhibitors</u> (e.g. sitagliptin), thiazolidinediones (e.g. pioglitazone) and <u>insulin</u>, and by alcohol. β-blockers may mask symptoms of hypoglycaemia. The efficacy of sulphonylureas is reduced by drugs that elevate blood glucose, e.g. <u>prednisolone</u>, <u>thiazide</u> and <u>loop diuretics</u>.

PRACTICAL PRESCRIBING

Prescription	There are several sulphonylureas to choose from. Those with a shorter duration of action and hepatic metabolism (e.g. gliclazide) are the easiest to use, particularly in elderly patients with impaired renal function. Gliclazide (standard release) is usually started at a dosage of 40–80 mg once daily. The dose is increased gradually until blood glucose is controlled, with higher doses (160–320 mg daily) being given as two divided doses. Gliclazide is also available as a modified release (MR) form. Note that gliclazide 30-mg MR tablets have an equivalent glucose-lowering effect to 80-mg standard-release tablets. It is important to prescribe these carefully to avoid dosing errors.
Administration	Sulphonylureas should be taken with meals (e.g. once daily at breakfast or twice daily at breakfast and evening meal).
Communication	Advise patients that a sulphonylurea has been prescribed as a long-term treatment to control blood sugar and reduce the risk of diabetic complications, such as kidney disease. Explain that tablets are not a replacement for **lifestyle measures** and should be taken in addition to a healthy diet and regular exercise. Warn them about **hypoglycaemia,** advising them to watch out for symptoms, such as dizziness, nausea, sweating and confusion. If hypoglycaemia develops, they should take something sugary (e.g. glucose tablets or a sugary drink), then something starchy (e.g. a sandwich), and seek medical advice if symptoms recur.
Monitoring	Assess blood glucose control by measuring **haemoglobin A_{1c} (HbA$_{1c}$)**. In treating type 2 diabetes with a single agent, the **target** HbA$_{1c}$ is usually <48 mmol/mol. Treatment is **intensified** by addition of a second agent if the HbA$_{1c}$ is >58 mmol/mol, and a new target of <53 mmol/mol is then set (balancing the risks of hyperglycaemia against the risks of treatment, particularly hypoglycaemia). Home capillary blood glucose monitoring is not routinely required, although measurement may be helpful to determine if any unusual symptoms are due to hypoglycaemia. Measurement of renal and hepatic function before treatment can determine the need for caution or identify contraindications to treatment.
Cost	Non-proprietary gliclazide 80 mg tablets are inexpensive, and considerably cheaper than newer antidiabetic drugs, e.g. DPP-4 inhibitors.

Clinical tip—During acute illness, insulin resistance increases and renal and hepatic function may become impaired. All oral hypoglycaemics become less effective at controlling blood glucose and side effects are more likely, e.g. hypoglycaemia with sulphonylureas. In hospital inpatients, insulin treatment may be required temporarily during severe illness. Insulin has a short half-life and its dosage can be adjusted more easily than can oral medication in response to acute fluctuations in blood glucose.

Tetracyclines

CLINICAL PHARMACOLOGY

Common indications	❶ **Acne vulgaris,** particularly where there are inflamed papules, pustules and/or cysts (*Propionibacterium acnes*). ❷ **Lower respiratory tract infections,** including **infective exacerbations of COPD** (e.g. *Haemophilus influenzae*), **pneumonia** and **atypical pneumonia** (mycoplasma, *Chlamydia psittaci, Coxiella burnetii* [Q fever]). ❸ Chlamydial infection, including **pelvic inflammatory disease.** ❹ Other infections, such as typhoid, anthrax, malaria and Lyme disease (*Borrelia burgdorferi*).
Spectrum of activity	Tetracyclines have a relatively **broad spectrum** of activity against many Gram-positive and Gram-negative organisms, including chlamydia, mycoplasma and spirochaetes. However, their utility may be limited by increasing bacterial resistance.
Mechanisms of action	Tetracyclines **inhibit bacterial protein synthesis.** They bind to the ribosomal 30S subunit found specifically in bacteria. This prevents binding of transfer RNA to messenger RNA, which prevents addition of new amino acids to growing polypeptide chains. Inhibition of protein synthesis is **bacteriostatic** (stops bacterial growth), which assists the immune system in killing and removing bacteria from the body. Tetracyclines were discovered in 1945 and have been widely used. Consequently, bacteria are increasingly **resistant**. A common mechanism is an efflux pump, which allows bacteria to pump out tetracyclines, preventing cytoplasmic accumulation.
Important adverse effects	Like most antibiotics, tetracyclines commonly cause **nausea, vomiting** and **diarrhoea,** although with a lower risk of *Clostridium difficile* infection than other broad-spectrum antibiotics (see <u>Penicillins, broad-spectrum</u>). **Hypersensitivity reactions** occur in about 1%, including immediate and delayed reactions (see <u>Penicillins</u>). As antibiotic structures are different, there is no cross-reactivity with penicillins or other β-lactam antibiotics. Tetracycline-specific side effects include: **oesophageal** irritation, ulceration and dysphagia; **photosensitivity** (an exaggerated sunburn reaction when skin is exposed to light); and **discolouration** and/or hypoplasia of **tooth enamel** in children. Rare, but potentially serious, adverse effects include **hepatotoxicity** and **intracranial hypertension,** the latter causing headache and visual disturbance.
Warnings	Tetracyclines bind to teeth and bones during fetal development, infancy and early childhood and so should not be prescribed during ✘**pregnancy,** ✘**breastfeeding** or for ✘**children ≤12 years of age.** They should be used with caution in ▲**renal impairment** as their antianabolic effects can raise serum urea and reduced excretion can increase the risk of adverse effects.
Important interactions	Tetracyclines bind to divalent cations. They should therefore not be given within 2 hours of <u>calcium</u>, <u>antacids</u> or <u>iron</u>, which will prevent antibiotic absorption. Tetracyclines can enhance the anticoagulant effect of <u>warfarin</u> by killing normal gut bacteria that synthesise vitamin K.

PRACTICAL PRESCRIBING

Prescription	Tetracyclines are primarily available for oral administration. The dose and frequency of administration vary between individual drugs, e.g. *doxycycline* 200 mg on day 1, then 100–200 mg orally daily, *lymecycline* 408–816 mg orally 12-hrly. As with other antibiotics, higher doses are prescribed for more severe or difficult-to-treat infections. The duration of treatment depends on the indication: for example, 5–7 days in **infective exacerbations of COPD,** 8 weeks in **acne.**
Administration	Tetracyclines are usually formulated as capsules or tablets. These should be swallowed whole with plenty of water while sitting or standing to stop them getting stuck in the oesophagus where they may cause ulceration.
Communication	Explain to patients that the aim of treatment is to get rid of infection and improve symptoms. Before prescribing, always check with patients personally or get a collateral history to ensure they have no **allergy** to tetracyclines. Warn them to seek medical advice if a rash or other unexpected symptoms develop. If an allergy develops during treatment, give the patient written and verbal advice not to take this antibiotic in the future and make sure that the allergy is clearly documented in the patient's medical records. Advise patients to take the treatment **during a meal** with a full glass of water when sitting or standing. They should **avoid indigestion remedies** and medicines containing iron or zinc 2 hours before and after taking the antibiotic. During treatment they should **protect their skin from sunlight,** even on cloudy days.
Monitoring	Check that infection resolves by resolution of symptoms, signs (e.g. reduction in inflamed papules, pustules and cysts in acne) and blood markers (e.g. resolution of inflammatory markers in respiratory infection) as appropriate.
Cost	Tetracyclines are inexpensive. For example, a 1-week course of doxycycline 100 mg for respiratory infection costs around £1.

Clinical tip—Demeclocycline is a tetracycline notable for its ability to increase serum sodium concentrations in patients with **syndrome of inappropriate antidiuretic hormone (SIADH).** It appears to do this by blocking the binding of antidiuretic hormone (ADH) to its receptor, although the mechanism is poorly understood. Other non-antibiotic properties of tetracyclines, including antiinflammatory, immune-modulating and neuroprotective effects, are being tested in clinical trials and may lead to new therapeutic applications in the future.

Thyroid hormones

CLINICAL PHARMACOLOGY

Common indications	❶ Primary hypothyroidism. ❷ Hypothyroidism secondary to hypopituitarism.
Mechanisms of action	The thyroid gland produces thyroxine (T_4), which is converted to the more active triiodothyronine (T_3) in target tissues. Thyroid hormones **regulate metabolism and growth.** Deficiency of these hormones causes hypothyroidism, with clinical features including lethargy, weight gain, constipation and slowing of mental processes. Hypothyroidism is treated by long-term replacement of thyroid hormones, most usually as **levothyroxine** (synthetic T_4). **Liothyronine** (synthetic T_3) has a shorter half-life and quicker onset (a few hours) and offset (24–48 hours) than levothyroxine. It is therefore reserved for emergency treatment of severe or acute hypothyroidism.
Important adverse effects	The adverse effects of levothyroxine are usually due to excessive doses, so are predictably similar to symptoms of hyperthyroidism. These include **gastrointestinal** (e.g. diarrhoea, vomiting, weight loss), **cardiac** (e.g. palpitations, arrhythmias, angina) and **neurological** (e.g. tremor, restlessness, insomnia) manifestations.
Warnings	Thyroid hormones increase heart rate and metabolism. They can therefore precipitate cardiac ischaemia in people with ▲**coronary artery disease,** in whom replacement should be started cautiously at a low dose and with careful monitoring. In ▲**hypopituitarism,** corticosteroid therapy must be initiated before thyroid hormone replacement to avoid precipitating an Addisonian crisis.
Important interactions	As gastrointestinal absorption of levothyroxine is reduced by antacids, calcium and iron salts, administration of these drugs needs to be separated by about 4 hours. An increase in levothyroxine dose may be required in patients taking **cytochrome P450 inducers,** e.g. phenytoin, carbamazepine. Levothyroxine-induced changes in metabolism can increase insulin or oral hypoglycaemic requirements in diabetes mellitus and enhance the effects of warfarin.

PRACTICAL PRESCRIBING

Prescription	**Levothyroxine** is prescribed for oral administration. For thyroid hormone replacement, a starting dose of 50–100 micrograms daily is recommended, except in the elderly or people with cardiac disease, who should start on 25 micrograms daily. The dose is adjusted monthly in 25–50-microgram increments according to monitoring (see below) to a usual maintenance dose of 50–200 micrograms once daily. Remember to write 'micrograms' in full to reduce the risk of dosing errors. **Liothyronine** may be prescribed for IV administration in emergency care. It should be used only after consultation with senior and specialist colleagues.
Administration	Levothyroxine is available in 25-, 50- and 100-microgram tablets, so a combination is often required for adequate dosing (e.g. patients requiring 175 micrograms will need to take one of each strength daily).
Communication	Explain to patients that treatment will **replace a natural hormone** that their body has stopped making and that this will give them more energy and make them feel better. Advise them that it may take some time (months in some cases) for them to feel 'back to normal'. It is important to emphasise (for most people) that **treatment is for life** and that they should not stop taking it. **Warn them of the signs of too much treatment** (e.g. shakiness, anxiety, sleeplessness, diarrhoea) and advise them to see a doctor if these occur, as their treatment may need to be reduced. If they take **calcium or iron replacement,** advise them to leave a gap of about 4 hours between these treatments and levothyroxine.
Monitoring	The aim of therapy is to relieve symptoms and return the patient to a euthyroid state. Initially you should review your patient monthly and dose changes should be guided by symptoms. **Thyroid function tests** should be measured 3 months after starting treatment or a change in dose. In primary hypothyroidism, **thyroid stimulating hormone (TSH)** is the main guide to dosing. It is elevated due to loss of negative feedback of T_4 on the pituitary. With adequate levothyroxine replacement, TSH should return to normal or low-normal concentrations. Stable patients should have annual clinical review and thyroid function tests.
Cost	Non-proprietary levothyroxine treatment costs around £4 per month.

Clinical tip—Patients may experience *hyper*thyroid symptoms (see Important adverse effects) soon after they begin taking levothyroxine. If this happens, continue therapy at a lower dose (rather than stopping it) and arrange to review the patient over the next 1–2 weeks to look for the re-emergence of *hypo*thyroid symptoms. Thyroid function tests will be unhelpful in guiding therapy at this early stage as it is likely that both TSH and T_4 concentrations will be raised: TSH because the levels of this hormone take some time to normalise (weeks) and T_4 because of the levothyroxine therapy.

Trimethoprim

CLINICAL PHARMACOLOGY

Common indications	Trimethoprim is a first-choice antibiotic for the treatment of: ❶ **Acute lower urinary tract infection (UTI)**. ❷ Prophylaxis of **recurrent UTI.** Alternatives include <u>nitrofurantoin, amoxicillin</u> and <u>cefalexin</u>. It is also an option for the treatment of **acne, respiratory tract infections** and **prostatitis**. Co-trimoxazole is used for treatment and prevention of **pneumocystis pneumonia** in immunosuppression, e.g. HIV infection.
Spectrum of activity	Trimethoprim *ought* to have broad activity against many Gram-positive and Gram-negative bacteria (particularly enterobacteria, e.g. *Escherichia coli*), but is increasingly **limited by resistance**. Combination with a sulfonamide (e.g. sulfamethoxazole, as co-trimoxazole) **extends the spectrum** to include activity against the fungus *Pneumocystis jirovecii.*
Mechanisms of action	Bacteria are unable to use external sources of folate, so need to make their own for essential functions such as DNA synthesis. Trimethoprim **inhibits bacterial folate synthesis,** slowing bacterial growth (bacteriostasis). Its clinical utility is reduced by **widespread bacterial resistance.** Mechanisms of resistance include reduced intracellular antibiotic accumulation and reduced sensitivity of target enzymes. Sulfamethoxazole, a sulfonamide, also inhibits bacterial folate synthesis, but at a different step in the pathway. Given together, the drugs cause more complete inhibition of folate synthesis.
Important adverse effects	Trimethoprim most commonly causes **GI upset** (nausea, vomiting and sore mouth) and **skin rash** (3–7%). Severe **hypersensitivity** reactions, including anaphylaxis, drug fever and erythema multiforme, occur rarely with trimethoprim, but more commonly with sulfonamides, which limits their use. As a folate antagonist, trimethoprim can impair haematopoiesis, causing **haematological disorders** such as megaloblastic anaemia, leucopenia and thrombocytopenia. It can also cause **hyperkalaemia** and elevation of plasma creatinine concentrations.
Warnings	Trimethoprim is contraindicated in the ✖**first trimester of pregnancy,** because, as a folate antagonist, it is associated with an increased risk of fetal abnormalities (e.g. neural tube defects, cleft lip/palate). It should be used cautiously in people with ▲**folate deficiency,** who are more susceptible to adverse haematological effects. As trimethoprim is mostly excreted unchanged into urine, it is useful in the treatment of UTIs, but is less suitable in ▲**renal impairment;** if it is used, a dose reduction is necessary. ▲**Neonates,** the ▲**elderly** and people with ▲**HIV infection** are particularly susceptible to adverse effects.
Important interactions	Use with ▲**potassium-elevating drugs** (e.g. <u>aldosterone antagonists</u>, <u>ACE inhibitors</u>, <u>ARBs</u>) predisposes to hyperkalaemia. Use with other ▲**folate antagonists** (e.g. <u>methotrexate</u>) and ▲**drugs that increase folate metabolism** (e.g. phenytoin) increases the risk of adverse haematological effects. Trimethoprim can enhance the anticoagulant effect of warfarin by killing normal gut flora that synthesise vitamin K.

PRACTICAL PRESCRIBING

Prescription	*Trimethoprim* is prescribed for oral administration. For **treatment of acute UTI** the usual dosage is 200 mg 12-hrly, with duration of treatment being determined by severity of infection. As **prophylaxis for recurrent UTI,** it may be prescribed at a lower dose (100 mg) less often (once at night) for a prolonged period. *Co-trimoxazole* can be prescribed for oral or IV administration. A weight-based dosage (120 mg/kg per day, oral or IV, in 2–4 divided doses) is given for 14–21 days to treat **pneumocystis infection.** A lower dose (e.g. 960 mg orally 3 times a week) is used for pneumocystis prophylaxis.
Administration	Oral trimethoprim and co-trimoxazole are available as tablets and in suspension. Intravenous co-trimoxazole must be diluted immediately before use (to prevent crystallisation) in 125–500 mL <u>sodium chloride</u> 0.9% or <u>glucose</u> 5% and infused slowly over 60–90 minutes.
Communication	Explain to patients that the aim of treatment is to get rid of infection and improve symptoms. Where antibiotics are for **prophylaxis**, emphasise that this is a long-term medication, rather than a course that should stop. Before prescribing, always check with patients personally or get a collateral history to ensure that they have no **allergy** to trimethoprim or Septrin® (the brand name for co-trimoxazole). As allergic reactions are common with these antibiotics, it is particularly important to warn patients to seek medical advice if a rash or other unexpected symptoms develop. If an allergy develops during treatment, give the patient written and verbal advice not to take this antibiotic in the future and make sure that the allergy is clearly documented in the patient's medical records.
Monitoring	Check that **acute infection** resolves by resolution of symptoms (e.g. reduction in dysuria), signs (e.g. resolution of pyrexia) and investigations (e.g. fall in inflammatory markers, sterile urine on repeat culture in selected cases) as appropriate. For **long-term treatment,** full blood count monitoring may be useful for early detection and treatment of haematological disorders (e.g. by replacing folate and/or stopping the antibiotic).
Cost	Both trimethoprim and co-trimoxazole have been on the market for many years and, as tablets, are inexpensive. Costs are increased by prescribing oral antibiotic suspensions (five-fold).

Clinical tip—Trimethoprim competitively inhibits creatinine secretion by the renal tubules. This commonly leads to a **small reversible rise in serum creatinine concentration** during trimethoprim treatment, without reduction in the glomerular filtration rate. For this reason, trimethoprim tends to be less effective for UTI in patients with renal impairment, as the increased serum concentration of creatinine completes with trimethoprim for secretion into the urinary tract.

Valproate (valproic acid)

CLINICAL PHARMACOLOGY

Common indications	❶ Seizure prophylaxis in **epilepsy.** Epilepsy is classified by seizure type which, in turn, guides antiepileptic drug choice. Valproate has a broad spectrum of antiepileptic activity, making it effective in **most seizure types.** It is a first-line choice for prophylaxis of generalised tonic–clonic seizures, absence seizures, focal seizures (with or without secondary generalisation) and myoclonic seizures. ❷ Selected cases of **established convulsive status epilepticus** that have not responded to adequate treatment with a <u>benzodiazepine</u>. ❸ **Bipolar disorder,** for the acute treatment of manic episodes and prophylaxis against recurrence.
Mechanisms of action	The mechanism of action of valproate is incompletely understood. It appears to be a weak **inhibitor of neuronal sodium channels,** stabilising resting membrane potentials and reducing neuronal excitability. It also **increases** the brain content of **γ-aminobutyric acid** (GABA), the principal inhibitory neurotransmitter, which regulates neuronal excitability.
Important adverse effects	The most common dose-related adverse events are **GI upset** (such as nausea, gastric irritation and diarrhoea), **neurological and psychiatric** effects (including tremor, ataxia and behavioural disturbances), **thrombocytopenia** and transient increase in **liver enzymes.** Hypersensitivity reactions include **hair loss,** with subsequent regrowth being curlier than original hair. Rare, **life-threatening, idiosyncratic** adverse effects include severe liver injury, pancreatitis, bone marrow failure and antiepileptic hypersensitivity syndrome (see <u>Carbamazepine</u>).
Warnings	Valproate should be avoided where possible in ✘**women of child-bearing age,** particularly around the time of ✘**conception** and in the ✘**first trimester of pregnancy.** It is the antiepileptic drug associated with the greatest risk of **fetal abnormalities,** including neural tube defects, craniofacial, cardiac and limb abnormalities and developmental delay. It should be avoided in patients with ▲**hepatic impairment** and dose reduction is required in patients with ▲**severe renal impairment.**
Important interactions	Valproate inhibits hepatic enzymes, increasing plasma concentration and risk of toxicity with ▲<u>lamotrigine</u> (by inhibition of glucuronidation) and ▲**drugs metabolised by cytochrome P450 (CYP) enzymes,** such as <u>warfarin</u>. Valproate is itself metabolised by CYP enzymes, so its concentration is reduced and risk of seizures may be increased by ▲**CYP inducers** (e.g. <u>carbamazepine</u>, phenytoin) and, through an uncertain mechanism, by ▲<u>carbapenems</u>. Adverse effects are increased by ▲**CYP inhibitors** (e.g. <u>macrolides</u>, protease inhibitors). The efficacy of antiepileptic drugs is reduced by ▲**drugs that lower the seizure threshold** (e.g. <u>antipsychotics</u>, <u>tramadol</u>).

PRACTICAL PRESCRIBING

Prescription	Valproate is formulated as a sodium salt, which is prescribed in epilepsy, and as valproic acid, licensed for bipolar disorders. Valproate dose is equivalent in the two formulations, but care is required when switching between them. The usual daily starting dose of valproate is 600 mg for **epilepsy** and 750 mg for **bipolar disorder,** taken in 1–3 divided doses. The dose is increased to a usual daily maintenance of 1–2 g.
Administration	Oral valproate is formulated as a bewildering array of normal or enteric-coated tablets, capsules, granules and oral solutions. Some formulations can be crushed (tablets) or mixed with food (granules), whereas modified-release and enteric-coated formulations should be swallowed whole without chewing. It is important to give the patient appropriate instructions for the formulation chosen. Valproate can be given IV (by slow injection or infusion) where oral administration is not possible.
Communication	For epilepsy, explain to patients that the aim of treatment is to **reduce frequency of seizures.** Warn patients that they may have some indigestion or tummy upset when starting valproate, but that these will settle in a few days and can be reduced by taking **tablets with food.** As the most serious potential adverse effects are unpredictable, patients should seek **urgent medical advice** for unexpected symptoms such as lethargy, loss of appetite, vomiting or abdominal pain (may indicate liver poisoning) or bruising, a high temperature or mouth ulcers (may indicate blood abnormalities). For women, discuss ✖**contraception and pregnancy** (see Clinical tip). Advise patients **not to drive** unless they have been seizure-free for 12 months, and for 6 months after changing or stopping treatment.
Monitoring	Monitor **efficacy** by comparing seizure frequency before and after starting treatment or dose adjustment. Monitor **safety** by patient report. Measurement of liver function (including prothrombin time) before and during the first 6 months of treatment may be useful. **Plasma valproate concentrations** (usually 40–100 mg/L) do not correlate well with therapeutic effect. They should therefore only be measured to check for adherence or toxicity.
Cost	Valproate is inexpensive (around £9 for a 100-pack of 500 mg tablets). However, cost increases with complexity of the formulation.

Clinical tip—Both epilepsy and its treatment can impact the outcome of pregnancy. As valproate has the most teratogenic risk, it should not be prescribed for ✖**girls or women of child-bearing age** unless there is no safer alternative. If unavoidable, the risks must be discussed fully with a specialist, and pregnancy excluded before starting treatment. The patient must use reliable contraception. If pregnancy is planned, folic acid 5 mg daily should be prescribed and all efforts made to switch to an alternative antiepileptic agent. For unplanned pregnancies during valproate treatment, advise the patient that there is at least a 90% chance of a normal baby. Prenatal fetal monitoring should be offered.

Vancomycin

CLINICAL PHARMACOLOGY

Common indications	**❶** Treatment of Gram-positive infection, e.g. **endocarditis,** where infection is severe and/or penicillins cannot be used due to resistance (e.g. meticillin-resistant *Staphylococcus aureus* [MRSA]) or allergy. **❷** Treatment of **antibiotic-associated colitis** caused by *Clostridium difficile* infection (usually second-line treatment where metronidazole is ineffective or poorly tolerated).
Spectrum of activity	Vancomycin has a **relatively narrow spectrum** of activity against **Gram-positive bacteria**, notably *Staphylococcus* spp. (including MRSA), *Streptococcus* spp. and *C. difficile*. Vancomycin-resistant enterococci (VRE) are of increasing concern. It has no activity against Gram-negative organisms.
Mechanisms of action	Vancomycin inhibits growth and cross-linking of peptidoglycan chains, **inhibiting synthesis of the cell wall of Gram-positive bacteria**, thus lysing and killing the bacteria (bactericidal). It is inactive against most Gram-negative bacteria, which have a different (lipopolysaccharide) cell wall structure. **Acquired resistance** to vancomycin is increasingly reported. One mechanism is modification of cell wall structure by bacteria to prevent vancomycin binding.
Important adverse effects	The most common adverse effect is pain and inflammation of the vein (**thrombophlebitis**) at the infusion site. If vancomycin is infused rapidly, severe adverse reactions can occur. These include a rate-related infusion reaction termed 'red man syndrome'. This is characterised by generalised erythema and, less commonly, may be associated with hypotension and bronchospasm. Although the mechanism involves mast cell degranulation, it is not due to antigen–antibody interaction. However, true allergy to vancomycin (**immediate or delayed hypersensitivity**) can also occur. Intravenous vancomycin can cause **nephrotoxicity,** including renal failure and interstitial nephritis, **ototoxicity,** with tinnitus and hearing loss, **neutropenia** and **thrombocytopenia.**
Warnings	Vancomycin treatment requires careful monitoring of plasma drug concentrations and dose adjustment to avoid toxicity. Particular caution, including dose reduction, should be taken when prescribing for people with ▲**renal impairment** and the ▲**elderly** (increased risk of hearing impairment).
Important interactions	Vancomycin increases the risk of ototoxicity and/or nephrotoxicity when prescribed with ▲aminoglycosides, ▲loop diuretics or ▲ciclosporin (an immunosuppressant drug).

PRACTICAL PRESCRIBING

Prescription	Vancomycin is a large hydrophilic molecule that is very poorly absorbed across lipid membranes. For **systemic infection**, vancomycin must therefore be given IV. The initial dosage regimen is determined by renal function and adjusted according to plasma drug concentration (see Monitoring). Antibiotic treatment may be required for several weeks for patients with severe or deep infection, e.g. **endocarditis** or **osteomyelitis.** For *C. difficile* **colitis,** vancomycin must be given orally, typically 125 mg 6-hrly for 10–14 days. The **indication**, **review date** and **duration** of treatment should be documented on all inpatient antibiotic prescriptions to aid antibiotic stewardship.
Administration	Oral vancomycin is formulated as capsules, although the powder used for injection can be taken as an oral solution (off license). Intravenous vancomycin is diluted and given by slow infusion to reduce the risk of 'red man syndrome' (e.g. 1 g in 250 mL sodium chloride 0.9% over 60 minutes).
Communication	Explain to patients that the aim of treatment is to get rid of infection and improve symptoms. Warn them to **report any ringing in the ears** or change in hearing during treatment, as this is only reversible if treatment is stopped promptly. Vancomycin treatment is relatively uncommon, so patients are unlikely to give a history of prior vancomycin allergy.
Monitoring	Where IV therapy is used, pre-dose (trough) **plasma vancomycin concentrations** should be measured during treatment. Vancomycin dosage should be adjusted to keep trough plasma concentrations above 10 mg/L to maintain therapeutic effect but below 15 mg/L to minimise toxicity. Efficacy is assessed by monitoring symptoms, signs (e.g. pyrexia) and inflammatory markers (white cell count, C-reactive protein). Safety monitoring should include daily **renal function**. **Platelet and leucocyte counts** should be monitored in prolonged courses.
Cost	A 10–14-day course of oral treatment for *C. difficile* colitis costs around £9 for metronidazole, £260 for vancomycin and £1350 for fidaxomicin. These **costs are part of the consideration when developing treatment pathways**. For example in the treatment of *C .difficile* colitis, National Institute for Health and Care Excellence (NICE) recommend metronidazole for the first episode of mild to moderate infection, vancomycin for recurrent, severe or metronidazole-resistant infection and fidaxomicin for recurrent infection in patients with multiple co-morbidities or where vancomycin is ineffective.

Clinical tip—Prescription of vancomycin and subsequent monitoring and dosage adjustment is complex. Furthermore, vancomycin treatment is relatively uncommon, so it can be difficult for a junior doctor to gain expertise in this field. Always consult local guidelines and contact microbiology or pharmacy colleagues to ensure vancomycin prescription is done safely and effectively.

Vitamins

CLINICAL PHARMACOLOGY

Common indications	❶ *Thiamine* (vitamin B₁) is used in the treatment and prevention of **Wernicke's encephalopathy** and **Korsakoff's psychosis,** which are manifestations of severe thiamine deficiency. ❷ *Folic acid* (the synthetic form of folate or vitamin B₉) is used in **megaloblastic anaemia** as a result of folate deficiency, and in the first trimester of pregnancy to reduce the risk of **neural tube defects.** ❸ *Hydroxocobalamin* (a synthetic form of cobalamin or vitamin B₁₂) is used in the treatment of **megaloblastic anaemia** and **subacute combined degeneration of the cord** as a result of vitamin B₁₂ deficiency. ❹ *Phytomenadione* (the plant form of vitamin K) is recommended for all newborn babies to prevent **vitamin K deficiency bleeding,** and is used to **reverse the anticoagulant effect of <u>warfarin</u>** (prothrombin complex concentrate should also be given in cases of major bleeding).
Mechanisms of action	Vitamins are organic substances required in small amounts for normal metabolic processes. **Vitamin deficiencies** and their associated clinical manifestations may be treated with a pharmaceutical form of the relevant vitamin; the mechanism of action is self-explanatory (see Common indications). In pregnancy and the preconception period, giving folic acid reduces the risk of congenital **neural tube defects.** As it is required for normal cell division, it may work by facilitating cell proliferation involved in neural tube closure, but this is not completely understood. ***Phytomenadione* reverses <u>warfarin</u>** by providing a fresh supply of vitamin K for the synthesis of vitamin K-dependent clotting factors by the liver.
Important adverse effects	When given IV, *phytomenadione* and high-dose *thiamine* may rarely cause **anaphylaxis.** Most other vitamin preparations are relatively non-toxic.
Warnings	In patients with ▲**co-existing vitamin B₁₂ and folate deficiency,** you should replace both vitamins simultaneously. This is because replacing folate alone may be associated with (and perhaps hasten) progression of the neurological manifestations of vitamin B₁₂ deficiency. The major concern is the risk of provoking subacute combined degeneration of the cord. *Phytomenadione* is less effective in reversing <u>warfarin</u> in patients with **severe liver disease,** as clotting factors are synthesised in the liver.
Important interactions	As noted above, vitamin K and <u>warfarin</u> have an antagonistic interaction which, initially, is desirable. However, attempting to restart warfarin after vitamin K has been given may result in erratic dosing requirements.

folic acid, thiamine, hydroxocobalamin, phytomenadione

PRACTICAL PRESCRIBING

Prescription	In hospital, patients at high risk of **thiamine deficiency** are best treated initially with a compound preparation of B and C vitamins, given by injection. *Pabrinex®* is the usual choice. It is prescribed in 'pairs' of ampules: for *prophylaxis* in high-risk patients the dose is 1 pair 12-hrly IV for 3 days; *treatment* doses are higher. Oral thiamine (e.g. 200 mg daily) is used in the longer term. To **prevent neural tube defects,** folic acid 400 micrograms daily should be started before conception ideally, or otherwise at the diagnosis of pregnancy, and continued until week 12. This can be purchased without prescription. Where there is high risk of neural tube defect (e.g. in epilepsy), a higher dose of 5 mg daily is used. This is also the dose used in **folate deficiency anaemia.** In **vitamin B$_{12}$ deficiency,** hydroxocobalamin is given by IM injection. Oral cyanocobalamin is an alternative, but as the problem is usually with vitamin B$_{12}$ absorption, it may be less effective. To prevent **vitamin K deficiency bleeding** in neonates, phytomenadione 1 mg IM is given once only (lower doses in preterm neonates). To treat **over-warfarinisation,** it is best to give a low dose of phytomenadione (e.g. 1 mg orally or IV). In cases of major bleeding, 10 mg IV is given. Consult a local protocol or the BNF for further guidance.
Administration	Each carton of *Pabrinex®* contains 2 ampules labelled No 1 and No 2. The contents of both ampules are added to a small bag (50–100 mL) of 0.9% <u>sodium chloride</u> or 5% <u>glucose</u>, mixed, and infused over 30 minutes. *Phytomenadione*, when given IV, should be injected very slowly.
Communication	It is always worth raising the issue of folic acid supplementation in a consultation with a woman of child-bearing age, due to the benefits of starting this in the preconception period.
Monitoring	Treatment of **thiamine deficiency** is monitored clinically. Treatment of **folate** and vitamin B$_{12}$ **deficiency** are monitored clinically and with full blood counts. The effect of **phytomenadione** on the international normalised ratio (INR) is evident 12–24 hours after administration. No monitoring is required after prophylactic use in neonates.
Cost	Most vitamin preparations are inexpensive.

Clinical tip—In patients taking warfarin, a high INR with no bleeding may be corrected with a small oral dose of vitamin K (e.g. 0.5–1 mg). This is preferred to higher doses which may make subsequent dosing erratic. The oral formulation of vitamin K usually stocked on wards (menadiol phosphate) is available only as 10 mg tablets, making small doses impractical. An alternative is to use phytomenadione solution intended for IV administration but to give it orally (off license, but endorsed by the BNF). It can be diluted as necessary (e.g. with sterile water) to allow the required dose to be measured out.

Warfarin

CLINICAL PHARMACOLOGY

Common indications	**❶ Venous thromboembolism** (VTE, the collective term for **deep vein thrombosis** and **pulmonary embolism**): Warfarin is an option for treatment and prevention of recurrence (secondary prevention) of VTE. Initial concomitant therapy with heparin is required as it takes several days for anticoagulation with warfarin to be fully established. Direct oral anticoagulants (DOACs) are alternatives for this indication. **❷ To prevent arterial embolism in patients with atrial fibrillation (AF) or prosthetic heart valves:** for non-valvular AF, DOACs are alternatives. For patients with prosthetic heart valves, treatment is short term after tissue valve replacement and lifelong for mechanical valve replacement.
Mechanisms of action	In simplistic terms, venous and intracardiac clot formation is driven largely by the coagulation cascade, while arterial thrombosis is more a phenomenon of platelet activation. The coagulation cascade is an amplification reaction between clotting factors that generates a fibrin clot. Warfarin inhibits hepatic production of vitamin K-dependent coagulation factors (factors II, VII, IX and X, and proteins C and S). It does this by **inhibiting vitamin K epoxide reductase,** the enzyme responsible for restoring vitamin K to its reduced form, necessary as a co-factor in the synthesis of these clotting factors.
Important adverse effects	The main adverse effect of warfarin is **bleeding.** In therapeutic use or minor over-warfarinisation, there is increased risk of bleeding from minor trauma (e.g. intracerebral haemorrhage after minor head injury) and existing abnormalities such as peptic ulcers. Severe over-warfarinisation can trigger spontaneous bleeding, such as epistaxis or retroperitoneal haemorrhage. Warfarin can be reversed with phytomenadione (vitamin K₁) or dried prothrombin complex.
Warnings	As there is a fine line between thrombosis and haemorrhage in patients taking warfarin, its risks and benefits must be carefully balanced. Warfarin is contraindicated in patients at ✖**immediate risk of haemorrhage,** including after trauma and in patients requiring surgery. Patients with ▲**liver disease** who are less able to metabolise the drug are at risk of over-warfarinisation. Warfarin should not be used in the first trimester of ✖**pregnancy** due to a risk of teratogenicity (cardiac and cranial abnormalities). It should also be avoided later in pregnancy due to the risk of peripartum haemorrhage.
Important interactions	The plasma concentration of warfarin required to prevent clotting is close to the concentration that causes bleeding (**low therapeutic index**). Small changes in hepatic warfarin metabolism by cytochrome P450 (CYP) enzymes can cause clinically significant changes in anticoagulation. ▲**CYP inducers** (e.g. phenytoin, carbamazepine, rifampicin) increase warfarin metabolism and risk of clots. ▲**CYP inhibitors** (e.g. fluconazole, macrolides) decrease warfarin metabolism and increase bleeding risk. Other **antibiotics** can increase the effect of warfarin by killing gut flora that synthesise vitamin K, but this is not usually a clinical problem.

PRACTICAL PRESCRIBING

Prescription	Warfarin is taken orally once a day. The dose is 5–10 mg on day 1, with the lower dose used for patients who are elderly, lighter or at increased bleeding risk (e.g. due to interacting medicines). Subsequent doses are guided by the **international normalised ratio (INR)** (see Monitoring). After starting warfarin, it takes several days for full anticoagulation to be achieved. Patients needing immediate anticoagulation usually start both heparin (fast onset of action) and warfarin. Heparin is stopped once the INR is in the target range. A single episode of VTE is treated with warfarin for 3–6 months. Lifelong warfarin may be required for recurrent VTE or AF, although the risk–benefit balance should be reviewed periodically.
Administration	Traditionally, warfarin is taken each day at around 18:00 hours for consistent effects on the INR taken the following morning. This may also help patients remember when to take it (around tea time). The comedian Paul O'Grady, who takes the drug, has been known to remind his afternoon radio listeners, 'It's time for our warfarin!'
Communication	Advise patients that warfarin treatment is a balance between benefits (preventing clots) and risks (bleeding). It is important for patients to understand how food, alcohol and other drugs can affect warfarin treatment. Patients receive an **anticoagulant book ('Yellow Book')**, which acts as an alert to their warfarin therapy and is used to record warfarin doses, blood test results, treatment indication and duration. For patients requiring **long-term anticoagulation for AF**, NICE recommends that patient preference should be taken into account when deciding between warfarin or DOACs (decision support tool, http://www.anticoagulation-dst.co.uk/). This is a relatively complex discussion, but some key issues are: **warfarin** is a well-established drug that requires regular blood tests (frequently to start with), and may interact with alcohol, drugs and foods; **DOACs** are newer drugs that do not require frequent blood tests and may interact with other drugs but not food.
Monitoring	The INR is the prothrombin time of a person on warfarin divided by that of a non-warfarinised 'control'. The **target INR range** varies by indication (e.g. 2.0–3.0 in AF and VTE, higher in metallic prosthetic cardiac valves). INR is measured daily in hospital inpatients and every few days in outpatients commencing warfarin. Once a stable dose of warfarin has been established, INR measurement is less frequent.
Cost	Warfarin drug costs are about £1/month per patient, but associated monitoring costs add to this. DOACs cost more, but need less monitoring.

Clinical tip—Dosing warfarin can be a challenge. Follow local guidelines if possible, and if in doubt seek advice from the anticoagulation service. Changes in INR lag behind changes in the warfarin dose. Look back over the last 48–72 hours to see what doses have led to the current INR. Avoid large dose swings wherever possible.

Z-drugs

CLINICAL PHARMACOLOGY

Common indications	Short-term treatment of **insomnia** which is debilitating or distressing, although non-pharmacological treatment (or treatment of the underlying cause, if applicable) is invariably preferable.
Mechanisms of action	The 'Z-drugs' have a similar mechanism of action to <u>benzodiazepines</u>, although they are chemically distinct. Their target is the γ-aminobutyric acid type A (GABA$_A$) receptor. The GABA$_A$ receptor is a chloride (Cl⁻) channel that opens in response to binding by GABA, the main inhibitory neurotransmitter in the brain. Opening the channel allows chloride to flow into the cell, making the cell more resistant to depolarisation. Like benzodiazepines, **Z-drugs facilitate and enhance binding of GABA to the GABA$_A$ receptor.** This has a widespread depressant effect on synaptic transmission. The clinical manifestations of this include reduced anxiety, sleepiness and sedation. Note that Z-drugs are not useful anticonvulsants, as they can be taken by the oral route only. Z-drugs have a shorter duration of action than most benzodiazepines.
Important adverse effects	All Z-drugs can cause **daytime sleepiness,** which may affect ability to drive or perform complex tasks the day after taking the medication. **Rebound insomnia** may occur when the drugs are stopped. Other **neurological effects** include headache, confusion, nightmares and (rarely) amnesia. As Z-drugs are chemically distinct from each other, their adverse effects differ. *Zopiclone* can cause **taste disturbance,** whereas *zolpidem* more commonly causes **GI upset.** Prolonged use of Z-drugs beyond 4 weeks can lead to **dependence,** with **withdrawal symptoms** on stopping, including headaches, muscle pains and anxiety. In **overdose,** Z-drugs cause **drowsiness, coma and respiratory depression.**
Warnings	Z-drugs should be used with caution in the ▲**elderly,** who are often more sensitive to drugs with neurological effects. They should not be prescribed for patients with ✖**obstructive sleep apnoea** or those with ✖**respiratory muscle weakness** or ✖**respiratory depression,** in whom they may worsen respiratory failure during sleep.
Important interactions	Z-drugs enhance the sedative effects of alcohol, <u>antihistamines</u> and benzodiazepines. They enhance the hypotensive effect of antihypertensive medications. As Z-drugs are metabolised by cytochrome P450 (CYP) enzymes, ▲**CYP inhibitors** (e.g. <u>macrolides</u>) can enhance sedation, whereas **CYP inducers** (e.g. phenytoin, rifampicin) can impair sedation.

PRACTICAL PRESCRIBING

Prescription	Z-drugs should only be prescribed at the lowest effective dose for the shortest possible period (generally no longer than 2 weeks). Typical doses are zopiclone 7.5 mg or zolpidem 10 mg, to be taken at bedtime. Starting doses should be halved for elderly patients.
Administration	Z-drugs are available for oral administration only, as tablets or capsules.
Communication	When treating insomnia, explain to patients that 'sleeping tablets' should only be used as a **short-term measure** to help them get over a bad patch. Discuss reasons why they are not sleeping and offer advice on 'sleep hygiene'. Advise them to take tablets **only when really needed,** as the body can get used to them if taken regularly. Warn patients that the maximum time they should use the tablets for is **2–4 weeks,** as if used for longer they may become dependent on them and may feel unwell when they stop taking them. Warn them **not to drive or operate complex or heavy machinery** after taking the drug and explain that sometimes sleepiness may persist the following day.
Monitoring	Efficacy and safety are monitored clinically.
Cost	Both zopiclone and zolpidem are available in non-proprietary preparations and are relatively inexpensive.

Clinical tip—The routine prescription of hypnotics, such as Z-drugs, is not recommended for the treatment of insomnia because of the potential for tolerance and dependence and because it does not address the underlying cause of insomnia. However, hypnotics can be useful as short-term treatment in *specific* circumstances: e.g. for an anxious patient wishing to get a good night's sleep prior to surgery, or for recently bereaved people for whom insomnia is a significant problem.

Fluids

Colloids (plasma substitutes)

CLINICAL PHARMACOLOGY

Common indications	❶ Colloids are used to **expand circulating volume** in states of **impaired tissue perfusion** (including **shock**). However, <u>compound sodium lactate</u> and <u>sodium chloride</u> 0.9% are usually preferable. ❷ In **cirrhotic liver disease,** albumin is used to prevent effective hypovolaemia in **large-volume paracentesis** (ascitic fluid drainage).
Mechanisms of action	Intravenous (IV) colloid preparations contain **comparatively large, osmotically active molecules,** such as albumin or modified gelatin, in solution or suspension. In principle, these molecules cannot readily cross a semipermeable membrane (including vascular endothelium) and their osmotic effect 'holds' the infused volume in the intravascular compartment. For example, under experimental conditions, 70–80% of a gelatin-based colloid remains in the plasma. Their effect in **expanding circulating volume** is therefore potentially greater than that of a crystalloid (a solution that *can* cross a semipermeable membrane). In practice, however, most patients requiring volume expansion (e.g. for sepsis) have 'leaky' capillaries, so loss of the colloid molecule (and therefore the associated fluid volume) into the interstitium is more rapid than under experimental conditions. There is no convincing evidence that colloids are clinically superior to crystalloids, and trials using starch-based colloids have demonstrated harm. Sodium-based crystalloids (e.g. <u>compound sodium lactate</u>, <u>sodium chloride</u> 0.9%) are therefore usually favoured. **Large-volume paracentesis** (generally defined as >5 L) in **cirrhotic liver disease** can produce adverse haemodynamic effects. It is customary to administer human albumin solution (HAS) to mitigate this, although the evidence supporting this practice is much debated.
Important adverse effects	Colloids contain sodium, diffusion of which into the interstitium promotes **oedema.** Excessive plasma volume expansion may increase left ventricular filling beyond the point of maximal contractility on the Starling curve, causing a fall in cardiac output and **pulmonary oedema.** Gelatins may cause **hypersensitivity reactions,** including anaphylaxis – another reason to prefer crystalloids, which are non-allergenic.
Warnings	Rapid infusion of IV fluid should be undertaken cautiously in patients with ▲**heart failure,** due to the risk of pulmonary oedema (see Adverse effects). This can present a tricky situation in practice if there is a pressing need for fluid resuscitation (e.g. due to sepsis). The way to deal with this is to reduce the *volume* of fluid challenges, but still to infuse them rapidly so that the effect of transient volume expansion is appreciated. In ▲**renal impairment,** it is vital to monitor fluid balance closely to avoid volume overload.
Important interactions	There are no clinically important interactions.

PRACTICAL PRESCRIBING

Prescription	Colloids are prescribed in the 'infusions' section of the drug chart. Synthetic colloids are usually prescribed by brand name. You need to specify the volume to be infused and the rate at which it is to be given. The rate may be described either in mL/hr or as the intended duration for infusion of the total volume. For example, if deemed appropriate to use a colloid in a patient with **shock,** you might prescribe 250 mL of Gelofusine® to be given over 5 minutes. In the context of **large-volume paracentesis,** you should consult with specialist colleagues regarding the need for albumin. A common regimen is to give 100 mL of albumin 20% solution for every 2 L of ascitic fluid drained.
Administration	Infusions may be administered simply through a giving set, in which case the flow is controlled with a roller valve and the rate estimated from the number of drips per minute. A pressure bag can be applied to help infuse the fluid more quickly if required. An infusion pump can be used to control the rate and volume precisely, although the maximum infusion rate is usually too slow for an effective fluid challenge. An alternative is to use a 50-mL syringe and a three-way tap to give the desired volume by successive injection of aliquots.
Communication	Explain that you advise treatment with fluid through a drip to (for example) improve blood pressure. Ask the patient to report any irritation, swelling or wetness around the cannula site, as this may indicate that the cannula is no longer functioning correctly.
Monitoring	Patients requiring expansion of circulating volume are sick and require close monitoring. It is vital to assess haemodynamic status (e.g. pulse, blood pressure, jugular venous pressure, capillary refill time, urine output) before and after infusion as a guide to further therapy. Similarly, close monitoring is required in the context of large-volume paracentesis to detect adverse haemodynamic consequences, whether due to ascitic fluid drainage or albumin administration.
Cost	Colloid solutions are considerably more expensive than crystalloids.

Clinical tip—In managing a severely ill patient requiring large-volume fluid therapy, it is a good idea to use warmed fluids if possible, to avoid causing hypothermia. A fluid-warming cabinet (hopefully containing some warm bags of fluid!) can usually be found in the operating department, emergency department, or intensive care unit.

Compound sodium lactate (Hartmann's solution)

CLINICAL PHARMACOLOGY

Common indications	❶ To **provide sodium and water** in patients unable to take enough orally. ❷ To **expand circulating volume** in states of **impaired tissue perfusion** (including **shock**). This may be done as a 'fluid challenge', where a bolus of fluid (e.g. 500 mL) is infused rapidly. <u>Sodium chloride</u> 0.9% and <u>colloids</u> are alternatives.
Mechanisms of action	Compound sodium lactate (more commonly known by its eponymous name, Hartmann's solution) is a balanced crystalloid solution. Its electrolyte composition approximates serum: one litre contains Na^+ 131 mmol, Cl^- 111 mmol, K^+ 5 mmol, Ca^{2+} 2 mmol and lactate 29 mmol. The infused lactate is readily metabolised, generating bicarbonate. This makes it a suitable choice for **providing sodium and water** in patients unable to take enough orally. As compound sodium lactate contains sodium in a concentration similar to extracellular fluid, the infused volume is largely retained in the extracellular water compartment. As intravascular water accounts for about 20% of extracellular water, about 20% of the infused volume will remain in vessels to **expand circulating volume** (a transiently greater increase may occur before distribution is complete). This makes it a viable choice for use in fluid resuscitation. Its main advantage over <u>sodium chloride</u> 0.9% is its lower chloride content, making it less likely to cause hyperchloraemic acidosis.
Important adverse effects	Compound sodium lactate contains sodium, diffusion of which into the interstitium promotes **oedema.** Excessive plasma volume expansion may increase left ventricular filling beyond the point of maximal contractility on the Starling curve, causing a fall in cardiac output and **pulmonary oedema**.
Warnings	Rapid infusion of IV fluid should be undertaken cautiously in patients with ▲**heart failure,** due to the risk of pulmonary oedema (see <u>Colloids</u> for further discussion). In **renal impairment,** it is vital to monitor fluid balance closely to avoid overload. Compound sodium lactate contains potassium 5 mmol/L; this does not cause meaningful hyperkalaemia (above 5 mmol/L), but the serum potassium concentration should be monitored as part of overall disease management. Compound sodium lactate is best avoided in ▲**severe liver disease** because there may not be sufficient capacity to metabolise lactate.
Important interactions	There are no clinically important interactions.

compound sodium lactate (Hartmann's solution)

PRACTICAL PRESCRIBING

Prescription	Compound sodium lactate is prescribed in the 'infusions' section of the drug chart. You need to specify the volume to be infused and the rate at which it is to be given. The rate may be described either in mL/hr or as the intended duration for infusion of the total volume. For example, in **patients unable to take sufficient fluid orally,** you might prescribe compound sodium lactate 500 mL at 100 mL/hr and glucose 5% 2 L at 100 mL/hr. Together, these would provide about 65 mmol/day of sodium and 2400 mL of water, representing a reasonable 'maintenance' fluid regimen. To **expand circulating volume,** you might prescribe compound sodium lactate 500 mL over 5 minutes.
Administration	Infusions may be administered simply through a giving set, in which case the flow is controlled with a roller valve and the rate estimated from the number of drips per minute. A pressure bag can be applied to help infuse the fluid more quickly if required. Preferably, however, an infusion pump should be used to control the rate precisely. The maximum rate of infusion using a pump is usually too slow for an effective fluid challenge. An alternative is to use a 50-mL syringe and a three-way tap to give the desired volume by successive injection of aliquots.
Communication	Explain that you are offering treatment with a drip because (for example) they are unable to take enough fluid by mouth. As appropriate, encourage the patient to drink more, explaining that this is much better than giving fluid artificially. Ask the patient to report any irritation, swelling or wetness around the cannula site, as this may indicate that the cannula is no longer functioning correctly.
Monitoring	In any patient receiving fluid infusions, fluid balance should be monitored and recorded (see Glucose). In the context of impaired tissue perfusion, it is vital to assess haemodynamic status (e.g. pulse, blood pressure, jugular venous pressure, capillary refill time, urine output) before and after infusion as a guide to further therapy.
Cost	Compound sodium lactate is inexpensive. However, the associated costs (including infusion equipment, consumables, staff time and treatment of complications) may be considerable.

Clinical tip—As it has a slightly lower sodium content and a substantially lower chloride content, compound sodium lactate is often preferable to sodium chloride 0.9%. There is much to be said for using it as your 'standard' sodium-based crystalloid solution. The main caveat is that it offers less flexibility in terms of potassium replacement (as this is fixed at 5 mmol/L, whereas sodium chloride and glucose are routinely available in combination with potassium chloride in concentrations of 20 and 40 mmol/L).

Glucose (dextrose)

CLINICAL PHARMACOLOGY

Common indications	❶ Glucose 5% is used to **provide water** in patients unable to take enough orally. ❷ Glucose 10%, 20% and 50% are used to treat **hypoglycaemia** when this is *severe or cannot be treated orally*. Glucagon is an alternative. ❸ Glucose 10%, 20% and 50% are used with <u>insulin</u> to treat **hyperkalaemia.** <u>Calcium gluconate</u> may also be given in this setting (to stabilise the myocardium). ❹ Glucose 5% is used for **reconstitution and dilution of drugs** intended for administration by injection or infusion. <u>Sodium chloride</u> 0.9% and sterile water are alternatives.
Mechanisms of action	Glucose ($C_6H_{12}O_6$) is a monosaccharide that is the principal source of energy for cellular metabolism. It exists in several isomeric configurations: D-glucose (dextrose) is most relevant in mammalian biology. Glucose 5% solution is primarily **a means of providing water**. The glucose content ensures it is *initially* isotonic with serum, so that it does not induce osmotic lysis of red cells on initial mixing with blood. Glucose is rapidly taken up by cells and metabolised, leaving 'free' *(hypotonic)* water that distributes across all body water compartments. Higher-concentration glucose solutions are used to treat **hypoglycaemia;** the mechanism for this is self-explanatory. In **hyperkalaemia,** soluble <u>insulin</u> is given to stimulate Na^+/K^+-ATPase and shift potassium into cells. In this context, glucose is given to prevent hypoglycaemia. As less than 10% of an infused glucose solution remains in the intravascular space, it not used to expand circulating volume.
Important adverse effects	**Glucose 50% is highly irritant to veins** and may cause local pain, phlebitis and thrombosis. Its use is now discouraged, unless it can be given via a central line. Glucose 20% is also irritant, but less so. **Hyperglycaemia** will occur if glucose administration exceeds its utilisation (more likely in patients with diabetes mellitus).
Warnings	Giving IV glucose to patients at risk of ▲**thiamine deficiency** can cause **Wernicke's encephalopathy.** If glucose is necessary (e.g. to treat hypoglycaemia), thiamine (as Pabrinex®; see <u>Vitamins</u>) must also be given. In ▲**renal failure,** close monitoring of fluid balance is essential to avoid overload. Administering hypotonic fluid to patients with ▲**hyponatraemia** (or those who are more susceptible to its effects, e.g. ▲**children** and patients with ▲**brain injuries**) may precipitate hyponatraemic encephalopathy.
Important interactions	Glucose and <u>insulin</u> have antagonistic effects, but are often administered concurrently (e.g. in patients requiring IV insulin infusions). The rate of glucose infusion should ideally be kept constant unless treatment for hypoglycaemia is required.

glucose 5%, glucose 10%, glucose 20%, glucose 50%

PRACTICAL PRESCRIBING

Prescription	Glucose 5% is generally prescribed in the 'infusions' section of the drug chart. 'Glucose', not 'dextrose', is the approved name for prescription writing. You need to specify the volume to be infused and the rate at which it is to be given. Rate may be specified either in mL/hr or as the duration for infusion of the total volume. In **patients unable to take enough fluid orally,** you might prescribe glucose 5% 2 L at 100 mL/hr (write two prescriptions, each for 1 L, corresponding to the two 1-L 'bags' that will be needed). To meet a typical adult's overall water and electrolyte requirement, potassium may be prescribed as a constituent of the glucose solution (e.g. 20 mmol per 1 L bag; see Potassium chloride), and a sodium-containing crystalloid (e.g. sodium chloride 0.9% 500 mL at 100 mL/hr) may be prescribed separately. For **severe hypoglycaemia,** you might prescribe glucose 10% 100 mL for infusion over 1–2 minutes. In **hyperkalaemia,** glucose (e.g. glucose 50% 50 mL, or glucose 20% 100 mL) is infused with Actrapid® 10 units over about 30 minutes. Refer to a local guide or the British National Formulary (BNF) for details of how to **reconstitute and dilute drugs.**
Administration	IV fluids are provided in bags of various volumes, the largest of which is 1 L. Infusions may be administered simply through a giving set, in which case the flow is controlled with a roller valve, and the rate estimated from the number of drips per minute. Alternatively, and preferably, an infusion pump can be used to control the rate and volume precisely.
Communication	For patients receiving IV fluid replacement, explain (if appropriate) that they should still try to take fluid by mouth, as this is much better than receiving it artificially though a drip. Patients with severe hypoglycaemia may be uncooperative, but should be strongly encouraged to accept treatment before unconsciousness supervenes.
Monitoring	Fluid balance should be monitored carefully in all patients receiving IV fluid therapy. This consists of measuring fluid input (including oral intake and infusions) and output (urine output and additional losses, e.g. from surgical drains), and calculating the net fluid balance (input minus output) for each 24-hour period. In the treatment of **hypoglycaemia** and **hyperkalaemia,** the plasma glucose and serum potassium concentrations should be monitored closely.
Cost	Glucose solutions are inexpensive. However, associated costs (including infusion equipment, consumables, staff time and treatment of complications) may be considerable.

Clinical tip—An alternative option for treating severe hypoglycaemia is **glucagon,** a natural hormone that stimulates hepatic glycogenolysis and gluconeogenesis. The usual dose is 1 mg IV or IM. This provides a useful option when IV access if not readily available. Glucagon is poorly effective if hepatic glycogen stores are depleted, e.g. in malnutrition.

Potassium chloride

CLINICAL PHARMACOLOGY

Common indications	❶ For **prevention of potassium depletion** in patients unable to take enough orally (see Clinical tip). ❷ For **treatment of established potassium depletion and hypokalaemia**. IV administration is necessary when this is severe (<2.5 mmol/L), symptomatic, or causing arrhythmias.
Mechanisms of action	The normal potassium requirement to **prevent potassium depletion** is about 1 mmol/kg/day in adults. In patients unable to tolerate dietary intake, who are instead receiving their sodium and water requirement by IV infusion, potassium may be provided intravenously. **Established potassium depletion** and **hypokalaemia** may be caused, for example, by diarrhoea, vomiting, drugs (e.g. loop and thiazide diuretics) and secondary hyperaldosteronism. In severe cases, hypokalaemia may result in arrhythmias (which may be life-threatening), muscle weakness and (in extreme cases) paralysis. IV potassium repletion in these scenarios may be life-saving. For the best effect, IV potassium is given with sodium chloride rather than glucose. This is because infusion of negatively-charged Cl⁻ ions promotes retention of K^+ in the serum, whereas glucose may promote insulin release with resultant stimulation of Na^+/K^+-ATPase, shifting potassium into cells. Hypokalaemia is often associated with hypomagnesaemia. When it is, it may be difficult to correct unless magnesium is also replaced. Always check the magnesium level and prescribe magnesium replacement if necessary (seek advice on how to do this).
Important adverse effects	The major risk of IV potassium infusion is overcorrection leading to **hyperkalaemia** and a resultant risk of **arrhythmias.** Close monitoring is essential to avoid this. Potassium-containing solutions are **irritant to veins** if infused rapidly or in too high concentration. For this reason, the infusion rate in a peripheral vein should generally not exceed 20 mmol/hr.
Warnings	It is unnecessary and potentially dangerous to prescribe potassium for the prevention of potassium depletion in patients with **renal impairment** or **oliguria,** as they have minimal potassium losses and are very susceptible to hyperkalaemia.
Important interactions	Intravenous potassium has an additive effect with other **potassium-elevating drugs,** including oral potassium supplements, aldosterone antagonists, potassium-sparing diuretics, angiotensin-converting enzyme (ACE) inhibitors and angiotensin-receptor blockers.

PRACTICAL PRESCRIBING

Prescription	Potassium chloride is not available as a 'stand-alone' solution on general wards. Instead, it is prescribed as an ingredient in sodium chloride and glucose solutions, in concentrations of 20 or 40 mmol/L, and in compound sodium lactate at a fixed concentration of 5 mmol/L. Although potassium chloride is added at the manufacturing stage, in prescriptions it is usually specified as an 'additive' (this is not necessary for compound sodium lactate). For example, you might write a prescription for 1 L of sodium chloride 0.9% and then, in the additives section, prescribe 'potassium 20 mmol'. The nurse would then select a ready-made 1-L bag of sodium chloride 0.9% with potassium chloride 0.15%. The potassium content of 20 mmol is usually printed on the bag in red ink.
Administration	For routine use in prevention of potassium depletion, there are no special considerations for the administration of potassium other than those for fluid replacement in general. In the treatment of established potassium depletion and hypokalaemia, when more rapid infusion (**max. 20 mmol/hr**) may be required, IV potassium should ideally be given into a large vein and under close monitoring. In intensive care units higher concentrations may be given via a central venous catheter.
Communication	In the context of established potassium depletion and hypokalaemia, advise patients that they have a low level of potassium in their blood, and without treatment this could upset their heart rhythm. You are therefore offering treatment with potassium via a drip. You will need to monitor them closely during this, including with blood tests. This is to ensure the low potassium level is corrected, but not overcorrected, because this too can be risky.
Monitoring	When prescribing potassium for patients unable to take adequate amounts orally, the serum potassium concentration should be monitored. The intensity of this depends on the clinical context. Close monitoring is necessary when treating established potassium depletion and hypokalaemia.
Cost	Cost is not a factor in prescribing decisions for hypokalaemia.

Clinical tip—In non-severe, asymptomatic hypokalaemia, it is usually preferable (and safer) to administer potassium replacement orally. A reasonable prescription might be for potassium chloride with potassium bicarbonate (Sando-K®, which contains potassium 12 mmol/tab) 2 tablets two or three times daily.

Sodium chloride

CLINICAL PHARMACOLOGY

Common indications	❶ Sodium chloride 0.9% and 0.45% are used to **provide sodium and water** in patients unable to take enough orally. ❷ Sodium chloride 0.9% is used to **expand circulating volume** in states of **impaired tissue perfusion** (including **shock**). <u>Compound sodium lactate</u> and <u>colloids</u> are alternatives. ❸ Sodium chloride 0.9% is used for **reconstitution and dilution of drugs** intended for administration by injection or infusion. <u>Glucose</u> solutions and sterile water are alternatives.
Mechanisms of action	The extracellular fluid (ECF) compartment is made up of intravascular water (about 20%) and interstitial water (about 80%). Sodium is partitioned into ECF by Na^+/K^+-ATPase on cell membranes, which pumps sodium out of cells in exchange for potassium. As the main cation in ECF, sodium is the principal determinant of its osmolality. Osmolality is tightly regulated within a narrow range, so an increase in body sodium content (e.g. due to administration of a sodium-containing fluid) leads to an increase in ECF volume. The amount by which it expands depends on the sodium concentration of the fluid relative to ECF. Sodium chloride 0.9% contains sodium 154 mmol/L, similar to that of ECF. Accordingly, ECF expands by approximately the same amount as the volume of sodium chloride 0.9% administered. This distributes between the intravascular and interstitial compartments, so about 20% of the volume administered remains in vessels to **expand circulating volume.** Sodium chloride 0.9% and 0.45% are also used to **provide sodium and water** if the patient's requirements cannot be met orally. The normal sodium requirement for adults is about 1 mmol/kg/day.
Important adverse effects	Diffusion of sodium and water into the interstitium promotes **oedema.** The concentration of chloride in sodium chloride 0.9% (154 mmol/L) is significantly higher than that of ECF (about 100 mmol/L). This may cause **hyperchloraemia** which, in turn, promotes **acidaemia.** Probably the best explanation for this is that as Cl^- concentration rises, so HCO_3^- concentration must fall (and/or H^+ and K^+ rise) to maintain electroneutrality. Excessive plasma volume expansion may increase left ventricular filling beyond the point of maximal contractility on the Starling curve, causing a fall in cardiac output and **pulmonary oedema**.
Warnings	Rapid infusion of IV fluid should be undertaken cautiously in patients with ▲**heart failure,** due to the risk of pulmonary oedema (see <u>Colloids</u> for further discussion). In **renal impairment,** it is vital to monitor fluid balance closely to avoid overload.
Important interactions	There are no clinically important interactions.

sodium chloride 0.9%, sodium chloride 0.45%

PRACTICAL PRESCRIBING

Prescription	Sodium chloride is prescribed in the 'infusions' section of the drug chart. Write 'sodium chloride 0.9%' rather than 'normal saline', since the latter is misleading and is not printed on product labelling. You need to specify the volume to be infused and the rate at which it is to be given. Rate may be specified either in mL/hr, or as the duration for infusion of the total volume. For example, in **patients unable to take sufficient fluid orally,** you might prescribe sodium chloride 0.9% 500 mL at 100 mL/hr and <u>glucose</u> 5% 2 L at 100 mL/hr. Together, these would provide about 77 mmol/day of sodium and 2400 mL of water, representing a reasonable 'maintenance' fluid regimen. To **expand circulating volume,** you might prescribe 500 mL of sodium chloride 0.9% to be given over 5 minutes. Refer to a local guide or the BNF for details of how to **reconstitute and dilute drugs.**
Administration	Infusions may be administered simply through a giving set, in which case the flow is controlled with a roller valve, and the rate estimated from the number of drips per minute. Alternatively, and preferably, an infusion pump can be used to control the rate and volume precisely. The maximum rate of infusion using a pump is usually too slow for an effective fluid challenge. An alternative is to use a 50-mL syringe and a three-way tap to give the desired volume by successive injection of aliquots.
Communication	Explain that you are offering treatment with a drip because (for example) they are unable to take enough fluid by mouth. If appropriate, encourage the patient to drink more, explaining that this is much better than giving fluid artificially. Ask the patient to report any irritation, swelling or wetness around the cannula, as this may indicate that the cannula is no longer functioning correctly.
Monitoring	In any patient receiving fluid infusions, fluid balance should be monitored and recorded (see <u>Glucose</u>). In the context of **impaired tissue perfusion,** it is vital to assess haemodynamic status (e.g. pulse, blood pressure, jugular venous pressure, capillary refill time, urine output) before and after infusion as a guide to further therapy.
Cost	Sodium chloride itself is inexpensive. However, associated costs (including infusion equipment, consumables, staff time and treatment of complications) may be considerable.

Clinical tip—When administering a fluid to **expand circulating volume,** consider using a blood product giving set. This permits a higher flow rate than a standard giving set.

Self-assessment and knowledge integration

Tags used to identify focus areas:

Systems

Blood	Blood
CVS	Cardiovascular system
GI	Gastrointestinal system
Endo	Endocrine and reproductive
Infection	Infection
IV fluids	Intravenous fluids
MSK	Musculoskeletal
Neuro	Neurological/psychiatry
Renal/GU	Renal/genitourinary tracts
Resp	Respiratory
Skin	Skin
Tox	Toxicology

Topics

Indications	Common indications
Mechanisms	Mechanisms of action
AEs	Important adverse effects
Warnings	Warnings
Interactions	Important interactions
Prescription	Prescription
Admin	Administration
Comm	Communication
Monitoring	Monitoring

Blood
Indications
Prescription

1. An 85-year-old woman is admitted to the acute medical unit with a urinary tract infection (UTI). Her past medical history includes a left-leg deep vein thrombosis (DVT) 5 years ago, for which she was treated with warfarin for 3 months. She has no risk factors for bleeding and her renal function is normal.

What is the most appropriate antithrombotic therapy while in hospital?

A. Aspirin 75 mg orally daily
B. Dalteparin 5000 units subcutaneous (SC) daily
C. Dalteparin 5000 units SC daily and warfarin orally to target international normalised ratio (INR) 2–3
D. Unfractionated heparin 5000 units SC 12-hourly (hrly)
E. Warfarin orally to target INR 2–3

Blood
AEs

2. A 75-year-old man is found to have acute haemolytic anaemia. He has a past medical history of glucose-6-phosphate dehydrogenase (G6PD) deficiency. It emerges that he has inadvertently been taking medicines from his wife's blister pack instead of his own. Her medications include allopurinol, levothyroxine, metformin, quinine and sitagliptin.

What drug is most likely to have precipitated haemolysis?

A. Allopurinol
B. Levothyroxine
C. Metformin
D. Quinine
E. Sitagliptin

Blood
AEs

3. An 86-year-old man is admitted to the emergency department with shock after a major gastrointestinal bleed. His wife advises that he is taking dabigatran for atrial fibrillation (AF).

What drug reverses the anticoagulant effect of dabigatran?

A. Andexanet α
B. Dried prothrombin complex
C. Idarucizumab
D. Phytomenadione (vitamin K_1)
E. Protamine

Blood
Interactions

4. A 77-year-old woman attends the anticoagulation clinic. She has a past medical history of AF and stroke. She takes warfarin and has been on a stable dosage for about 2 years. Last month, she was briefly admitted to hospital following a seizure. This was ascribed to cerebrovascular disease and she was put on an 'antiepileptic medicine'. She does not know its name and has not brought a list of her medications. Her INR today is 1.6 (target 2–3).

What drug is most likely to interact with warfarin to lower the INR?

A. Carbamazepine
B. Diazepam
C. Gabapentin
D. Pregabalin
E. Valproate

Blood

Monitoring

5. A 31-year-old woman develops a DVT when she is 16 weeks pregnant and requires anticoagulation with a low molecular weight heparin (LMWH) for the rest of her pregnancy.

What test would be most useful to determine if her anticoagulation is adequate?

A. Activated partial thromboplastin ratio
B. Antifactor Xa assay
C. INR
D. Plasma fibrinogen concentration
E. Platelet count

CVS

Indications

6. A 52-year-old man sees his general practitioner (GP) with episodic chest pain that occurs on exertion. His GP makes a diagnosis of stable angina.

What treatment would be most likely to prevent further chest pain?

A. Aspirin
B. Bisoprolol
C. Glyceryl trinitrate
D. Ramipril
E. Simvastatin

CVS

Indications

7. A 68-year-old man is discharged from hospital following treatment for a non-ST-elevation myocardial infarction. He has made a good recovery and has no symptoms. His current medications are aspirin, clopidogrel, bisoprolol and atorvastatin.

What additional drug is most likely to reduce the risk of further cardiovascular events?

A. Amiloride
B. Digoxin
C. Glyceryl trinitrate
D. Ramipril
E. Warfarin

CVS

Indications

8. A 72-year-old woman with a previous diagnosis of heart failure (New York Heart Association class III) complains of ankle swelling and is slightly more breathless than usual. Her current medications are bisoprolol, bumetanide and ramipril. Recent blood tests have showed mild hypokalaemia with a serum potassium concentration around 3.1 mmol/L (normal 3.5–4.7).

What drug should be added to her treatment?

A. Amiloride
B. Furosemide
C. Indapamide
D. Isosorbide mononitrate
E. Spironolactone

CVS

Indications

9. A 76-year-old man is found to have atrial fibrillation. He is asymptomatic. He has a past medical history of hypertension, hypercholesterolaemia and heart failure (New York Heart Association class II). He takes furosemide, ramipril and simvastatin, and has no allergies. Physical examination is normal except for a heart rate of approximately 120 beats/min with an irregular rhythm.

What is the most appropriate drug for ventricular rate control?

A. Amiodarone
B. Bisoprolol
C. Digoxin
D. Doxazosin
E. Verapamil

CVS

Mechanisms

10. An 82-year-old woman with ischaemic heart disease and cardiac failure is treated with bisoprolol, furosemide, ramipril, simvastatin and spironolactone.

Which of her medications acts by inhibiting a membrane transport protein?

A. Bisoprolol
B. Furosemide
C. Ramipril
D. Simvastatin
E. Spironolactone

CVS

Mechanisms

11. A 54-year-old man is found to have supraventricular tachycardia. Metoprolol is given in an effort to restore sinus rhythm.

What receptor is the main target of metoprolol?

A. α_1-adrenoceptor
B. α_2-adrenoceptor
C. β_1-adrenoceptor
D. β_2-adrenoceptor
E. β_3-adrenoceptor

CVS
Interactions

12. An 81-year-old man presents with syncope. He has a past medical history of hypertension, angina and chronic obstructive pulmonary disease (COPD). His usual oral medications are amlodipine, diltiazem, indapamide, ramipril and simvastatin. Two days ago, he saw a doctor who did not have access to his full medical records, but advised him that he should be taking a β-blocker. Bisoprolol was prescribed.

On examination, his heart rate is 45 beats/min. His blood pressure is 96/60 mmHg. The ECG shows third-degree heart block.

What medication is most likely to interact with bisoprolol to cause heart block?

A. Amlodipine
B. Diltiazem
C. Indapamide
D. Ramipril
E. Simvastatin

CVS
AEs

13. A 63-year-old woman presents to the practice nurse complaining of swollen ankles. Her past medical history includes hypertension, type 2 diabetes and COPD. Her medication includes amlodipine, chlortalidone, metformin, gliclazide and tiotropium. Examination is unremarkable save for slight pitting oedema of her ankles. The practice nurse suspects an adverse drug reaction.

What drug is most likely to be contributing to her peripheral oedema?

A. Amlodipine
B. Chlortalidone
C. Gliclazide
D. Metformin
E. Tiotropium

CVS
Neuro
AEs

14. A 42-year-old woman is admitted to hospital after collapsing on the train. The ambulance service recorded broad-complex tachycardia on an electrocardiogram (ECG), which spontaneously terminated. The pharmacist is concerned that her hospital admission may be due to an adverse effect of her medication, which includes amitriptyline.

To whom should this event be reported?

A. British National Formulary (BNF)
B. Care Quality Commission (CQC)
C. Manufacturer of the drug
D. Medicines and Healthcare Products Regulatory Agency (MHRA)
E. National Institute for Health and Care Excellence (NICE)

CVS

Warnings

15. A 59-year-old woman is attending the pre-operative assessment clinic before having a hysterectomy. Her past medical history includes hypercholesterolaemia, hypertension and a transient ischaemic attack (TIA). Her regular medications are amlodipine, atorvastatin, clopidogrel, indapamide and ramipril.

What medicine should she be advised to stop taking 1 week before the procedure?

A. Amlodipine
B. Atorvastatin
C. Clopidogrel
D. Indapamide
E. Ramipril

CVS

Prescription

16. A 48-year-old man has started taking isosorbide mononitrate immediate-release tablets 20 mg twice daily for prevention of angina symptoms.

What are the most appropriate times of day for him to take the tablets?

A. 12pm and 12am
B. 12pm and 8pm
C. 8am and 12pm
D. 8am and 3pm
E. 8am and 8pm

CVS

Admin

17. A young man collapses at a wedding reception. He was seen fumbling with a cartridge-like device before he collapsed, but had not been able to use it. On examination, he is unresponsive. His breathing is noisy; this improves slightly with a head-tilt-chin-lift manoeuvre. His face appears flushed and his lips are swollen. A carotid pulse is palpable but it is thready.

An ambulance has been called but has not arrived. The cartridge-like device is handed to you. It is labelled 'EpiPen® Auto-Injector'.

How should this be administered?

A. Intramuscularly into the anterolateral thigh
B. Intramuscularly into the triceps muscle
C. Intravenously into any available peripheral vein
D. Subcutaneously into the anterior abdominal wall
E. Subcutaneously into the tissue overlying the triceps muscle

CVS

Monitoring

18. A 58-year-old woman who started taking simvastatin 3 months ago is asked to attend a follow-up visit with her GP.

What blood test should be performed to monitor for side effects of statins?

A. Creatine kinase
B. Liver profile
C. Fasting lipid profile
D. Full blood count
E. Thyroid function tests

CVS

Monitoring

19. A 68-year-old man has started taking eplerenone for heart failure following a myocardial infarction.

What test should be performed in the first 1–2 weeks of therapy to identify possible adverse effects?

A. Echocardiogram
B. Electrocardiogram
C. Serum brain natriuretic peptide
D. Serum potassium
E. Serum troponin

CVS

Comm

20. A 50-year-old Caucasian man attends a blood pressure check with his practice nurse. He was noted to have high blood pressure at a routine health check last month. As his blood pressure remains high, a decision is made to start antihypertensive treatment with ramipril.

What common side effect should the nurse discuss with him?

A. Blurred vision
B. Diarrhoea
C. Dry cough
D. Headache
E. Urinary retention

Endo

Indications

Monitoring

21. A 55-year-old man attends the general practice for a planned review. Three months ago, he was found to have type 2 diabetes, and has since made concerted efforts to follow lifestyle advice. You advise him to have a blood test to measure haemoglobin A_{1c} (HbA$_{1c}$) concentration.

What HbA$_{1c}$ threshold best describes the level at which pharmacological therapy should be offered?

A. 28 mmol/mol (4.7%)
B. 48 mmol/mol (6.5%)
C. 53 mmol/mol (7.0%)
D. 58 mmol/mol (7.5%)
E. 64 mmol/mol (8.0%)

Endo

Indications

22. A 56-year-old woman was diagnosed with type 2 diabetes 3 months ago. She has a body mass index (BMI) of 27 kg/m^2 and no known allergies. Despite lifestyle changes, her blood glucose control is poor and her haemoglobin A_{1c} is below target. She has normal renal function. Her GP advises her to commence pharmacological therapy.

What drug would be the most appropriate initial therapy?

A. Acarbose
B. Gliclazide
C. Insulin
D. Metformin
E. Sitagliptin

Endo

Mechanisms

23. A 45-year-old man with type 2 diabetes is taking metformin.

What is the main means by which metformin lowers blood glucose concentration?

A. Increased pancreatic insulin secretion
B. Increased peripheral insulin sensitivity
C. Increased urinary glucose excretion
D. Reduced hepatic glucose output
E. Reduced intestinal glucose absorption

Endo

Mechanisms

24. An 84-year-old woman has started taking anastrozole, after being found to have advanced breast cancer.

What best describes the mechanism of action of anastrozole?

A. 5α-reductase inhibition
B. Aromatase inhibition
C. Inhibition of ergosterol synthesis
D. Luteinising hormone (LH)/follicle-stimulating hormone (FSH) suppression
E. Selective oestrogen receptor modulation

Endo

AEs

25. A 78-year-old man is admitted to the emergency department with loss of consciousness and is found to have a blood glucose concentration of 1.2 mmol/L. His usual medications are bendroflumethiazide, bisoprolol, gliclazide, metformin and prednisolone.

What drug is most likely to have caused his hypoglycaemia?

A. Bendroflumethiazide
B. Bisoprolol
C. Gliclazide
D. Metformin
E. Prednisolone

Endo

AEs

26. A 50-year-old man presents to review the results of recent blood tests. He has a past medical history of type 2 diabetes and hypertension. He takes metformin 1 g twice daily and ramipril 10 mg daily.

Investigations: Creatinine 148 μmol/L (60–110), estimated glomerular filtration (eGFR) 44 mL/min/1.73 m^2 (>60)

What complication is more likely if metformin is taken in the context of renal impairment?

A. Diabetic ketoacidosis
B. Hypersensitivity reaction
C. Lactic acidosis
D. Megaloblastic anaemia
E. Respiratory alkalosis

Endo

AEs

27. A 59-year-old man with type 2 diabetes is found to have suboptimal glycaemic control. He takes metformin 1 g twice daily. He is content to start a second medication, but says he cannot accept an increased risk of hypoglycaemia.

What drug is most likely to increase the risk of hypoglycaemic attacks?

A. Empagliflozin
B. Gliclazide
C. Metformin
D. Pioglitazone
E. Sitagliptin

Endo

AEs

28. A 70-year-old woman presents with abdominal pain and shock. A surgical cause is suspected, and she is placed 'nil by mouth' while arrangements for an emergency laparotomy are made. She has a past medical history of polymyalgia rheumatica. She has taken prednisolone 5 mg daily for several years, but none in the last 3 days because of nausea.

What is the most appropriate option for immediate steroid replacement?

A. Budesonide
B. Fludrocortisone
C. Fluticasone
D. Hydrocortisone
E. Prednisolone

Endo

AEs

29. A 28-year-old woman is started on tamoxifen for locally advanced oestrogen-receptor positive breast cancer.

What is the most appropriate advice to give her regarding potential side effects?

A. It can stimulate milk production from her breasts
B. It causes infertility
C. It is safe to take during pregnancy
D. There is an increased risk of cancer of the lining of the womb
E. There is an increased risk of ovarian cancer

Endo

AEs

30. A 58-year-old man with type 2 diabetes is taking metformin and gliclazide. Despite this, his blood glucose is poorly controlled and his GP advises him to commence saxagliptin, a dipeptidylpeptidase-4 inhibitor. His medical history includes COPD, congestive cardiac failure, fatty liver, gout and pancreatitis.

Which medical condition is a relative contraindication to dipeptidylpeptidase-4 inhibitor treatment?

A. COPD
B. Congestive cardiac failure
C. Fatty liver
D. Gout
E. Pancreatitis

Endo

Interactions

31. A 72-year-old woman is admitted with a suspected pulmonary embolism (PE) and requires a computerised tomography (CT) pulmonary angiogram with contrast. She is taking alendronic acid, atorvastatin, diltiazem, metformin and ramipril.

What drug should be withheld now and for 48 hours after the procedure?

A. Alendronic acid
B. Atorvastatin
C. Diltiazem
D. Metformin
E. Ramipril

Endo

Interactions

32. A 34-year-old woman has started taking tamoxifen following a mastectomy for locally advanced oestrogen-receptor positive breast cancer. Her past medical history includes anxiety, hay fever and schizophrenia. Her current medications are codeine, fluoxetine, loratadine, propranolol and risperidone.

What drug is most likely to reduce the efficacy of tamoxifen?

A. Codeine
B. Fluoxetine
C. Loratadine
D. Propranolol
E. Risperidone

Endo
Neuro
Interactions

33. A 25-year-old woman presents to her GP to request a combined oral contractive pill. She has a past medical history of epilepsy, which is well controlled on lamotrigine 200 mg daily and levetiracetam 1 g 12-hrly. After appropriate assessment and counselling, a preparation containing ethinylestradiol 30 micrograms and levonorgestrel 150 micrograms per tablet (Microgynon 30®) is prescribed.

What modification, if any, is most likely to be needed to her antiepileptic treatment?

A. Decrease levetiracetam dosage
B. Decrease lamotrigine dosage
C. Increase levetiracetam dosage
D. Increase lamotrigine dosage
E. No changes required to antiepileptic therapy

Endo
Comm

34. A 66-year-old woman with a new diagnosis of type 2 diabetes sees her GP to commence treatment with an oral hypoglycaemic drug. She has been researching options on the internet and asks the GP what the difference is between metformin and a sulphonylurea.

What statement about metformin compared with a sulphonylurea is most correct?

A. It causes more weight gain
B. It is associated with a lower risk of abdominal side effects
C. It is associated with a lower risk of death from cardiovascular complications
D. It is associated with an increased risk of hypoglycaemia
E. It is more expensive

GI
Indications
Mechanisms
AEs

35. A 24-year-old woman is vomiting following an evacuation of retained products of conception, performed under general anaesthesia. She was given cyclizine 50 mg intravenous (IV) 30 minutes ago but this has not improved her symptoms.

Her past medical history is notable for a severe illness involving fever and muscles spasms, which was thought to have been precipitated by a prochlorperazine injection.

What is the most appropriate treatment for her nausea and vomiting?

Self-assessment and knowledge integration

A. Chlorpromazine
B. Cyclizine
C. Haloperidol
D. Metoclopramide
E. Ondansetron

GI

Indications

Prescription

36. A 48-year-old woman who has peptic ulcers caused by *Helicobacter pylori* infection presents to her GP to commence treatment. She is allergic to benzylpenicillin, which caused an anaphylactic reaction.

What is the most appropriate 1-week oral treatment regimen?

A. Lansoprazole, amoxicillin and clarithromycin
B. Lansoprazole, amoxicillin and metronidazole
C. Omeprazole and clarithromycin
D. Omeprazole and metronidazole
E. Omeprazole, clarithromycin and metronidazole

GI

Indications

Mechanisms

37. An 86-year-old woman has been taking codeine phosphate to treat a sprained wrist. Co-incidentally, she has noticed that this has improved the diarrhoea she usually suffers from as a result of diverticular disease.

Although her wrist has now healed, she is keen to continue taking the codeine, as not having to open her bowels so regularly has considerably improved her quality of life. However, the codeine does makes her feel a little 'light headed', which she finds unpleasant.

What alternative opioid would be better to treat her diarrhoea?

A. Loperamide
B. Morphine (immediate release)
C. Morphine (modified release)
D. Oxycodone (modified release)
E. Pethidine

GI

Indications

38. A 62-year-old man with a background of alcoholic cirrhosis is admitted to the acute medical unit with confusion. A diagnosis of hepatic encephalopathy is made. His wife reports that he had been complaining of constipation in the days leading up to admission.

What laxative should be prescribed?

A. Docusate sodium
B. Ispaghula husk
C. Lactulose
D. Macrogol
E. Senna

GI
Indications
Warnings

39. A 50-year-old man complains of severe itch. He has had this for several days and it affects his whole body. He was admitted yesterday with progressive ascites as a result of cirrhotic liver disease. He is taking furosemide, spironolactone, lactulose and phosphate enemas. He has no allergies.

On examination of his skin, there are multiple spider naevi over his upper body and excoriation marks over his arms, trunk and thighs.

What is the most appropriate initial pharmacological treatment?

A. Chlorphenamine orally
B. Codeine phosphate orally
C. Hydrocortisone topically
D. Loratadine orally
E. Prednisolone orally

GI
Mechanisms

40. An 85-year-old woman is advised to take ranitidine for dyspepsia.

What best describes the mechanism of action of ranitidine?

A. Antagonism of histamine H_1 receptors in gastric parietal cells
B. Antagonism of histamine H_1 receptors in the vagus nerve
C. Antagonism of histamine H_2 receptors in gastric parietal cells
D. Antagonism of histamine H_2 receptors in gastric chief cells
E. Antagonism of histamine H_2 receptors in the vagus nerve

GI
AEs
Monitoring

41. A 55-year-old man is seen in the gastroenterology clinic to discuss the management of his ulcerative colitis (UC). Apart from his inflammatory bowel disease, he has no other medical problems. A decision is made to start azathioprine. The benefits and risks of treatment are discussed.

What blood test will he need to have each week in the first month of treatment?

A. Full blood count
B. Liver function
C. Thyroid function
D. Renal function
E. Serum glucose

GI
AEs

42. A 55-year-old woman with psoriatic arthritis was admitted to hospital 12 days ago with severe cellulitis. On admission, her liver function was normal but she has now developed cholestatic jaundice.

Her medications are flucloxacillin, methotrexate, morphine, paracetamol and simvastatin.

Which drug is most likely to have caused her cholestatic jaundice?

A. Flucloxacillin
B. Methotrexate
C. Morphine
D. Paracetamol
E. Simvastatin

GI

Interactions

43. A 44-year-old man complains of heartburn. His past medical history includes asthma, epilepsy and hypothyroidism. His current medications are beclomethasone, carbamazepine, levothyroxine, montelukast and salbutamol. His GP recommends a trial of Gaviscon® in the first instance.

What medicine should he be advised to separate from Gaviscon® by at least 2 hours?

A. Beclomethasone
B. Carbamazepine
C. Levothyroxine
D. Montelukast
E. Salbutamol

Infection

Renal/GU

Indications

Warnings

44. A 22-year-old woman complains of dysuria. Her GP diagnoses an uncomplicated UTI. Her only medication is the combined oral contraceptive pill and she has not missed any doses of this. She has no allergies.

What is the most appropriate treatment?

A. Cefotaxime
B. Ciprofloxacin
C. Clarithromycin
D. Gentamicin
E. Trimethoprim

Infection

Skin

Indications

45. A 72-year-old woman is admitted to hospital with severe cellulitis of her right leg. She has no allergies.

What is the most appropriate treatment?

A. Amoxicillin and clarithromycin
B. Benzylpenicillin and flucloxacillin
C. Cefotaxime and aciclovir
D. Co-amoxiclav and metronidazole
E. Co-amoxiclav and gentamicin

Infection

Resp

Indications

46. An 83-year-old woman is admitted to the acute medical unit with a diagnosis of mild community-acquired pneumonia (CURB-65 score 1). Her mobility is poor, but she has no active co-morbidities, does not usually take any medications and has no allergies.

What would be the most appropriate antibiotic to treat her infection?

A. Cefotaxime
B. Ciprofloxacin
C. Doxycycline
D. Ertapenem
E. Flucloxacillin

Infection

Indications

Mechanisms

47. A 75-year-old man is being treated for a UTI. He has no other medical problems and takes no regular medicines. He has no allergies. The results of his urine microscopy have returned. The bacterial sensitivities suggest any β-lactam antibiotic would be suitable.

What antibiotic should be prescribed?

A. Amoxicillin
B. Ciprofloxacin
C. Clarithromycin
D. Doxycycline
E. Metronidazole

Infection

Indications

48. A 60-year-old woman is admitted with fever, confusion and seizures. A decision is made to treat her empirically for herpes simplex viral encephalitis.

What is the most appropriate treatment?

A. Aciclovir
B. Amoxicillin
C. Ceftriaxone
D. Dexamethasone
E. Fluconazole

Infection

Indications

49. A 77-year-old man with multiple sclerosis is admitted as an emergency with urinary sepsis. He has a long-term suprapubic catheter for the treatment of urinary retention. Urine cultures grew *Pseudomonas aeruginosa*.

What antibiotic is most likely to be active against this organism?

A. Amoxicillin
B. Cephalexin
C. Ciprofloxacin
D. Nitrofurantoin
E. Trimethoprim

Infection

Mechanisms

50. Hospital guidelines indicate that patients who are immunocompromised, e.g. by neutropenia, who develop infection should be treated with bactericidal rather than bacteriostatic antibiotics.

What antibiotic has a consistently bactericidal mechanism of action?

A. Amoxicillin
B. Chloramphenicol
C. Clarithromycin
D. Doxycycline
E. Trimethoprim

Infection

Mechanisms

51. A 44-year-old man needs antibiotic treatment for infection with a penicillinase-producing strain of *Staphylococcus aureus*.

What antibiotic is this organism most likely to be resistant to?

A. Benzylpenicillin
B. Co-amoxiclav
C. Flucloxacillin
D. Piperacillin with tazobactam
E. Vancomycin

Infection

AEs

Warnings

52. A 54-year-old man has a history of a severe anaphylactic reaction to penicillin. He now requires antibiotics for treatment of sepsis of uncertain cause.

What antibiotic is most likely to be safe in the context of a severe penicillin allergy?

A. Cefotaxime
B. Ciprofloxacin
C. Co-amoxiclav
D. Ertapenem
E. Tazocin®

Infection

AEs

Monitoring

53. A 53-year-old man with severe *Haemophilus influenzae* epiglottitis, who has a history of severe allergy to all β-lactam antibiotics, is started on IV chloramphenicol.

Which test should be performed regularly to monitor treatment safety?

A. Audiometry
B. C-reactive protein
C. Full blood count
D. Liver function
E. Renal function

Infection

Neuro

AEs

54. A 56-year-old man notices tinnitus and dizziness after discharge from hospital where he was treated for severe pneumonia. During this admission (which included a spell in the intensive care unit), his antibiotic treatment included courses of doxycycline, co-amoxiclav, clarithromycin, piperacillin with tazobactam and gentamicin.

Which antibiotic is most likely to have caused this adverse effect?

A. Clarithromycin
B. Co-amoxiclav
C. Doxycycline
D. Gentamicin
E. Piperacillin with tazobactam

Infection

AEs

55. A 68-year-old woman is found to have cellulitis. She has a past medical history of hypertension, leg cramps and urge incontinence. Her medication comprises bendroflumethiazide, oxybutynin and quinine sulfate. She is allergic to penicillin, which causes a rash. The doctor begins to prescribe clarithromycin, but is alerted to a possible interaction by the electronic prescribing system.

What is the main risk of prescribing clarithromycin in this case?

A. Hyperkalaemia
B. QT-interval prolongation
C. Renal impairment
D. Myopathy
E. Seizures

Infection

Warnings

56. A hospital antibiotic committee recommends the narrow-spectrum penicillin benzylpenicillin rather than the broad-spectrum penicillin amoxicillin as first-line antibiotic therapy for community-acquired pneumonia. It is to be prescribed with doxycycline.

What is the main advantage of narrow-spectrum over broad-spectrum antibiotics?

A. Easier to administer
B. Less likely to give rise to antibiotic resistance
C. Less likely to trigger an allergic reaction
D. More likely to be effective against β-lactamase-producing organisms
E. More likely to be effective where the pathogen is unknown

Infection

Resp

Warnings

57. A 4-year-old boy is found to have pneumonia.

What antibiotic is contraindicated at this age?

A. Amoxicillin
B. Cefotaxime
C. Co-amoxiclav
D. Clarithromycin
E. Doxycycline

Infection
Resp
Interactions
Comm

58. A 72-year-old woman is advised to take doxycycline 100 mg daily and prednisolone 30 mg daily for an exacerbation of COPD. Her usual medication is aspirin 75 mg daily, ferrous sulfate 200 mg twice daily, furosemide 40 mg daily, lansoprazole 30 mg daily and ramipril 5 mg daily.

What medicine should she be advised to separate from doxycycline by at least 2 hours?

A. Aspirin
B. Ferrous sulfate
C. Furosemide
D. Lansoprazole
E. Ramipril

Infection
Interactions
Comm

59. A 29-year-old man who has been advised to take antibiotics asks his doctor if he can drink alcohol while on treatment.

What antibiotic should not be taken with alcohol?

A. Amoxicillin
B. Clarithromycin
C. Doxycycline
D. Metronidazole
E. Trimethoprim

Infection
Interactions

60. A 58-year-old man attends his GP with a 2-day history of cough productive of green sputum, fever and shortness of breath on exertion. His medical history includes atrial fibrillation, hypertension and hypercholesterolaemia. His regular medications are bisoprolol, indapamide, ramipril, simvastatin and warfarin. He is allergic to penicillin and doxycycline. His GP diagnoses a lower respiratory tract infection (LRTI) and prescribes clarithromycin.

What drug should be held while he is taking clarithromycin to avoid a significant drug interaction?

A. Bisoprolol
B. Indapamide
C. Ramipril
D. Simvastatin
E. Warfarin

Infection
Admin

61. A 92-year-old man with severe fluid overload requires treatment with IV antibiotics. The cardiologist has recommended that these be given as low-volume bolus injections rather than by infusion if possible.

Which antibiotic can be administered as an IV bolus injection?

A. Amoxicillin
B. Clarithromycin
C. Doxycycline
D. Gentamicin
E. Vancomycin

Infection
Renal/GU
Monitoring

62. A 47-year-old woman is being treated with once-daily gentamicin for pyelonephritis. She received her first dose 21 hours ago. Her next dose is due in 3 hours and the nurse has called you to ask if any tests need to be performed before it is given.

What test should be performed 18–24 hours after the first dose of gentamicin?

A. Audiometry
B. C-reactive protein (CRP) concentration
C. Estimated glomerular filtration rate (eGFR)
D. Serum creatinine concentration
E. Serum gentamicin concentration

Infection
Monitoring
Prescription

63. A 54-year-old woman who presented with fever and left flank pain is found to have pyelonephritis. Co-amoxiclav 1.2 g IV 8-hrly is started. After 48 hours of antibiotics, her pain has improved and her temperature is 37.2°C.

Her blood tests show C-reactive protein (CRP) 88 mg/L (admission 206, normal <4), white cell count (WCC) 10 × 10⁹/L (admission 15, normal 4–11) and normal renal function. *Escherichia coli* was cultured from urine, sensitive to nitrofurantoin, co-amoxiclav and piperacillin–tazobactam, but resistant to trimethoprim. Renal ultrasound showed no obstruction or collection.

What is the most appropriate next step in management?

A. Continue IV co-amoxiclav
B. Stop antibiotics
C. Switch to oral co-amoxiclav
D. Switch to oral nitrofurantoin
E. Switch to IV piperacillin with tazobactam

Infection
Comm

64. A 19-year-old man has had seven episodes of genital herpes in the past year. He asks if he can start aciclovir tablets to reduce the frequency of attacks.

What is the most appropriate advice to give him regarding suppressive treatment with aciclovir?

A. He should take the treatment as soon as he notices the onset of symptoms

B. He should wash his hands before and after handling the tablets

C. He will need to continue the treatment indefinitely

D. It will clear his body of the virus within 6 months

E. It will not completely stop spread of infection to sexual partners

IV fluids

Indications

Prescription

65. A 75-year-old man who has long-term hypoxic brain injury is admitted to hospital because his gastrostomy feeding tube has become blocked. It is due to be replaced sometime the next day. You are asked to prescribe IV fluid to cover the next 24–36 hours.

He weighs 80 kg. He is not dehydrated. His serum potassium concentration and renal function are normal.

What is the most appropriate fluid regimen to prescribe at this stage?

A. 500 mL glucose 5% over 12 h;
500 mL sodium chloride 0.9% over 12 h

B. 1 L glucose 5% over 12 h;
1 L sodium chloride 0.9% over 12 h

C. 1 L sodium chloride 0.9% over 10 h;
1 L sodium chloride 0.9% over 10 h;
1 L glucose 5% with potassium chloride 40 mmol over 10 h

D. 1 L glucose 5% with potassium chloride 40 mmol over 8 h;
1 L glucose 5% with potassium chloride 40 mmol over 8 h;
500 mL sodium chloride 0.9% over 8 h

E. 1 L glucose 5% with potassium chloride 20 mmol over 8 h;
1 L glucose 5% with potassium chloride 20 mmol over 8 h;
1 L glucose 5% with potassium chloride 20 mmol over 8 h

IV fluids

Indications

Prescription

66. A 35-year-old woman is found to be hypotensive. She was admitted 6 hours ago with acute pancreatitis. Analgesia and IV fluids were administered and she was transferred to the ward. Over the past hour, her heart rate has been 100–110 beats/min and her blood pressure around 85/50 mmHg. She has not passed any urine since admission. Her serum potassium concentration is 5.1 mmol/L (normal 3.5–4.7).

What is the most appropriate option for initial fluid resuscitation?

A. Glucose 5% 500 mL IV over 10 minutes
B. Human albumin solution (HAS) 5% 250 mL IV over 10 minutes
C. Sodium chloride 0.9% 500 mL IV over 10 minutes
D. Sodium chloride 0.9% with potassium 20 mmol/L 500 mL IV over 10 minutes
E. Sterile water 500 mL IV over 10 minutes

MSK

Neuro

Mechanisms

67. A 66-year-old woman with severe chronic pain takes amitriptyline, ibuprofen, morphine, omeprazole and senna.

Which of her medications acts by inhibiting synthetic enzyme function?

A. Amitriptyline
B. Ibuprofen
C. Morphine
D. Omeprazole
E. Senna

MSK

Tox

AEs

68. A 63-year-old woman, who is an inpatient, complains of headache, nausea and sore mouth. She was admitted 2 weeks ago with a fracture of her left femoral neck. She has a past medical history of rheumatoid arthritis.

Blood tests reveal new renal and liver impairment and pancytopenia. Reviewing her drug chart, you notice that her methotrexate has been prescribed daily instead of weekly.

What is the most appropriate immediate treatment for her methotrexate toxicity?

A. Activated charcoal
B. Folic acid
C. Folinic acid
D. Granulocyte colony stimulating factor (G-CSF)
E. Haemodialysis

MSK

CVS

Warnings

69. A 63-year-old man with gout, hypertension and hypercholesterolaemia complains of swelling and pain in his left big toe. His GP makes a diagnosis of acute gout. His regular medications are allopurinol, amlodipine, indapamide, ramipril and simvastatin.

What drug could be stopped or substituted to reduce the risk of future attacks of gout?

A. Allopurinol
B. Amlodipine
C. Indapamide
D. Ramipril
E. Simvastatin

MSK

Warnings

70. A 62-year-old woman is found to have gout. Her past medical history includes asthma and hypertension. Her current medications are bendroflumethiazide, salbutamol and Symbicort®. She is intolerant to aspirin as it exacerbates her asthma.

What treatment for gout is most strongly contraindicated in this case?

A. Codeine
B. Colchicine
C. Naproxen
D. Paracetamol
E. Prednisolone

Neuro

Indications

71. A 45-year-old woman is seen in her GP surgery with a 6-month history of moderate depression. Attempts to treat this with cognitive-behavioural therapy have proved unsuccessful. There are no psychotic features and she is assessed to be at low risk of self-harm. She has no other medical problems.

What is the most appropriate treatment?

A. Amitriptyline
B. Citalopram
C. Mirtazapine
D. Olanzapine
E. Psychological interventions only

Neuro

Indications

Prescription

72. A 40-year-old man is brought to the emergency department because of a fit. He is accompanied by a friend who says the fit started about 25 minutes ago. On examination, there are findings consistent with an ongoing clonic seizure. The capillary blood glucose concentration is 5.9 mmol/L. No antiepileptic treatment has been administered so far.

What is the most appropriate immediate treatment?

A. Carbamazepine 200 mg by nasogastric tube
B. Chlordiazepoxide 30 mg by nasogastric tube
C. Lorazepam 4 mg by slow IV injection
D. Phenytoin 20 mg/kg by IV infusion
E. Valproate 10 mg/kg by slow IV injection

Neuro

Indications

73. A 31-year-old woman with a past psychiatric history of bipolar disorder presents with a 2-month history of tiredness, reduced appetite and a general dissatisfaction with life. The psychiatrist makes a diagnosis of moderate bipolar depression and recommends pharmacological treatment. She is not currently taking any mood-stabilising medication and is concerned about the risk of precipitating a manic episode.

What is the most appropriate treatment?

A. Gabapentin
B. Lamotrigine
C. Lithium
D. Sertraline
E. Valproate

Neuro

Indications

74. A 55-year-old man attends his GP complaining that he has been unable to sleep for weeks. He has recently lost his job and is worried about his finances. He would like to take something to help him sleep as he has a job interview in a few days.

What drug may be offered as a short-term measure to treat his insomnia?

A. Diazepam
B. Midazolam
C. Propofol
D. St John's wort
E. Zopiclone

Neuro

Indications

75. A 55-year-old man presents to his GP complaining of pain in his right foot. He describes a prickling, burning sensation that has been present for some weeks, particularly at night, and is interfering with sleep. He has a past medical history of type 2 diabetes, for which he takes metformin. He also takes paracetamol regularly but this is insufficient.

What is the most appropriate treatment at this stage?

A. Amitriptyline
B. Carbamazepine
C. Ibuprofen
D. Morphine
E. Tramadol

Neuro

Mechanisms

76. A 50-year-old woman with bipolar disorder is advised to take lamotrigine.

What is the most likely molecular site of action of lamotrigine?

A. Calcium channels
B. γ-aminobutyric acid (GABA) receptors
C. Potassium channels
D. Sodium channels
E. Synaptic vesicles

Neuro

Mechanisms

77. A 75-year-old man with generalised tonic–clonic seizures secondary to cerebrovascular disease is advised to take levetiracetam.

What is the most likely molecular site of action of levetiracetam?

A. Calcium channels
B. γ-aminobutyric acid (GABA) receptors
C. Potassium channels
D. Sodium channels
E. Synaptic vesicles

Neuro

Warnings

78. A 72-year-old woman has become aggressive on a general medical ward after being admitted with a significant urinary tract infection and delirium. Her medical problems include hypertension and type 2 diabetes. On admission, it was noted that her corrected QT interval was slightly prolonged. As she has been hitting the nursing staff with her walking stick repeatedly and is endangering herself and other patients a decision is made to administer a drug to calm her.

What drug should be avoided because of her prolonged QT interval?

A. Diazepam
B. Haloperidol
C. Lorazepam
D. Propofol
E. Zopiclone

Neuro

AEs

79. A 20-year-old woman with epilepsy, who suffers from generalised tonic–clonic seizures of undetermined aetiology, is advised to take lamotrigine.

What symptom should prompt her to seek urgent medical attention?

A. Difficulty concentrating
B. Headache
C. Nausea
D. Rash
E. Tiredness

Neuro

Warnings

80. A 34-year-old man presents to the emergency department following a tonic–clonic seizure. In the course of this, he knocked over a kettle of boiling water and sustained a significant burn injury to his right arm, which will need to be cleaned once adequate analgesia is established. He had a past medical history of focal epilepsy, for which he takes carbamazepine.

What analgesic is most strongly contraindicated in this setting?

A. Codeine
B. Morphine
C. Naproxen
D. Paracetamol
E. Tramadol

Neuro

Warnings

81. A 58-year-old woman complains of fizzing shapes in her vision, followed by a headache and nausea. Her past medical history includes asthma, ischaemic heart disease, osteoporosis, psoriasis and type 2 diabetes. Her doctor diagnoses migraine with aura and considers prescribing sumatriptan.

What is the main contraindication to prescribing sumatriptan in this case?

A. Asthma
B. Ischaemic heart disease
C. Osteoporosis
D. Psoriasis
E. Type 2 diabetes

Neuro

Interactions

82. A 56-year-old man, who is an inpatient, has a 2-minute generalised tonic–clonic seizure. He was admitted 1 week ago with chest pain caused by a pulmonary embolus. Dalteparin, warfarin, paracetamol and ibuprofen had been started. Three days ago, he was found to have hospital-acquired pneumonia, and meropenem was added. He has a past medical history of epilepsy. He takes sodium valproate (Epilim Chrono®) 500 mg 12-hrly. He is allergic to penicillin (it brings him out in hives).

What medication is most likely to have interacted with valproate to increase the risk of seizures?

A. Dalteparin
B. Ibuprofen
C. Meropenem
D. Paracetamol
E. Warfarin

Neuro

Monitoring

83. A 46-year-old woman with bipolar disorder is advised to take olanzapine and fluoxetine.

What monitoring option should be assessed at baseline and intermittently during therapy?

A. Albumin, bilirubin and INR
B. Haemoglobin and whi
C. Serum sodium and potassium
D. Thyroid stimulating hormone (TSH), triiodothyronine (T_3) and thyroxine (T_4)
E. Weight, lipid profile and haemoglobin A_{1c}

Neuro

Comm

84. An 84-year-old man is reviewed in the dementia clinic with his carer. He has been taking donepezil for 6 months following a diagnosis of dementia. Despite maximum dose, there has been a continued significant decline in his cognitive function.

What is the most appropriate advice to give him and his carer?

A. Donepezil does not work for everyone and so he should stop taking it
B. Full effects of treatment may not be seen for up to a year and so he should continue treatment
C. Splitting the dose (taking half in the morning and half at night) may improve efficacy
D. Switch to taking donepezil at night to improve efficacy
E. They should switch to rivastigmine

Renal/GU

Indications

Prescription

85. A 72-year-old woman is found to be hypokalaemic. She had an elective right knee arthroplasty 3 days ago. Over the last 24 hours she has developed vomiting and abdominal pain. Viral gastroenteritis is suspected, as other patients on the ward have been affected by the same symptoms.

On examination, her pulse is 88 beats/min and her blood pressure is 156/90 mmHg. Her mucous membranes are dry. Her serum potassium concentration is 2.3 mmol/L (3.5–4.7). The rest of her serum biochemistry is normal. The ECG shows small T waves.

What is the most appropriate initial treatment?

A. Co-amilofruse 5/40 1 tablet orally
B. Potassium chloride 40 mmol in 1 L of sodium chloride 0.9% IV over 2 hours
C. Potassium chloride 40 mmol in 1 L of glucose 5% IV over 1 hour
D. Potassium chloride/bicarbonate (Sando-K®) 3 tablets orally
E. Ramipril 5 mg orally

Renal/GU

Indications

86. A 69-year-old woman has persistent hyperkalaemia despite treatment with IV fluids, insulin and glucose. She was admitted 2 days earlier with diarrhoea and vomiting, which had caused an acute kidney injury. Preparations are being made for urgent haemodialysis.

What other medication may be considered to control hyperkalaemia while waiting for haemodialysis?

A. Calcium gluconate
B. Calcium polystyrene sulfonate (Calcium Resonium®)
C. Gliclazide
D. Ipratropium bromide
E. Salbutamol

Renal/GU

Mechanisms

87. A 73-year-old woman is advised to take oxybutynin to improve her symptoms of urinary urgency and urge incontinence.

What best describes the mechanism by which oxybutynin should improve her symptoms?

A. Agonism at the β_2-adrenoceptor
B. Antagonism at the α_1-adrenoceptor
C. Antagonism at the muscarinic M_3 receptor
D. Antagonism at the nicotinic acetylcholine receptor
E. Inhibition of 5α-reductase

Renal/GU

AEs

88. A 48-year-old man is found to be hyperkalaemic. One month ago he was admitted to hospital with a non-ST-elevation myocardial infarction, for which he underwent percutaneous intervention. His medications, which were all started during the recent hospital admission, comprise aspirin, clopidogrel, atorvastatin, bisoprolol and ramipril.

What drug is most likely to cause hyperkalaemia?

A. Aspirin
B. Atorvastatin
C. Bisoprolol
D. Clopidogrel
E. Ramipril

Renal/GU

AEs

Indications

89. A 92-year-old woman, who lives in a residential home for people with dementia, is found confused and wandering. Her caregivers think that this was precipitated by a medicine for 'overactive bladder', which was started last week. Unfortunately, they cannot find the drug in her room as she has been hiding things, and the GP surgery is closed.

What drug is most likely to have caused her confusion?

A. Finasteride
B. Furosemide
C. Solifenacin
D. Tamsulosin
E. Trimethoprim

Renal/GU

AEs

90. A 61-year-old man with benign prostatic enlargement is advised to take tamsulosin to improve urinary flow.

What side effect is most likely to occur when starting this new drug?

A. Bronchospasm
B. Postural hypotension
C. Erectile dysfunction
D. Gynaecomastia
E. Prostate cancer

Renal/GU
Warnings

91. An 82-year-old man with COPD is breathless and has recurrent exacerbations. His past medical history includes an episode of urinary retention secondary to benign prostatic enlargement.

What treatment should be used with caution in this patient?

A. Salbutamol
B. Salmeterol
C. Seretide®
D. Symbicort®
E. Tiotropium

Renal/GU
Infection
Warnings

92. A 33-year-old man with severe renal impairment requires antibiotic treatment for sepsis.

What antibiotic can generally be used without dosage reduction in severe renal impairment?

A. Benzylpenicillin
B. Co-amoxiclav
C. Gentamicin
D. Metronidazole
E. Vancomycin

Renal/GU
Interactions

93. A 67-year-old man presents to the GP to discuss his medication. For several years he has been taking sildenafil for erectile dysfunction. He has previously found this to be an effective and tolerable treatment, but says it has recently been causing headaches.

He has a past medical history of COPD. In addition, he was recently found to have atrial fibrillation. His treatment has been adjusted frequently over the past few weeks. His regular treatment now comprises digoxin, diltiazem, simvastatin, tiotropium and warfarin. Examination is normal other than for an irregular pulse at a rate of 80–90 beats/min.

What drug is most likely to interact with sildenafil to provoke side effects?

A. Digoxin
B. Diltiazem
C. Simvastatin
D. Tiotropium
E. Warfarin

Renal/GU
Interactions

94. A 60-year-old man is advised to take sildenafil as required for erectile dysfunction. His medical problems include hypertension and COPD. His medication includes doxazosin, indapamide, ramipril, and salbutamol and tiotropium inhalers.

What drug should he avoid taking at the same time of day as sildenafil?

A. Doxazosin
B. Indapamide
C. Ramipril
D. Salbutamol
E. Tiotropium

Resp

Indications

95. A 12-year-old boy sees his GP following hospital admission for an acute asthma attack. He has made a good recovery and is now asymptomatic.

What is the most appropriate treatment to prevent future asthma attacks?

A. Beclometasone
B. Formoterol
C. Chlorphenamine
D. Ipratropium
E. Salbutamol

Resp

Mechanisms

96. A 72-year-old man with hypertension, COPD and irritable bowel syndrome sees his GP for a medication review. His medicines are amlodipine, doxazosin, fluticasone, hyoscine butylbromide, ipratropium and salmeterol.

What receptors are most likely to have been activated by this treatment?

A. α_1-adrenoceptors
B. α_2-adrenoceptors
C. β_1-adrenoceptors
D. β_2-adrenoceptors
E. Muscarinic receptors

Resp

AEs

97. A 62-year-old man with COPD complains that one of his medications is causing a dry mouth. He is taking aminophylline, fluticasone, salbutamol, salmeterol and tiotropium.

What is the most likely cause of his dry mouth?

A. Aminophylline
B. Fluticasone
C. Salbutamol
D. Salmeterol
E. Tiotropium

Tox

Indications

98. A 31-year-old man presents 7 hours after a paracetamol overdose. His only symptoms are nausea and epigastric discomfort. He has no relevant past medical history and takes no regular medication. The serum paracetamol concentration is above the treatment line on the paracetamol poisoning treatment graph.

What is the most appropriate treatment?

265

A. Acetylcysteine
B. Activated charcoal
C. Cyclizine
D. Omeprazole
E. Naloxone

Tox

Indications

99. A 68-year-old man is brought to the emergency department because he has become increasingly drowsy over the past 24 hours. He has had diarrhoea for the preceding week. His medical problems include chronic back pain, epilepsy and depression. Regular medications include diazepam, morphine, fluoxetine, paracetamol and sodium valproate. On examination, he has a Glasgow Coma Score (GCS) of 9 (scale range 3–15) and a respiratory rate of 8 breaths/min. His pupils are pinpoint. He appears dehydrated and blood tests reveal an acute kidney injury. Drug toxicity as a result of reduced renal elimination is suspected.

What is the most appropriate initial treatment?

A. Acetylcysteine
B. Activated charcoal
C. Flumazenil
D. Naloxone
E. Sodium bicarbonate

Tox

AEs

100. A 24-year-old woman is receiving an IV infusion of acetylcysteine for paracetamol poisoning. Thirty minutes into the infusion, she develops a rash. On examination, her heart rate is 95 beats/min and her blood pressure is 117/78 mmHg. She has a widespread urticarial rash.

What is the most appropriate immediate management?

A. Continue acetylcysteine and give chlorphenamine
B. Continue acetylcysteine and give ranitidine
C. Temporarily stop acetylcysteine and give adrenaline
D. Temporarily stop acetylcysteine and give chlorphenamine
E. Temporarily stop acetylcysteine and give ranitidine

Answers and explanations

1. B. Dalteparin 5000 units subcutaneous (SC) daily. All patients admitted to hospital should be assessed for the risk of developing venous thromboembolism (VTE). Pharmacological prophylaxis should be prescribed if there are any thrombotic risk factors, provided the patient is not at risk of bleeding. This patient's thrombotic risk factors include her age, history of deep venous thrombosis (DVT) and likely immobility during her acute illness. The usual choice is a <u>low molecular weight heparin</u> (LMWH) prescribed at a 'prophylactic dose', such as dalteparin 5000 units SC daily or enoxaparin 40 mg SC daily.

LMWH is preferred over <u>unfractionated heparin</u> (UFH) because its effect is more predictable. However, it is eliminated by the kidneys so is less appropriate in patients with renal impairment. In these cases, UFH may be used. <u>Aspirin</u> is usually employed to prevent *arterial* thromboembolism: for example, after a stroke. Its role in the prophylaxis of venous thrombosis is limited. <u>Warfarin</u> is used in the treatment of *established* VTE to prevent clot extension and recurrence. In this context, it is often initially combined with a LMWH. However, it is not employed routinely in inpatients to prevent VTE.

2. D. Quinine. While glucose-6-phosphate dehydrogenase (G6PD) deficiency is rare in northern Europe, it is common in southern Europe, parts of Africa, Asia and Oceania. Because of its X-linked inheritance pattern, it is more common in men. G6PD is an oxidative enzyme, which if inhibited (in the context of a deficiency state) leads to haemolysis of red blood cells. Food triggers of acute haemolysis classically include fava beans. Drug causes in the top 100 list include <u>aspirin</u>, <u>nitrofurantoin</u>, <u>quinolones</u>, <u>sulfonylureas</u> and <u>quinine</u>. There is significant variation between individuals in their response to different drugs, and many other drugs have not been tested for their effects on G6PD.

3. C. Idarucizumab. Dabigatran is a direct oral anticoagulant (DOAC) that directly inhibits thrombin, preventing conversion of fibrinogen to fibrin. Idarucizumab is a humanised monoclonal antibody fragment that binds to dabigatran and its metabolites, reversing its effects. Andexanet α is a recombinant, modified form of human factor Xa that reverses drugs that inhibit factor Xa, whether directly (e.g. rivaroxaban) or indirectly (e.g. <u>heparins and fondaparinux</u>). It has demonstrated efficacy in clinical trials and, at the time of writing, is under review by medicines regulators for its marketing authorisation.

Anticoagulation with warfarin can be reversed by <u>phytomenadione</u>, which replenishes vitamin K_1 for the synthesis of new clotting factors. In major bleeding, dried prothrombin complex can be used to replace factors IX, VII and X directly.

Protamine is a highly cationic peptide that forms a stable complex with heparin molecules, reversing their anticoagulant effect. It is most effective against unfractionated heparin but also binds low molecular weight heparins. It is ineffective against fondaparinux.

4. A. Carbamazepine. <u>Warfarin</u> is metabolised by cytochrome P450 (CYP) enzymes. <u>Carbamazepine</u> is an 'inducer' of certain CYP enzymes; that is, it interacts with the regulatory regions of the genes to increase their transcription. The resulting increase in the amount of enzyme allows warfarin to be metabolised more rapidly. This means that less warfarin is available to inhibit clotting factor production, so its anticoagulant effect is diminished and the international normalised ratio (INR) falls. This puts the patient at risk of thromboembolic complications. <u>Valproate</u> is a CYP *inhibitor,* so its effect would be to *increase* the INR. <u>Gabapentin and pregabalin</u> have few drug interactions. Diazepam is a <u>benzodiazepine</u> which is used to treat acute seizures but is not used for chronic seizure prophylaxis. It does not interact with warfarin.

The term 'cytochrome P450' refers to a family of enzymes. At undergraduate level you would not be expected to know about the individual members of this family, so it is reasonable to consider them collectively. Moreover, there is some cross-talk between the family members. For example, carbamazepine is a major inducer of CYP3A4 (the CYP enzyme that, in general, makes the greatest contribution to drug metabolism), but like most other CYP3A4 inducers, it also induces CYP2C9 (the most important contributor to warfarin metabolism).

5. B. Antifactor Xa assay. Low molecular weight heparins (LMWHs), e.g. dalteparin, promote binding of antithrombin to factor Xa, inhibiting the final part of the clotting cascade to prevent production of a fibrin clot. LMWH-related anticoagulation can be quantified with an antifactor Xa assay. This is not required routinely, but it may be useful when the LMWH effect is less predictable, such as in pregnancy, renal impairment and significantly abnormal body weight. Platelet count and serum potassium should be measured in patients receiving LMWH for >4 days to monitor for side effects (heparin-induced thrombocytopenia, hyperkalaemia), but this is not an indicator of anticoagulation.

In patients undergoing anticoagulation with <u>unfractionated heparin (UFH)</u>, careful monitoring of the activated partial thromboplastin time (APTT) is required. This is expressed as the activated partial thromboplastin ratio (APTR), calculated as the patient's APTT divided by that of a normal control. The rate of infusion is adjusted to achieve a target APTR of 1.5–2.5, representing sufficient but not excessive anticoagulation. <u>Warfarin</u> is monitored using the international normalised ratio (INR), the ratio of the patient's prothrombin time to that of a normal control. The target INR in most indications is 2.0–3.0. Fibrinogen is an acute phase protein and a marker of disseminated intravascular coagulation (a disordered clotting state usually associated with severe acute illness). It is not a useful measure of therapeutic anticoagulation.

6. B. Bisoprolol. Angina occurs when, as a result of narrowed atheromatous coronary arteries, insufficient blood is supplied to the myocardium to meet its oxygen demand. β-blockers, such as bisoprolol, are first choice drugs for the prevention of angina. They work by slowing the heart rate and reducing cardiac contractility, which in turn reduces myocardial work and oxygen demand. <u>Calcium channel blockers</u> and long-acting <u>nitrates</u> are alternatives. Short-acting <u>nitrates</u>, such as glyceryl trinitrate, are taken during an attack of angina to relieve chest pain.

They can be taken before exercise to reduce the risk of angina, but are less effective in preventing angina than regularly administered alternatives.

Aspirin, ACE inhibitors and statins do not directly prevent angina. A statin should be offered to all patients with ischaemic heart disease to reduce the risk of future coronary events. ACE inhibitors and aspirin should be offered to people who have atherosclerotic disease (e.g. ischaemic heart disease, cerebrovascular disease) to reduce the risk of recurrent events or death.

7. D. Ramipril. Clinical trials have shown that angiotensin-converting enzyme (ACE) inhibitors (e.g. ramipril), antiplatelet agents (e.g. aspirin, clopidogrel), β-blockers and statins significantly reduce the risk of recurrent events or death following a myocardial infarction. These drugs should be prescribed in combination for secondary prevention of cardiovascular events in all patients following myocardial infarction unless contraindicated.

The other drugs have no role in secondary prevention following myocardial infarction. Amiloride is a potassium-sparing diuretic, used to reduce potassium losses in patients taking other diuretics (loop or thiazide diuretics). Digoxin is a cardiac glycoside. It is an option for rate control in atrial fibrillation (AF), particularly in people with heart failure. Glyceryl trinitrate is a nitrate which is used to relieve angina by reducing myocardial work and oxygen demand; however, it does not prevent myocardial infarction. Warfarin is an anticoagulant. It is used to reduce the risk of intracardiac thrombus formation and therefore of systemic embolism in patients with AF.

8. E. Spironolactone. This patient needs treatment to control her symptoms of heart failure (ankle swelling and shortness of breath), and to normalise her serum potassium concentration, since hypokalaemia is associated with a risk of dangerous arrhythmias. Spironolactone is an aldosterone antagonist which competitively blocks the aldosterone receptor, causing increased sodium and water excretion and potassium retention in the distal renal tubules. Although aldosterone antagonists are relatively weak diuretics, they can improve symptoms and reduce mortality in patients with moderate heart failure. They also increase the serum potassium concentration. Eplerenone is an alternative aldosterone antagonist; it is significantly more expensive but is a useful option if spironolactone is not tolerated due to endocrine side effects.

Furosemide (a loop diuretic, like bumetanide which she is already taking) and indapamide (a thiazide-like diuretic) could improve symptoms by increasing sodium and water excretion. However, both drugs may further reduce the serum potassium concentration by increasing renal potassium excretion. Nitrates are used in the treatment of acute, but not chronic, heart failure and will not address the hypokalaemia. Amiloride (a potassium-sparing diuretic) can increase the serum potassium concentration but is a weak diuretic that will have little impact on symptoms and offers no prognostic benefits in heart failure.

9. B. Bisoprolol. There are two basic approaches to managing chronic atrial fibrillation (AF). One is 'rhythm control', which seeks to restore normal sinus rhythm either by electrical cardioversion, antiarrhythmic drugs, or both. The other is 'rate control', in which the abnormal heart rhythm is accepted as permanent, and efforts are focused simply on preventing ventricular rate from running too fast. In most cases, rate control is just as effective as rhythm control and considerably simpler.

The ideal agent for ventricular rate control in AF is either a β-blocker (e.g. bisoprolol) or a non-dihydropyridine calcium channel blocker (e.g. verapamil or diltiazem). In practice, a β-blocker is used in most patients. This would be a particularly appropriate choice for this patient because of his history of heart failure: β-blockers are indicated in heart failure to improve prognosis, whereas verapamil and diltiazem should be avoided.

Digoxin can be used for rate control in AF but, on its own, it is less effective than a β-blocker or calcium channel blocker and potentially more toxic. Likewise, although amiodarone is an effective agent for both rate and rhythm control in AF, it is much too toxic for first-line use. Doxazosin is an α-blocker used in hypertension and benign prostatic enlargement; it has no role in AF.

10. B. Furosemide. Furosemide is a loop diuretic which inhibits the $Na^+/K^+/2Cl^-$ co-transporter in the ascending limb of the loop of Henle, preventing transport of sodium, potassium and chloride ions from the renal tubular lumen into the epithelial cell.

Bisoprolol and spironolactone are receptor antagonists that block $β_1$-adrenoceptors and aldosterone receptors, respectively (see β-blockers and Aldosterone antagonists). Ramipril and simvastatin are enzyme inhibitors. Ramipril is an ACE inhibitor, preventing conversion of angiotensin I to angiotensin II. Simvastatin, a statin, inhibits 3-hydroxy-3-methyl-glutaryl coenzyme A (HMG CoA) reductase, preventing the synthesis of cholesterol.

11. C. $β_1$-adrenoceptor. Metoprolol is a β-blocker that is relatively selective for the $β_1$-adrenoceptor. Blockade of this receptor reduces the force of myocardial contraction and decreases the speed of electrical conduction in the heart. By prolonging the refractory period of the atrioventricular (AV) node and slowing conduction in the atria, it can terminate some supraventricular tachycardias and reduce the ventricular rate in atrial fibrillation.

$β_2$-adrenoceptors are found in smooth muscle, such as in the bronchial tree; $β_3$-adrenoceptors are found in adipose tissue. Blockade of these receptors is not clinically useful in the management of supraventricular tachycardias. Metoprolol does not have any effect on α-adrenoceptors.

12. B. Diltiazem. Diltiazem, like verapamil, is a non-dihydropyridine calcium channel blocker. Non-dihydropyridine calcium channel blockers are relatively cardioselective: they reduce the rate and force of cardiac contraction, and interfere with conduction at the atrioventricular (AV) node. These effects are similar to those of β-blockers. Non-dihydropyridine calcium channel blockers and β-blockers should not be combined except under the close supervision of a specialist, as their effects on the heart are additive. Together, they can cause heart block, cardiogenic shock, and even asystole. This patient has third-degree heart block: that is, transmission between the atria and ventricles is completely blocked and the chambers are now beating independently. This serious interaction highlights the dangers of prescribing drugs without a full and accurate medication history.

13. A. Amlodipine. Ankle swelling is a common adverse effect of treatment with dihydropyridine calcium channel blockers. It is understood to be due to preferential dilatation of the pre-capillary arterioles, relative to post-capillary venules, causing increased pressure in the capillary bed and therefore greater filtration of fluid from vessels to the interstitium. Chlortalidone is a thiazide-like diuretic. It does not cause oedema and, in other situations, might be expected to improve it. However, calcium channel blocker-induced oedema does not respond well to diuresis, because it is not due to increased extracellular fluid (ECF) volume. Drugs with a venodilation effect, notably ACE inhibitors and angiotensin receptor antagonists, may help. The oral diabetes agents gliclazide (a sulphonylurea) and metformin, and the inhaled antimuscarinic drug tiotropium, do not cause oedema.

14. D. Medicines and Healthcare Products Regulatory Agency (MHRA). In the UK, suspected adverse effects of medicines should be reported to the medicines regulator (the MHRA) by health professionals or the public using the Yellow Card scheme. All serious suspected adverse drug reactions should be reported. In this context, 'serious' is defined as a reaction that caused death or was life threatening, caused or prolonged hospital admission, resulted in significant disability or incapacity, or was considered in any other way 'medically significant'. In addition, all reactions (regardless of seriousness) to drugs undergoing intensive surveillance (identified by a ▼black triangle) should be reported, as should all reactions occurring in children.

The Care Quality Commission (CQC) is the UK regulator of health and social care organisations. The National Institute for Health and Care Excellence (NICE) is a non-departmental public body that provides guidance and advice on health and social care matters (notably the use of medicines and other medical technologies) in the UK. The British National Formulary (BNF) is a prescribing reference manual published jointly by the BMJ Group and the Pharmaceutical Press.

15. C. Clopidogrel. Clopidogrel is an antiplatelet agent. It is used to reduce the risk of future strokes in patients with a history of cerebrovascular disease. As it irreversibly inhibits platelet aggregation, its effect takes 7–10 days to wear off (reflecting the lifespan of circulating platelets). If surgery is planned in patients who take antiplatelet and anticoagulant medications, an assessment should be made about their risk of bleeding from surgery and their risk of thrombosis. In this case, it is probably advisable to withhold the patient's antiplatelet drug for the week before surgery, assuming her other vascular risk factors are well controlled. Antiplatelet drugs should not be stopped within 6–12 months of insertion of a coronary artery stent without first discussing this with a cardiologist.

16. D. 8am and 3pm. Isosorbide mononitrate is a nitrate that is used to control angina. Nitrates are associated with tachyphylaxis, a phenomenon in which they become less effective with continued use. To minimise this, it is helpful to have a 'nitrate-free period' overnight, when the patient is inactive. In this example, dosing at 8am and 3pm ensures the patient receives the peak activity of the drug during active daytime hours, with a nitrate-free period overnight. An alternative strategy could be to use a modified-release preparation, taken once daily in the morning.

17. A. Intramuscularly into the anterolateral thigh. Adrenaline (epinephrine) is the most important treatment for anaphylaxis. People who have experienced an anaphylactic reaction should be provided with an adrenaline auto-injector for self-administration in the event of a recurrent attack. The EpiPen® (adult form) is designed to deliver 300 micrograms of adrenaline as an intramuscular (IM) injection. It should be administered into the anterolateral thigh. You do this by removing the blue safety cap then jabbing the orange end of the device firmly against the outer thigh, holding it there for about 10 seconds. It can be given through clothing if necessary. Of note, not all the contents of the glass cartridge will be injected; the device contains 2 mg of adrenaline (as a 1 mg/mL solution) and delivers only 0.3 mg (0.3 mL) of this.

Injection into smaller muscles is less desirable, as absorption is not as reliable, but they can be used if necessary. The SC route should not be used, as absorption is too slow. Adrenaline must not be administered intravenously unless cardiac arrest supervenes.

18. B. Liver profile. Around 1 in 200 patients taking a statin will develop elevated liver enzymes or significant muscle side effects (myopathy, rhabdomyolysis). Early detection of this allows treatment to be adjusted, minimising the risk of long-term harm. A liver profile should be measured before starting statin treatment and again at 3 months. The statin should be stopped if liver transaminase levels increase to greater than three times the upper limit of normal.

Patients should be advised to report new muscle aches and pains to their doctor. However, there is no need to check creatine kinase levels unless these occur. Thyroid function should be checked *before* a statin is started, as untreated hypothyroidism is a reversible cause of hyperlipidaemia and can increase the risk of adverse effects from statins. A lipid profile may be a useful marker of *efficacy*, rather than safety, although in current guidelines target levels are specified only for secondary prevention.

19. D. Serum potassium. Eplerenone is an aldosterone antagonist. It acts by inhibiting the effects of aldosterone. This leads to increased sodium and water excretion and potassium retention. Patients are therefore at risk of developing hyperkalaemia. Serum potassium concentrations should be checked before and within 1–2 weeks of starting aldosterone antagonists, and whenever a dose adjustment is made.

20. C. Dry cough. Dry cough is a common side effect associated with ACE inhibitor therapy. It is due to increased levels of bradykinin, which is usually inactivated by ACE. Where it is problematic, an angiotensin receptor blocker may be offered as an alternative. These blockers do not inhibit ACE.

21. B. 48 mol/mol. Haemoglobin A_{1c} (HbA$_{1c}$) is used in three main ways:
1. To **diagnose** diabetes mellitus.
2. To set a **target** level of glycaemic control with an existing therapeutic regimen (e.g. to guide dosage titration).
3. To **trigger intensification** of treatment, by offering another agent.
Diagnostic and therapeutic decisions are commonly made at three key HbA$_{1c}$ levels (**48, 53** and **58 mmol/mol**), which are therefore worth committing to memory. Remember these in units of mmol/mol because, although percentage values are easier to recall, they are no longer quoted (because of a drive for international harmonisation).

HbA$_{1c}$ values ≥**48 mmol/mol** can support a **diagnosis** of diabetes mellitus. Patients treated by lifestyle measures should **target** HbA$_{1c}$ levels <48 mmol/mol, and drug treatment should be started if this is not achieved. Patients taking a single agent should also target HbA$_{1c}$ <48 mmol/mol, but in those on two or more agents the target is **<53 mmol/mol** (recognising that treatment with two agents carries more risks and burdens, which may offset its glycaemic control benefits). The trigger for **intensification** of pharmacological treatment (i.e. adding another agent) is HbA$_{1c}$ ≥**58 mmol/mol**.

22. D. Metformin. Metformin is the first-line choice for type 2 diabetes because it lowers blood glucose without causing weight gain or hypoglycaemia, it is associated with decreased risk of cardiovascular mortality and it is cheap. The place in therapy of dipeptidylpeptidase-4 (DPP-4) inhibitors (e.g. sitagliptin) as second-line alternatives or add-on treatment to metformin is determined by their favourable effects on body weight and relatively low risk of hypoglycaemia compared with alternatives, e.g. sulphonylureas. However, they have not been shown to have cardiovascular benefits and are comparatively expensive.

Sulphonylureas (e.g. gliclazide) lower blood glucose by stimulating pancreatic insulin secretion. This is associated with weight gain and an increased risk of hypoglycaemia. Sulphonylureas are therefore used as second- or third-line agents where blood glucose is not controlled on metformin alone. Insulin has similar adverse effects and is reserved for people with type 2 diabetes where oral hypoglycaemics in combination are ineffective.

Acarbose inhibits intestinal α-glucosidases, delaying the digestion and absorption of starch and sucrose. Its effects on blood glucose are small compared with other oral hypoglycaemic drugs and it doesn't feature in the NICE guidelines for the management of type 2 diabetes. It is not among the top 100 most frequently prescribed drugs.

23. D. Reduced hepatic glucose output. The main mechanism by which metformin lowers blood glucose is through a reduction in hepatic glucose output (from gluconeogenesis). It may also improve peripheral insulin sensitivity (and therefore glucose uptake) but this is probably less important to its glucose-lowering effect. Other minor contributors to its glucose-lowering effect include weight loss and reduced dietary intake.

24. B. Aromatase inhibition. Anastrozole is a <u>sex hormone antagonist</u>. It acts by inhibiting aromatase, which prevents the peripheral conversion of androstendedione to oestendione. This reduces the amount of oestendione that can be converted to oestradiol (the active form of oestrogen). Reducing oestradiol decreases the amount able to bind oestrogen-receptor positive breast cancers, reducing tumour growth. Tamoxifen is another example of a sex hormone antagonist used in breast cancer treatment, but it acts as a selective oestrogen receptor modulator.

5α-reductase inhibitors, e.g. finasteride, are used in the treatment of benign prostatic enlargement. <u>Antifungals</u> such as fluconazole inhibit ergosterol synthesis. <u>Oestrogens and progestogens</u> suppress luteinising hormone (LH)/follicle-stimulating hormone (FSH) secretion.

25. C. Gliclazide. <u>Sulphonylureas</u> (e.g. gliclazide) lower blood glucose by stimulating pancreatic insulin secretion. Hypoglycaemia is a potentially serious adverse effect, which is more likely with high treatment doses, where drug metabolism is reduced, where risk of hypoglycaemia is increased and where other glucose-lowering medications are prescribed.

<u>Metformin</u> lowers blood glucose by reducing hepatic glucose output and doesn't usually cause hypoglycaemia. <u>Bendroflumethiazide</u> and <u>prednisolone</u> both raise blood glucose and can reduce the efficacy of glucose-lowering agents. <u>β-blockers</u> may mask symptoms of hypoglycaemia such as sweating, shaking, tachycardia and anxiety, which are mediated by sympathoadrenal activation.

26. C. Lactic acidosis. The molecular mechanism of metformin is complex and not fully understood. It inhibits complex I of the mitochondrial electron transport chain, causing a change in cellular redox state with an increase in lactate:pyruvate ratio. Metformin has rarely been associated with a state of severe metabolic acidosis and high serum lactate concentration (together termed **lactic acidosis**). This is a serious condition that may be life threatening. The extent to which this is *caused by,* as opposed to *associated with*, metformin is controversial. Clinical trial and population data suggest that metformin does not increase the risk in stable patients taking standard doses. However, in supratherapeutic concentrations (due to overdose or renal impairment, since metformin is eliminated by the kidneys), meformin may be a contributory factor.

Metformin does not cause respiratory alkalosis or diabetic ketoacidosis. The risk of hypersensitivity reactions is unlikely to be altered by renal impairment. Metformin may interfere with vitamin B_{12} absorption and therefore cause or contribute to megaloblastic anaemia, but renal failure is unlikely to modulate this effect significantly.

27. B. Gliclazide. Gliclazide, a <u>sulphonylurea</u>, acts by stimulating pancreatic insulin secretion. Its adverse effects are predictable from the actions of insulin, including hypoglycaemia and weight gain. All the other drugs are oral antihyperglycaemic agents with a low risk of hypoglycaemia. Empagliflozin is a sodium–glucose co-transporter 2 (SGLT-2) inhibitor, which inhibits reabsorption of glucose from the proximal renal tubule. This lowers blood glucose, but as insulin secretion is not stimulated, and normal homeostatic responses to hypoglycaemia are intact, the risk of hypoglycaemia is low. <u>Metformin</u> acts mainly by reducing hepatic glucose output and, to a lesser extent, improving peripheral insulin sensitivity. Pioglitazone is a thiazolidinedione. It activates the γ subclass of nuclear peroxisome proliferator-activated receptors (PPARγ), promoting expression of genes which enhance insulin sensitivity. It does not increase insulin secretion and so does not increase the risk of hypoglycaemia, but it does promote weight gain. Thiazolidinediones increase the risk and severity of heart failure. This concern, among other factors, has been associated with reduced prescribing of this drug class. Sitagliptin, a <u>DPP-4 inhibitor</u>, targets the enzyme that inactivates incretins. Incretins promote insulin secretion, but only when the blood glucose concentration is normal or elevated, so hypoglycaemia is not induced.

28. D. Hydrocortisone. Medically administered <u>systemic corticosteroids</u>, like endogenous corticosteroids, suppress hypothalamic secretion of corticotropin-releasing hormone (CRH) and pituitary secretion of adrenocorticotropic hormone (ACTH). When taken chronically, prolonged suppression of ACTH release leads to adrenocortical atrophy. If the exogenous steroid is then stopped abruptly, or if the stress of an intercurrent illness necessitates increased corticosteroid secretion, the atrophied adrenal glands may be unable to meet this need. The resulting state of acute adrenal insufficiency (an 'Addisonian crisis') may cause hypotension and various non-specific symptoms (e.g. confusion, weakness, nausea, abdominal pain).

In this case, it is possible that acute adrenal insufficiency explains the patient's presentation. Parenteral corticosteroid replacement must be given urgently. If she does have a 'surgical abdomen', she still requires intensified corticosteroid therapy to cover the associated physiological stress. A typical choice for acute steroid replacement is **hydrocortisone 100 mg IV**. Fludrocortisone is a mineralocorticoid that will not address the acute need for glucocorticoid replacement. Budesonide and fluticasone (see <u>Corticosteroids, inhaled</u>) and prednisolone are glucocorticoids, but they cannot be administered IV. Fluid resuscitation (e.g. with <u>sodium chloride 0.9%</u>) should also be given urgently.

29. D. There is an increased risk of cancer of the lining of the womb.
Tamoxifen is a <u>sex hormone antagonist</u>, which can lead to endometrial changes including a small risk of endometrial cancer, but not ovarian cancer. Patients should be advised to report vaginal bleeding to their doctor. Other side effects include *suppression* of lactation and increased risk of venous thromboembolism. Tamoxifen does not cause infertility, and is in fact a treatment option in anovulatory infertility. It is not safe in pregnancy, as it increases the risk of abnormal fetal development.

30. E. Pancreatitis. A rare adverse effect of <u>DPP-4 inhibitors</u> is acute pancreatitis, affecting 0.1–1% people taking these drugs. DPP-4 inhibitors should therefore be used with caution in people with a previous history of pancreatitis. Patients should be advised to stop taking the drug and seek urgent medical attention if they develop symptoms that could indicate acute pancreatitis (e.g. severe and persistent stomach pain which may reach through to the back).

None of the other conditions listed require caution or are contraindications to DPP-4 inhibitor therapy. As many DPP-4 inhibitors are renally excreted, a dose reduction may be required for people with moderate to severe renal impairment.

31. D. Metformin. Metformin must be withheld before and for 48 hours after injection of IV contrast media (e.g. for computerised tomography [CT] scans, coronary angiography) when there is an increased risk of renal impairment because of contrast nephropathy. This can lead to metformin accumulation and lactic acidosis.

32. B. Fluoxetine. Tamoxifen is a <u>sex hormone antagonist</u>. It is a prodrug that requires activation by a cytochrome P450 (CYP) enzyme, CYP2D6. CYP2D6 is also involved in the metabolism of other drugs, including codeine (also a prodrug, which is metabolised by CYP2D6 to morphine), loratadine, propranolol and risperidone. Fluoxetine, a <u>selective serotonin reuptake inhibitor (SSRI)</u>, is a potent inhibitor of CYP2D6. For the prodrugs tamoxifen and codeine, inhibition of CYP2D6 results in lower plasma levels of active metabolites. This can result in reduced efficacy. For drugs that are inactivated by CYP2D6, such as propranolol (a β-blocker), risperidone (a <u>second-generation antipsychotic</u>) and loratadine (an <u>antihistamine</u>), the interaction may increase the risk of adverse effects.

33. D. Increase lamotrigine dosage. <u>Lamotrigine</u> is metabolised by glucuronidation. Other drugs, including <u>oestrogens</u> such as ethinylestradiol, can induce more rapid lamotrigine glucuronidation. This reduces lamotrigine concentrations and may lead to a loss of seizure control. If contraception with a systemic oestrogen is considered appropriate (alternative contraception, e.g. with an intrauterine device, may be preferable), a pre-emptive increase to the dosage of lamotrigine should be considered. This may be supported by plasma lamotrigine concentration measurement.

34. C. It is associated with a lower risk of death from cardiovascular complications. In comparative studies, <u>metformin</u> was associated with a lower risk of cardiovascular death than <u>sulphonylureas</u> despite a similar reduction in blood glucose. Another class of oral antihyperglycaemic agent that appears to lower cardiovascular risk are SGLT-2 inhibitors (not yet in the top 100 most frequently prescribed drugs). No such effect has been demonstrated for <u>DPP-4 inhibitors</u> or <u>thiazolidinediones</u>.

<u>Metformin</u> lowers blood glucose without causing hypoglycaemia or weight gain. By contrast, <u>sulphonylureas</u> lower blood glucose by stimulating pancreatic insulin secretion, hence causing hypoglycaemia and weight gain. The most common reason that metformin is not tolerated is abdominal side effects, such as nausea, cramps and diarrhoea.

Both sulphonylureas and metformin cost around 3p per tablet, considerably cheaper than newer antidiabetic drugs, e.g. <u>DPP-4 inhibitors</u> such as sitagliptin, which cost £1–2 per dose.

35. E. Ondansetron. Predicting which antiemetic will work in which patient is not easy. In practice, drug selection is often based on pragmatic considerations such as familiarity and availability, and then adjusted according to the patient's response. With the patient having already had cyclizine (an <u>antiemetic</u> that acts by <u>histamine H₁-receptor antagonism</u>), it would now be best to offer her a drug from a different class. This choice is influenced by her past reaction to prochlorperazine, which sounds like neuroleptic malignant syndrome (NMS). NMS is a serious condition that may be precipitated by drugs that have an antidopaminergic effect, including <u>phenothiazine antiemetics</u> (e.g. prochlorperazine, chlorpromazine), <u>dopamine antagonist antiemetics</u> (e.g. metoclopramide) and <u>antipsychotics</u> (including haloperidol, which is sometimes also used as an antiemetic). The risk of recurrence of NMS with re-exposure is unclear, but it would be prudent to avoid these drug classes where suitable alternatives exist. Ondansetron is an antiemetic that works by <u>serotonin 5-HT₃-receptor antagonism</u>; it is not associated with NMS.

36. E. Omeprazole, clarithromycin and metronidazole. *Helicobacter pylori* is a Gram-negative bacterium which causes peptic ulcer disease. Effective treatment requires combination therapy with two antibiotics and a <u>proton pump inhibitor (PPI)</u> for 1 week. Treatment with a single antibiotic may be ineffective and may cause the bacteria to develop resistance.

The various regimens considered acceptable for *H. pylori* eradication, including recommended drug doses, are set out in a helpful table in the BNF. Options for proton pump inhibition include lansoprazole, omeprazole and pantoprazole. The antibiotics are selected from amoxicillin (a <u>broad-spectrum penicillin</u>), clarithromycin (a <u>macrolide</u>) and <u>metronidazole</u>. As this patient has previously had an anaphylactic reaction to benzylpenicillin, amoxicillin is contraindicated and clarithromycin with metronidazole should be used. You should note that the doses recommended for antibiotics when used in *H. pylori* eradication may differ from those used in other indications.

37. A. Loperamide. Loperamide is an <u>antimotility drug</u> used in selected cases of diarrhoea. Pharmacologically, it is an <u>opioid</u> similar to pethidine, but unlike other opioids it does not cross the blood–brain barrier. This means it is devoid of central nervous system (CNS) effects, including analgesia, but retains the peripheral effects such as reducing gut motility. The antimotility effects are mediated by opioid μ-receptor agonism in the myenteric plexus of the gastrointestinal (GI) tract.

While the other opioids in this list will have similar antimotility effects, they are likely also to cause CNS effects which, in this context, are undesirable.

38. C. Lactulose. One of the main substances involved in the pathogenesis of hepatic encephalopathy is ammonia. Lactulose is an <u>osmotic laxative</u> that reduces absorption of ammonia by increasing the transit rate of colonic contents and by acidifying the stool, which inhibits the proliferation of ammonia-producing bacteria. This makes it an important treatment for patients with, or at risk of, hepatic encephalopathy, regardless of whether they are constipated. In these circumstances, the aim should be for patients to produce three loose stools each day. The other drugs are all laxatives that will treat the patient's constipation but will not be as beneficial in treating his encephalopathy.

39. D. Loratadine orally. Pruritus is a common problem in liver disease. Non-pharmacological measures such as warm baths may be helpful but are often insufficient. First-line pharmacological treatment is usually with an <u>antihistamine</u>. When prescribing for patients with advanced liver disease, it is important to avoid using sedating drugs wherever possible. This is because sedation can precipitate hepatic encephalopathy. Chlorphenamine is a first-generation antihistamine with pronounced sedative effects. By contrast, loratadine is a second-generation antihistamine which, by virtue of not crossing the blood–brain barrier, does not cause sedation.

 <u>Topical corticosteroids</u> are sometimes used for inflammatory lesions associated with pruritus (e.g. eczema), but they are not an option for generalised pruritus. <u>Systemic corticosteroids</u> are not used for pruritus. As an <u>opioid</u> agonist, codeine phosphate may *cause* itch. Furthermore, its sedative effects may be problematic.

40. C. Antagonism of histamine H$_2$ receptors in gastric parietal cells. Ranitidine is a <u>histamine H$_2$-receptor blocker</u>. Histamine is released from paracrine cells in the stomach and binds to H$_2$ receptors on gastric parietal cell walls. Acting through second messenger systems, this activates the proton pumps that are responsible for gastric acid secretion. By blocking H$_2$ receptors, ranitidine increases the pH of the stomach contents and thereby reduces symptoms of gastritis and gastro-oesophageal reflux.

41. A. Full blood count. The most serious dose-related adverse effect of azathioprine is bone marrow suppression, which results most significantly in leucopenia and an increased risk of infection. For safety, full blood count should be monitored weekly for the first 4 weeks after initiation or dose alteration and 3-monthly thereafter.

42. A. Flucloxacillin. Cholestatic jaundice is a rare, but potentially serious, adverse effect of flucloxacillin (a <u>penicillinase-resistant penicillin</u>). It can occur even when treatment has been completed and is a contraindication to future use of this drug.

 Although <u>paracetamol</u>, <u>methotrexate</u> and simvastatin (a <u>statin</u>) can all cause liver toxicity, they do not generally cause cholestatic jaundice. Paracetamol in overdose causes hepatocellular necrosis, which can be fatal if untreated. Methotrexate can cause hepatitis as part of a hypersensitivity reaction or if taken in overdose. Chronic use of methotrexate can cause hepatic cirrhosis. Statins can cause a rise in liver enzymes (transaminases) and, less frequently, drug-induced hepatitis. <u>Morphine</u> does not cause hepatotoxicity, but it is metabolised in the liver so dose reduction is required in people with liver failure.

43. C. Levothyroxine. Gaviscon® is a compound <u>alginate</u> which also contains the <u>antacid</u> calcium carbonate. The divalent cation (Ca^{2+}) in calcium carbonate can bind many drugs in the gut and reduce their absorption. Examples include <u>tetracyclines</u>, digoxin, iron, bisphosphonates and thyroid hormones such as levothyroxine. In order to minimise this interaction, a 2-hour gap is advised between taking Gaviscon® and other medicines.

44. E. Trimethoprim. First-line options for an uncomplicated urinary tract infection (UTI) include trimethoprim, nitrofurantoin and amoxicillin (a broad-spectrum penicillin). Remember that when prescribing trimethoprim, you should make sure that the patient is not pregnant. Trimethoprim is potentially teratogenic in the first trimester. Nitrofurantoin should be avoided in the latter stages of pregnancy.

Cefotaxime, a third-generation cephalosporin, and gentamicin, an aminoglycoside, have to be given intravenously, so are not indicated for outpatient treatment of an uncomplicated UTI. However, cefaclor, an orally active second-generation cephalosporin, can be used as second- or third-line oral treatment for UTI (i.e. where first-line antibiotics do not work), and is an option for UTIs occurring in pregnancy. Ciprofloxacin is a quinolone that can be used as second- or third-line oral treatment for UTI or for complicated UTIs, but should not be used as a first-line treatment, as bacteria can easily become resistant to it. Unless their use is essential, quinolones should be avoided in pregnancy and in children as they may cause arthropathy. Macrolides, such as clarithromycin, have little activity against the Gram-negative organisms that commonly cause UTI, such as *Escherichia coli*. They are not known to be harmful in pregnancy.

45. B. Benzylpenicillin and flucloxacillin. In the clinical setting, antibiotics are chosen based on a 'best guess' as to the likely causative organism and antibiotic sensitivities. When infection is severe, being wrong with this guess and prescribing inadequate antibiotic treatment can be life threatening, so combination antibiotics are often prescribed to cover all likely eventualities.

Skin and soft tissue infections are most commonly caused by *Staphylococcus aureus* and group A streptococci (e.g. *Streptococcus pyogenes*). These bacteria are usually sensitive to flucloxacillin (a penicillinase-resistant penicillin) and benzylpenicillin (a 'standard' penicillin), respectively. As such, this combination is appropriate for severe cellulitis.

Amoxicillin (a broad-spectrum penicillin) and clarithromycin (a macrolide) are used in severe pneumonia to cover typical and atypical organisms, respectively. Cefotaxime (a cephalosporin) and aciclovir (an antiviral drug) are used in suspected intracranial infection to cover bacterial meningitis and viral encephalitis, pending a diagnosis from lumbar puncture. Co-amoxiclav (amoxicillin with clavulanic acid) and metronidazole are used in intraabdominal sepsis to cover Gram-negative aerobic and anaerobic gut organisms. Co-amoxiclav and gentamicin (an aminoglycoside) are used in complicated UTIs to cover Gram-negative organisms.

46. C. Doxycycline. A wide spectrum of organisms can cause community-acquired pneumonia, including *Streptococcus pneumoniae* (Gram positive), *Haemophilus influenzae* (Gram negative) and 'atypical' organisms such as *Mycoplasma pneumoniae* and *Legionella pneumophila*. The 'best guess' antibiotic for pneumonia therefore should ideally have a broad spectrum of activity to cover all these possibilities. Doxycycline (a <u>tetracycline</u>) is suitable because it covers Gram-positive, Gram-negative and atypical organisms.

Flucloxacillin is incorrect because it is a <u>penicillinase-resistant penicillin</u> with a narrow spectrum of activity, principally focused against *S. aureus*. The <u>quinolone</u> antibiotics, including ciprofloxacin, are generally reserved for second- or third-line therapy to preserve their usefulness, as bacteria easily acquire resistance to them. Ciprofloxacin is mostly effective against Gram-negative organisms, including *Pseudomonas aeruginosa*. Moxifloxacin and levofloxacin have greater activity against Gram-positive organisms and are therefore preferred for pneumonia. Ertapenem (a <u>carbapenem</u>) and cefotaxime (a <u>cephalosporin</u>) are broad-spectrum antibiotics given by injection. They are reserved for severe infections and those associated with resistant organisms, such as hospital-acquired pneumonia in people with underlying chronic lung disease.

47. A. Amoxicillin. <u>Penicillins</u>, <u>cephalosporins</u> and <u>carbapenems</u> are all β-lactam antibiotics, so-called because they share a common 'β-lactam ring' in their chemical structure. Of the drugs listed as options here, only amoxicillin is a β-lactam. Ciprofloxacin is a <u>quinolone</u>, clarithromycin is a <u>macrolide</u>, doxycycline is a <u>tetracycline</u> and <u>metronidazole</u> is a nitroimidazole (it is the only commonly used example from this class).

48. A. Aciclovir. Aciclovir is an antiviral which acts by inhibiting herpes-specific DNA polymerase. It is the antiviral of choice in suspected cases of herpes simplex encephalitis, and should be given intravenously in these circumstances. In relation to intracranial infection, amoxicillin, a broad-spectrum penicillin, should be given to patients at risk of *Listeria monocytogenes* meningitis (the very young and the very old). Ceftriaxone, a <u>cephalosporin</u>, has broad-spectrum antibiotic activity and is a first-line treatment for bacterial meningitis. Dexamethasone, a systemic <u>glucocorticoid</u>, can improve outcomes in patients with suspected pneumococcal meningitis. Fluconazole is an <u>antifungal</u> that can be used to treat invasive fungal infections under specialist guidance. In practice, whilst you might start empirical treatment with most of these antimicrobials to cover for bacterial or fungal meningitis, only aciclovir is used to treat suspected herpes simplex encephalitis.

49. C. Ciprofloxacin. UTIs are most commonly caused by *E. coli* and other Gram-negative organisms (*Klebsiella* and *Proteus* species) and Gram-positive *Staphylococcus saprophyticus*. First-line antibiotic choice is usually <u>nitrofurantoin</u> or <u>trimethoprim</u>, and second-line options include <u>amoxicillin</u> and <u>cephalexin</u>.

Patients with long-term catheters have reduced bladder defence against infection. This facilitates growth of organisms that don't usually infect healthy bladders. *Pseudomonas aeruginosa* is a Gram-negative organism well suited to colonising catheters. It forms biofilms that enable the bacteria to evade the host's defence and survive in environments where they wouldn't otherwise be successful.

P. aeruginosa is resistant to most broad-spectrum antibiotics. <u>Ciprofloxacin</u> is unusual among orally administered antibiotics in that it is effective against *P. aeruginosa*. Otherwise, IV antibiotics such as <u>antipseudomonal penicillins</u>, third- and fourth-generation <u>cephalosporins</u>, <u>carbapenems</u> or <u>aminoglycosides</u> can be used. *P. aeruginosa* rapidly becomes resistant to antibiotics during treatment. This may be slowed or prevented by using more than one antibiotic class in combination.

50. A. Amoxicillin. *Bactericidal antibiotics* kill bacteria, whereas bacteriostatic antibiotics prevent bacterial growth. Bactericidal antibiotics include those that disrupt bacterial cell walls (e.g. all penicillins, cephalosporins, carbapenems, vancomycin) or inhibit DNA synthesis (e.g. quinolones, metronidazole, nitrofurantoin). *Bacteriostatic antibiotics* generally are those that inhibit protein synthesis (e.g. macrolides, tetracyclines, trimethoprim). Chloramphenicol is generally considered to be bacteriostatic, but in high concentrations and with highly susceptible organisms it can be bactericidal.

In theory, bactericidal antibiotics should be more effective than bacteriostatic antibiotics. In practice, there is no clinically significant difference in efficacy. Bactericidal antibiotics may be considered necessary in deep-seated infections where antibiotic penetrance is poor (e.g. vegetations in endocarditis, osteomyelitis) or in situations where there is immunocompromise (e.g. neutropenia) or need for infection to be eradicated as rapidly as possible (e.g. meningitis).

51. A. Benzylpenicillin. Penicillinases are a type of β-lactamase enzyme produced by most staphylococci. They inactivate <u>penicillins</u> (e.g. benzylpenicillin) by breaking their β-lactam ring.

Flucloxacillin, a <u>penicillinase-resistant penicillin</u>, is more likely to be active against penicillinase-producing staphylococci because it has an acyl side chain that protects its β-lactam ring. It is the antibiotic of choice for straightforward staphylococcal infections. <u>Vancomycin</u> does not contain a β-lactam ring, so is naturally resistant to penicillinases. It is reserved for more severe Gram-positive infections or those resistant to penicillins (e.g. meticillin-resistant *S. aureus* [MRSA]). The compound preparations co-amoxiclav (see <u>Penicillins, broad</u>) and piperacillin–tazobactam (<u>Penicillins, antipseudomonal</u>) contain β-lactamase inhibitors. This improves their activity against penicillinase-producing staphylococci and, more importantly, β-lactamase-producing Gram-negative organisms.

52. B. Ciprofloxacin. Around 0.05% penicillin-treated patients develop a life-threatening immunoglobulin E (IgE)-mediated anaphylactic reaction to <u>penicillin</u>, including some or all of hypotension, bronchial and laryngeal oedema and oropharyngeal angioedema. As the reaction is to the basic penicillin structure, people who are allergic to one penicillin will be allergic to all. This man should therefore NOT receive co-amoxiclav (contains the <u>broad-spectrum penicillin</u> amoxicillin) or Tazocin® (contains the <u>antipseudomonal penicillin</u> piperacillin). As <u>cephalosporins and carbapenems</u> share structural similarities to penicillins, cross-reactivity can occur in penicillin-allergic patients. Cefotaxime and ertapenem are therefore also contraindicated in this patient. They may be used with caution in patients with a history of less severe penicillin allergy (e.g. rash).

Ciprofloxacin is a quinolone antibiotic. There is no cross-sensitivity between quinolones and penicillins; therefore ciprofloxacin is the least likely to precipitate further anaphylaxis.

53. C. Full blood count. Patients taking systemic chloramphenicol commonly develop dose-dependent bone marrow suppression which is fully reversible if the drug is withdrawn. Idiosyncratic aplastic anaemia is a rare adverse effect of systemic chloramphenicol, which can be fatal. During systemic therapy, **blood counts** should be monitored closely and a change in treatment considered if there is any change indicative of marrow suppression.

Prolonged chloramphenicol therapy can cause optic neuritis but **does not affect hearing** (unlike aminoglycoside treatment, which may be ototoxic). **C-reactive protein** (CRP) is a marker of severity of infection and can be used to monitor treatment efficacy, but not safety. Neither hepatotoxicity nor nephrotoxicity are recognised side effects of chloramphenicol treatment, so **liver and renal function do not need to be monitored** to ascertain safety. However, chloramphenicol is metabolised by the liver, so dose reduction and serum concentration measurement may be required in hepatic impairment. It inhibits liver enzymes, so can increase plasma concentrations of warfarin, antiepileptics and sulphonylureas.

54. D. Gentamicin. Aminoglycosides (e.g. gentamicin) accumulate in cochlear and vestibular hair cells where they trigger apoptosis and cell death. This can cause deafness, tinnitus and vertigo. Macrolides (e.g. clarithromycin) can also cause tinnitus and hearing loss, but this is rare and is usually associated with long-term therapy. Other drugs that cause ototoxicity include vancomycin and loop diuretics.

55. B. QT-interval prolongation. The QT interval is the time between the beginning of the QRS complex and the end of the T-wave. It mostly reflects the time taken for the ventricles to repolarise. The QT interval is said to be prolonged if, after correction for heart rate (by dividing it by the square root of the RR interval), it exceeds 0.44 seconds in men or 0.46 seconds in women. This is associated with an increased risk of a life-threatening arrhythmia called torsades de pointes, a form of ventricular tachycardia.

There are several causes of a prolonged QT interval. Drug causes include antiarrhythmics (e.g. amiodarone), antipsychotics (e.g. haloperidol), macrolide antibiotics (e.g. clarithromycin) and quinine. Combining drugs with QT-prolonging effects can be dangerous (clarithromycin with quinine sulfate for this patient) and should be avoided. A resource for checking which drugs prolong the QT interval can be found at www.qtdrugs.org (last checked 12/04/2018).

This patient is not taking any drugs that increase the potassium concentration, and is not at risk of seizures. Had she been taking a statin, there would have been a risk that clarithromycin could precipitate myopathy.

56. B. Less likely to give rise to antibiotic resistance. *Narrow-spectrum antibiotics* are active against a narrow group of bacterial types, e.g. benzylpenicillin against certain Gram-positive organisms and Gram-negative cocci. They are prescribed for infections where the organism has been identified and its sensitivity demonstrated on bacterial culture. They can also be used as part of an empirical (best guess) regimen where a particular organism is very likely: e.g. *Streptococcus pneumoniae* in community-acquired pneumonia.

Broad-spectrum antibiotics are active against a wide range of bacterial types: e.g. amoxicillin against a wide range of Gram-positive and Gram-negative organisms, including Gram-negative bacilli. They are prescribed empirically where the causative organism is unknown and the infection has diverse microbial causes. They are particularly used in patients with severe infection where failing to treat the causative organism effectively could have fatal consequences.

As narrow-spectrum antibiotics kill fewer normal microorganisms in the body than broad-spectrum antibiotics, they are **less likely to generate new antibiotic resistance** and **less likely to cause superinfection**, e.g. *Clostridium difficile* colitis. The spectrum of action doesn't affect the ease of administration or likelihood of allergy (e.g. if someone is penicillin allergic they will react to both benzylpenicillin and amoxicillin, as their allergy is to the basic penicillin structure).

57. E. Doxycycline. Tetracyclines (e.g. doxycycline) bind to calcium in developing teeth and bone. This can cause discolouration and/or hypoplasia of tooth enamel and, theoretically, could affect the developing skeleton. They should not be prescribed for women who are pregnant or breastfeeding or to children who have not yet formed their secondary dentition (under 12 years of age). The other antibiotics can be used in children if clinically indicated.

58. B. Ferrous sulfate. Tetracyclines bind to divalent cations. They should therefore be separated by at least 2 hours from doses of calcium, antacids or iron (e.g. ferrous sulfate). The interaction reduces absorption of both drugs, although the risk of subtherapeutic antibiotic concentrations is generally the greatest concern.

59. D. Metronidazole. People taking metronidazole who drink alcohol may experience an unpleasant reaction, including flushing, headache, nausea and vomiting. This reaction is thought to be due to inhibition of the enzyme acetaldehyde dehydrogenase, preventing clearance of the intermediate alcohol metabolite—acetaldehyde—from the body. Alcohol should be avoided during and for 48 hours after metronidazole treatment.

Chronic excessive alcohol consumption can reduce absorption of doxycycline (a tetracycline), but this is less likely and less severe than the interaction with metronidazole. The other antibiotics listed here do not interact with alcohol. Nevertheless, this might be a good opportunity to discuss 'safe' alcohol consumption (the Chief Medical Officers' low risk unit guidelines recommend no more than 14 units per week).

60. D. Simvastatin. The metabolism of statins is reduced by cytochrome P450 inhibitors, such as amiodarone, diltiazem, itraconazole, macrolides and protease inhibitors. This leads to accumulation of the statin in the body, which may put patients at increased risk of adverse effects. To reduce the risk, simvastatin can be safely held for 1 week. There is also a potential interaction with warfarin, although the risk of stroke from atrial fibrillation precludes stopping it. The international normalised ratio (INR) should be checked more often during treatment.

61. A. Amoxicillin. Amoxicillin (a <u>broad-spectrum penicillin</u>) is formulated for IV administration and can be given safely as a slow bolus injection or IV infusion (providing the patient is not allergic to penicillin). Clarithromycin (a <u>macrolide</u>), gentamicin (an <u>aminoglycoside</u>) and <u>vancomycin</u> all require slow IV infusion rather than bolus injection to minimise toxicity. As bolus injections, clarithromycin can cause phlebitis and arrhythmias; gentamicin can cause ototoxicity; and vancomycin can cause anaphylactoid reactions. Doxycycline (a <u>tetracycline</u>) is only available for oral administration.

In practice, antibiotic choice will be determined principally by the diagnosis (and therefore likely organisms and their sensitivities) and the severity of infection. The fluid volume associated with its administration would be an additional but secondary consideration.

62. E. Serum gentamicin concentration. Gentamicin, an <u>aminoglycoside</u>, is a potentially dangerous drug. Its dosing should be guided by measurement of the serum gentamicin concentration. There are several approaches to monitoring once-daily gentamicin therapy and you should consult local policies. However, the most common method is to measure the 'trough' concentration: that is, the lowest concentration expected during the dosage interval. This is taken 18–24 hours after the last dose, and should be <1 mg/L to minimise the risk of toxicity.

The other tests are less time critical and, generally, measurement so soon after the start of treatment is unlikely to be particularly informative. Audiometry may be used in prolonged aminoglycoside therapy to monitor its effects on hearing, since aminoglycosides are ototoxic. C-reactive protein (CRP) is an inflammatory marker which can be used to monitor for resolution of infection. Impaired renal function is common in severe infections and influences gentamicin dosing regimens. It is assessed using the estimated glomerular filtration rate (eGFR) and the serum creatinine concentration, from which eGFR is derived. The eGFR may be more informative than serum creatinine concentration, but it can be misleading when the renal function is unstable.

63. C. Switch to oral co-amoxiclav. A key component of good antibiotic management (stewardship) is daily review of all antimicrobial prescriptions in secondary care. At 48 hours after starting antibiotic treatment there are five prescribing decision options:
- Stop antibiotics if there is no evidence of infection.
- Switch antibiotics from IV to oral administration.
- Change antibiotics – ideally to a narrower spectrum if improving (or broader if no improvement or deterioration).
- Continue and review again at 72 hours.
- Set up outpatient parenteral antimicrobial therapy where a longer course of IV treatment is required.

For patients receiving IV antibiotics, switch to an oral agent should be considered if they are improving clinically and haemodynamically stable; they have a temperature

<38°C for 48 hours; they show a trend to normalisation of C-reactive protein (CRP) and white cell count (WCC); they can tolerate and absorb oral medications; and they don't have immunosuppression or deep-seated infection (e.g. abscess) requiring prolonged IV therapy. Intravenous-to-oral switch is good practice as it reduces treatment complications and duration of inpatient stay as well as drug and administration costs.

Our patient meets the criteria for IV-to-oral switch. Her urine cultures grew *E. coli* sensitive to <u>co-amoxiclav</u> and so it would be reasonable to switch to an oral preparation of this drug. She is not deteriorating or failing to improve, so does not need to switch to a broader- spectrum antibiotic (<u>piperacillin with tazobactam</u>). Although her infection is sensitive to the narrower-spectrum antibiotic nitrofurantoin, this is only effective for lower UTIs where it has been concentrated in the urine and so would be inappropriate for her clinical infection of pyelonephritis. For pyelonephritis, the treatment duration should usually be 10–14 days.

64. E. It will not completely stop spread of infection to sexual partners.
Suppressive treatment with aciclovir, an <u>antiviral drug</u>, aims to prevent recurrences of genital herpes. It should be considered in patients suffering from six or more episodes a year. It should be taken daily, rather than just when symptomatic. Patients should wash their hands before and after using *topical* aciclovir. The treatment is usually continued for 1–2 years, after which it is stopped and the patient is monitored for recurrence. Aciclovir acts by inhibiting viral replication, but it does not clear the virus from the body completely. Consequently, there is always a risk of spreading infection to sexual partners, including 'asymptomatic shedding'.

65. D. 1 L glucose 5% with potassium chloride 40 mmol over 8 hours; 1 L glucose 5% with potassium chloride 40 mmol over 8 hours; 500 mL sodium chloride 0.9% over 8 hours. The patient described in this scenario requires IV fluid therapy to cover his normal daily fluid and electrolyte requirements (often referred to as 'maintenance requirements'). For stable adult patients these are, roughly:
• Water 30 mL/kg/day
• Sodium 1 mmol/kg/day
• Potassium 1 mmol/kg/day
These requirements can be met using a combination of <u>glucose</u> 5% (which effectively just provides water), <u>sodium chloride</u> 0.9% (which provides water and sodium) and <u>potassium</u> chloride (which is given as an 'additive' in the other fluids). There are numerous ways of arriving at the appropriate amounts, but option D is a reasonable one. This will provide 2.5 L/day of water, 77 mmol/day of sodium and 80 mmol/day of potassium.

The other options are less satisfactory: option A provides only 1 L of water and no potassium; option B provides too much sodium and no potassium; option C provides too much sodium; and option E does not provide any sodium at all.

Different approaches need to be taken if patients have already built up a fluid deficit (i.e. they are dehydrated); if they have additional ongoing fluid losses (e.g. because of diarrhoea); or they have an electrolyte abnormality, oliguria or renal impairment.

66. C. Sodium chloride 0.9% 500 mL IV over 10 minutes. This patient is sick and requires urgent review by a senior clinician. While arranging this, it would be appropriate to start fluid resuscitation. Intravenous fluid solutions containing sodium at a concentration similar to that in extracellular fluid (ECF), such as <u>sodium chloride 0.9%</u> and <u>compound sodium lactate</u>, are retained in the extracellular compartment. This means that, after distribution, a reasonable proportion (about 20%) of the fluid remains in the circulation, thus making these solutions a viable option for fluid resuscitation. Fluids containing a supra-physiological concentration of potassium (e.g. sodium chloride 0.9% with potassium 20 mmol/L) are never used for fluid resuscitation due to the risk of inducing hyperkalaemia. However, compound sodium lactate, which contains a physiological concentration of potassium (5 mmol/L), may be used.

<u>Glucose</u> 5% is widely used for simple fluid replacement but is a poor choice for fluid resuscitation. This is because it distributes throughout total body water, leaving only about 7% in the circulation. Human albumin solution (HAS) is a <u>colloid</u> which is preferentially retained in the plasma. However, there is little evidence that the use of a colloid rather than a crystalloid makes any difference to clinical outcomes, and colloids are considerably more expensive. Moreover, albumin is not usually stocked on general wards: the time required to source it from elsewhere in the hospital is likely to be prohibitive to use in this setting. Sterile water is not used in fluid therapy because it is hypotonic, so can cause osmolysis of cells: it is, however, used for reconstitution and dilution of drugs.

The volume of fluid required for an initial fluid challenge is usually in the range 200–500 mL, infused rapidly (e.g. over 10 minutes). In patients with adequate cardiac reserve, 500 mL of sodium chloride 0.9% or compound sodium lactate is reasonable. If a colloid is to be used, options include HAS and synthetic colloids, such as a modified gelatin. The initial volume is usually lower than that used for crystalloids (e.g. 100–250 mL infused rapidly).

67. B. Ibuprofen. Ibuprofen is a <u>non-steroidal antiinflammatory drug</u> (NSAID) that inhibits the enzyme cyclooxygenase, preventing conversion of arachidonic acid to prostaglandins.

Amitriptyline and omeprazole inhibit membrane transport proteins. Amitriptyline is a <u>tricyclic antidepressant</u> that inhibits transporters responsible for removing serotonin and noradrenaline from the synaptic cleft. Omeprazole is a <u>proton pump inhibitor</u> that inhibits H^+/K^+-ATPase in gastric parietal cells, preventing the secretion of gastric acid. Morphine is a <u>strong opioid</u> that activates opioid μ (mu) receptors in the central nervous system. Senna is a <u>stimulant laxative</u> that acts as an irritant in the gut to increase water and electrolyte secretion from the colonic mucosa.

68. C. Folinic acid. <u>Methotrexate</u> inhibits the enzyme dihydrofolate reductase, which converts dietary folic acid to tetrahydrofolate (FH4). FH4 is required for DNA and protein synthesis. Folinic acid is readily converted to FH4 (without the need for dihydrofolate reductase) and is therefore useful in methotrexate toxicity. <u>Folic acid</u> cannot be used, as in the absence of dihydrofolate reductase activity it cannot be converted to FH4 and is therefore not metabolically useful.

Activated charcoal is only useful where poisons have been recently ingested (e.g. within 1 hour). Toxicity in this case has occurred over weeks. Haemodialysis is not useful in removing methotrexate from the circulation, although may be necessary when managing the associated renal failure. Granulocyte colony stimulating factor (G-CSF) has been used in the treatment of neutropenia as a result of methotrexate toxicity, but is not routinely part of initial management.

Methotrexate toxicity may be very serious and its management is complex. Advice should be sought from a poisons centre.

69. C. Indapamide. Gout is caused by deposition of uric acid in joints. The first metatarsophalangeal joint (of the big toe) is the most commonly affected site. The likely precipitant in this patient is indapamide, a thiazide-like diuretic, which reduces uric acid excretion by the kidneys. Other drug causes of gout include *low-dose aspirin*, some anticancer drugs (by increasing uric acid production with tumour breakdown), and alcohol.

Allopurinol prevents gout by reducing uric acid production through xanthine oxidase inhibition. It should not be started or stopped in acute gout, where sudden fluctuations in uric acid levels can worsen attacks. Calcium channel blockers (e.g. amlodipine), ACE inhibitors (e.g. ramipril) and statins (e.g. simvastatin) do not cause or worsen gout.

70. C. Naproxen. The most appropriate treatment for acute gout is an antiinflammatory. NSAIDs, e.g. naproxen, are the usual first-line choice in the absence of contraindications. In this case, however, they are strongly contraindicated by the patient's history of aspirin-induced bronchospasm. Colchicine is an alternative option. It should be avoided in renal and hepatic impairment, and it has some important drug interactions (e.g. with the antibiotic fusidic acid). Where NSAIDs and colchicine are contraindicated or not tolerated, a short course of oral corticosteroids (e.g. prednisolone) is a useful option. Codeine, a weak opioid, may provide her some pain relief, but it does not have any antiinflammatory action.

71. B. Citalopram. Antidepressants are indicated for moderate and severe depression, and for mild depression that has not responded adequately to psychological interventions, as in this case. A selective serotonin reuptake inhibitor (SSRI), such as citalopram, is first choice in most patients. Amitriptyline (a tricyclic antidepressant) and mirtazapine (an antagonist of pre-synaptic α_2-adrenoceptors) are also effective antidepressants, but as they cause more side effects they are generally reserved for cases in which SSRIs are deemed unsuitable. Olanzapine is a second-generation antipsychotic which is not indicated for non-psychotic depression.

72. C. Lorazepam 4 mg by slow IV injection. Broadly, status epilepticus may be defined as a state of unrelenting seizure activity. It is a life-threatening condition that requires urgent treatment. First-line pharmacological treatment is with a benzodiazepine, which in a hospital setting should be administered intravenously. The ideal choice is lorazepam because of its long duration of effect. In adults, this is usually given in an initial dose of 4 mg by slow IV injection, which may be repeated once if the seizure does not terminate. Diazepam is a reasonable alternative if lorazepam is unavailable. Chlordiazepoxide is also a long-acting benzodiazepine, but it is not available in an IV formulation, so is not suited to use in status epilepticus. If the seizure cannot be controlled with a benzodiazepine, an antiepileptic drug should be given: options include levetiracetam, valproate and phenytoin. If this is unsuccessful, the patient should be anaesthetised and managed in the intensive care unit. Carbamazepine has no role in the acute management of status epilepticus.

73. B. Lamotrigine. Options for treating episodes of bipolar depression include the second-generation antipsychotics olanzapine (with or without the selective serotonin reuptake inhibitor [SSRI] fluoxetine) and quetiapine, and the antiepileptic drug lamotrigine. Lamotrigine is unusual in that it does not increase the risk of mania, which probably makes it the best choice in this patient.

Gabapentin is an anticonvulsant that is also efficacious in neuropathic pain. It is not used in bipolar disorder. Lithium has long been used as a mood stabiliser in bipolar disorder, but its antidepressant effect is slow to develop. This makes it a less suitable choice in acute depressive episodes, but in patients already established on lithium it should be continued and the dosage optimised. Sertraline is an SSRI; evidence for its efficacy in bipolar depression is limited and it may increase the risk of mania. Valproate is an antiepileptic drug which is efficacious in bipolar disorder, but because of the risk of precipitating mania other options are preferable for acute depressive episodes.

74. E. Zopiclone. Zopiclone is a relatively short-acting sedative that is useful for the short-term treatment of insomnia. Its use in this scenario is justifiable given the acute and disabling nature of the patient's insomnia. It would be prudent to discuss with the patient that zopiclone should not be taken for a prolonged period, as there is potential for dependence to develop. Diazepam is a benzodiazepine with a long half-life. Feelings of sleepiness can persist for many hours after taking the drug and so it would not be appropriate given his impending job interview. Propofol and midazolam are both relatively short-acting IV sedatives with a much more profound effect than zopiclone. They should only be used in a hospital setting.

75. A. Amitriptyline. Amitriptyline, a tricyclic antidepressant, is a first-line option for treating neuropathic pain, most suitable if nocturnal pain and sleep interference are problematic. Gabapentin and pregabalin are alternative first-line options, particularly where tricyclics are contraindicated, e.g. because of cardiovascular disease or epilepsy. Carbamazepine is used in trigeminal neuralgia, but other drugs are better studied in other neuropathic pain syndromes. The opioids tramadol and morphine may be considered if first-line treatments are insufficient. NSAIDs such as ibuprofen, are not effective in the management of neuropathic pain.

76. D. Sodium channels. Lamotrigine is an antiepileptic drug with efficacy in bipolar depression. At a molecular level, its mechanism of action appears to centre on inactivation of voltage-sensitive sodium channels, impeding repetitive neuronal firing that is characteristic of seizures. It may have additional actions (including on excitatory neurotransmitter release and calcium channel function), but these are not fully understood. Like most other agents used in bipolar disorder, the mechanism by which its molecular effects give rise to its mood-stabilising properties is uncertain.

77. E. Synaptic vesicles. <u>Levetiracetam</u> is an antiepileptic drug effective in focal, generalised and myoclonic seizures. Its mechanism of action is not fully understood, but at a molecular level it appears to target a membrane glycoprotein called synaptic vesicle protein 2A (SV2A): through this, it probably interferes with synaptic vesicle function, and therefore the release of neurotransmitters during depolarisation. Mechanisms of antiepileptic activity exhibited by other drugs include voltage-sensitive sodium channel inhibition (<u>carbamazepine</u>, <u>lamotrigine</u>, phenytoin), voltage-sensitive calcium channel inhibition (<u>gabapentin, pregabalin</u>) and modulation of the γ-aminobutyric acid$_A$ (GABA$_A$) receptor (<u>benzodiazepines</u>). Some antiepileptic drugs have multiple actions (e.g. <u>valproate</u>).

78. B. Haloperidol. Haloperidol is a <u>first-generation (typical) antipsychotic</u>. One of the many adverse effects of this drug class is prolongation of the QT interval. First-generation antipsychotics should therefore be avoided in this patient, as should other drugs that prolong the QT interval, including <u>amiodarone</u>, <u>quinine</u>, <u>macrolide antibiotics</u> and <u>selective serotonin reuptake inhibitors</u>. Combining QT-prolonging drugs may have an additive effect, increasing the risk.

79. D. Rash. Although benign rashes are a common adverse effect of treatment with the antiepileptic agent <u>lamotrigine</u>, they may rarely be the first symptom of a hypersensitivity reaction. As these hypersensitivity reactions (Stevens–Johnson syndrome, toxic epidermal necrolysis, or drug reaction with eosinophilia and systemic symptoms) are serious and potentially life threatening, urgent medical review should be sought. The period of highest risk is the first 8 weeks of treatment, and rashes are more common with high initial doses. Rashes that occur later in therapy (after 2–3 months) are less likely to represent a hypersensitivity reaction to lamotrigine.

80. E. Tramadol. You need to be particularly careful when prescribing for patients with epilepsy, for two main reasons. First, antiepileptic drugs (including <u>lamotrigine, carbamazepine</u> and <u>valproate</u>) have many potential drug interactions that may result in drug toxicity (either of the antiepileptic drug or the other interacting drug) or loss of seizure control. Secondly, there are a number of drugs that can lower the seizure threshold, including <u>antidepressants</u>, <u>antipsychotics</u>, and <u>opioids</u>, particularly tramadol. The other opioids may have an effect on seizure threshold, but this is much less significant. In the context of severe pain, their benefits are likely to outweigh their risks. Naproxen (an <u>NSAID</u>) and <u>paracetamol</u> are not known to affect seizure threshold or interact with carbamazepine.

81. B. Ischaemic heart disease. <u>Serotonin 5-HT$_1$-receptor agonists</u>, such as sumatriptan, are an effective treatment for migraine symptoms. However, as they act through vasoconstriction, they can cause angina and, rarely, myocardial infarction. They are therefore contraindicated in patients with established cardiovascular disease.

82. C. Meropenem. Drug interactions are a common problem with many antiepileptic agents, including valproate, carbamazepine, lamotrigine and phenytoin. Valproate has a particularly serious interaction with carbapenem antibiotics, characterised by a rapid (within days) and profound (near-complete) reduction in serum valproate concentrations. This may lead to a loss of seizure control. Concurrent administration should be avoided if possible. If treatment with a carbapenem is essential in a patient taking valproate, the serum valproate concentration should be monitored closely. The mechanism of the interaction is unclear.

83. E. Weight, lipid profile and haemoglobin A_{1c} (HbA_{1c}). Olanzapine is a second-generation antipsychotic drug. Metabolic effects, such as weight gain, diabetes mellitus and lipid changes, are among the most common adverse effects of second-generation antipsychotics. Monitoring weight, lipid profile and HbA_{1c} at the baseline, 12 weeks into therapy, then annually, is therefore advised. Weight is monitored more intensively at the start of treatment (e.g. weekly for the first 6 weeks). Fluoxetine is an selective serotonin reuptake inhibitor which does not have specific safety monitoring requirements.

84. A. Donepezil does not work for everyone and so he should stop taking it. Patients taking donepezil should be reviewed regularly and where no benefit is seen after 3 months of treatment, it should be stopped. Decisions on changing treatment should involve patients and their carers. Although adverse effects of donepezil may be reduced by changing the time of day the drug is taken, this is unlikely to influence efficacy. Switching to a different cholinesterase inhibitor is unlikely to be beneficial.

85. B. Potassium chloride 40 mmol in 1 L of sodium chloride 0.9% IV over 2 hours. Hypokalaemia is a potentially dangerous electrolyte abnormality because of its association with arrhythmias. A serum potassium concentration <2.5 mmol/L is generally deemed to be 'severe', and this warrants IV treatment. On a general ward, this is administered through a peripheral cannula using a potassium-containing fluid, as illustrated in the correct option.

Option A is a combination of a loop diuretic (furosemide) and a potassium-sparing diuretic (amiloride). If hypokalaemia occurs during treatment with furosemide, exchanging it for co-amilofruse may resolve this. It is not a suitable treatment of other causes of hypokalaemia. In option C, the rate of potassium administration is too fast (it should generally not exceed 20 mmol/hr). Option D, giving potassium orally, is the preferred treatment for *non-severe* hypokalaemia. Option E, an ACE inhibitor, does have a potassium-elevating effect, but is not an appropriate treatment for acute hypokalaemia. Indeed, ACE inhibitors should be avoided whenever there is a risk of acute kidney injury, such as in patients who have become dehydrated.

86. E. Salbutamol. Like <u>insulin</u>, β_2-agonists stimulate Na^+/K^+-ATPase pumps on cell surface membranes, promoting a shift of K^+ from the extracellular to intracellular compartment. This makes nebulised salbutamol a useful adjunct in the treatment of hyperkalaemia. However, its potassium lowering effect is relatively short-lived. <u>Calcium gluconate</u> is used in hyperkalaemia to prevent arrhythmias but does not lower the serum potassium concentration. Calcium polystyrene sulfonate is a cation exchange resin that promotes loss of potassium through the gut. It is occasionally used to control chronic hyperkalaemia in chronic kidney disease (CKD), but its onset is too slow to be useful in acute hyperkalaemia. The <u>sulphonylurea</u> gliclazide, unlike insulin, is not useful in reducing serum potassium as the time required for absorption precludes its use in an urgent/emergency setting and the amount of insulin stimulated from the pancreas is unpredictable.

Other options to 'buy time' while awaiting definitive treatment of hyperkalaemia include sodium bicarbonate (if there is associated metabolic acidosis), and giving insulin and glucose as a continuous (rather than intermittent) infusion. Severe hyperkalaemia is a complex, life-threatening condition. Senior and specialist advice is essential.

87. C. Antagonism at the muscarinic M_3 receptor. Oxybutynin is an <u>antimuscarinic</u> drug that blocks muscarinic acetylcholine receptors, including the M_3 receptor that predominates in the bladder. This inhibits the procontractile effect of parasympathetic stimulation, causing relaxation of the bladder smooth muscle and increasing bladder capacity. This makes it a useful option for treatment for urge incontinence and overactive bladder symptoms.

α_1-<u>blockers</u> (e.g. doxazosin) and <u>5α-reductase inhibitors</u> (e.g. finasteride) are used to treat symptoms of benign prostatic enlargement. They have no role in the treatment of overactive bladder. β_2-<u>agonists</u> are used to induce smooth muscle relaxation in the airways; they are not used for overactive bladder. The nicotinic acetylcholine receptor is involved in neuromuscular transmission in skeletal muscle. Antagonists of this receptor are used in anaesthetic practice to induce muscle relaxation.

88. E. Ramipril. <u>ACE inhibitors</u> (e.g. ramipril) commonly cause an increase in the serum potassium concentration. This can usually be tolerated provided it does not exceed 6.0 mmol/L. Other drugs with a significant potassium-elevating effect include <u>angiotensin-receptor blockers</u>, <u>aldosterone-receptor antagonists</u>, oral and IV <u>potassium</u> supplements and potassium-sparing diuretics. <u>β-blockers</u> and <u>aspirin</u> can also increase the potassium concentration, but this effect is not usually significant. <u>Statins</u> and <u>clopidogrel</u> do not cause hyperkalaemia.

89. C. Solifenacin. Solifenacin is an <u>antimuscarinic</u> drug used to treat urinary urgency and urge incontinence. Side effects of antimuscarinics include dry mouth, blurred vision, constipation and confusion. Elderly patients, especially those with dementia, are particularly vulnerable to these side effects. The reasons for susceptibility to confusion are complex but include alteration in drug distribution and metabolism as well as increased sensitivity to their neurological effects. Where possible, alternative therapies should be used.

The other drugs listed are unlikely to have been started in this case. Finasteride is a 5α-reductase inhibitor and tamsulosin is an α-blocker; they are both used in men with benign prostatic enlargement, but not in overactive bladder. They are not known to cause confusion. Furosemide is a loop diuretic used in states of fluid overload such as heart failure, and does not directly cause confusion (although over-diuresis leading to dehydration might). Trimethoprim is an antibiotic that acts by interfering with bacterial folate synthesis. It is commonly used to treat UTIs but not overactive bladder. It causes confusion very rarely.

90. B. Postural hypotension. Tamsulosin (an α-blocker) blocks α_1-adrenoceptors in the smooth muscle of the prostate gland, increasing urinary flow and relieving obstructive symptoms. As α_1-adrenoceptors are also found in the smooth muscle of blood vessels, α-blockers can cause hypotension, particularly postural hypotension. Patients taking other antihypertensive medication should be especially vigilant to these effects and may need to omit their usual treatment when starting an α-blocker. Bronchospasm and erectile dysfunction are adverse effects of β-blockers (not α-blockers). Tamsulosin does not cause gynaecomastia or prostate cancer.

91. E. Tiotropium. Tiotropium is a long-acting antimuscarinic bronchodilator. Its side effects include urinary retention in people susceptible to this. It should therefore be avoided or used cautiously in patients with a history of urinary retention, or risk factors such as benign prostatic enlargement.

Salbutamol and salmeterol are, respectively, short- and long-acting β_2-agonists. Seretide® and Symbicort® are compound β_2-agonist–corticosteroid inhalers (see Corticosteroids, inhaled).

92. D. Metronidazole. Metronidazole is metabolised and eliminated by the liver. Dosage reduction is therefore required in severe hepatic impairment rather than renal impairment.

Many other antibiotics are eliminated by the kidney. In patients with renal impairment, antibiotics may therefore accumulate, increasing the risk of adverse effects. However, there is always a balance to be struck between the risk of drug toxicity and the risk of undertreating the infection. As such, renal impairment does not necessarily contraindicate the drug's use, but it does mandate a more cautious approach to drug selection and dosing regimens.

In severe renal impairment, dose reductions are required with penicillins such as benzylpenicillin and co-amoxiclav because of the risk of neurological toxicity, including fits; aminoglycosides such as gentamicin, which may cause ototoxicity and nephrotoxicity; and vancomycin, which may also cause nephrotoxicity and ototoxicity, as well as blood disorders such as neutropenia and thrombocytopenia.

93. B. Diltiazem. Sildenafil is a phosphodiesterase (type 5) inhibitor. It is metabolised by a member of the cytochrome P450 (CYP) enzyme family called CYP3A4. Diltiazem is a calcium channel blocker that inhibits CYP3A4 activity. If the drugs are taken together, the metabolism of sildenafil will be reduced such that the patient is exposed to higher sildenafil concentrations. This increases the chance of dose-related adverse effects, such as headache. A reduced dose of sildenafil is recommended in patients taking CYP inhibitors, other examples of which include amiodarone and macrolide antibiotics.

Diltiazem can also interact with digoxin, since they both reduce conduction at the AV node. This interaction may be exploited therapeutically, as in this case, to slow the ventricular rate in patients with AF. There are no other clinically significant interactions between the drugs listed.

94. A. Doxazosin. Sildenafil is a phosphodiesterase inhibitor that causes (among other things) vascular smooth muscle relaxation and vasodilatation. Doxazosin is an α-blocker, which also has a vasodilator effect. Concomitant use may cause hypotension and collapse. A gap of 4 hours should be left between taking sildenafil and α-blockers.

95. A. Beclometasone. Corticosteroids such as beclometasone suppress inflammation in the airways, reducing the risk of asthma attacks. Topical administration by inhaler reduces systemic side effects.

Ipratropium (an antimuscarinic) and salbutamol (a β_2-agonist) are short-acting bronchodilators. They are used to relieve breathlessness in acute attacks. They may also be taken before activities that are expected to provoke symptoms, such as exercise. However, they have no role as a regular treatment to prevent attacks. Formoterol is a long acting β_2-agonist (LABA). It is taken regularly to improve lung function, but it does not address the underlying pathology (inflammation). For this reason, it must not be given without an inhaled corticosteroid, and so would be an inappropriate choice at this stage. Antihistamines (e.g. chlorphenamine) can improve symptoms of histamine-mediated allergic disease, such as hay fever and skin itching, but do not prevent or control airways inflammation in asthma.

96. D. β_2-adrenoceptors. β_2-adrenoceptors are activated by salmeterol, a long acting β_2-agonist bronchodilator.

Doxazocin is an α-blocker, which antagonises α_1-adrenoceptors. Ipratropium and hyoscine butylbromide block muscarinic receptors (see Antimuscarinics, bronchodilators and Antimuscarinics, cardiovascular and GI uses, respectively). Amlodipine is a calcium channel blocker. Fluticasone is an inhaled corticosteroid which activates glucocorticoid receptors to influence gene transcription.

97. E. Tiotropium. Tiotropium is a long-acting antimuscarinic bronchodilator which inhibits parasympathetic stimulation of salivation, causing a dry mouth. None of the other drugs listed cause a dry mouth, although inhaled fluticasone (an inhaled corticosteroid) can cause oral thrush, the risk of which is reduced by rinsing and gargling after inhalation.

98. A. Acetylcysteine. Acetylcysteine is a specific antidote for paracetamol poisoning. It is highly effective if started within 8–10 hours of the overdose. The decision about whether to administer acetylcysteine is guided by the nature of the overdose and the serum paracetamol concentration. If it was a single overdose taken at a known time, you should measure the paracetamol concentration 4 or more hours after the time of ingestion, then compare this with a paracetamol poisoning treatment graph found in the BNF. If the concentration is above the treatment line, acetylcysteine is indicated. If the overdose was staggered (i.e. the time between the first and last doses was more than 1 hour) or its timing is uncertain, you cannot interpret the paracetamol concentration. You then need to make a decision based on the amount of paracetamol ingested. If this exceeds 75 mg/kg, treatment with acetylcysteine is likely to be necessary.

Activated charcoal is given in paracetamol poisoning only if the patient presents within 1 hour of the overdose. Cyclizine is an antiemetic (see Antiemetics, histamine H₁-receptor antagonists). It may be an appropriate symptomatic treatment for the patient's nausea, but it is not as important as acetylcysteine at this stage. Omeprazole is a proton pump inhibitor, which is not indicated in this case. Naloxone is a specific antidote for opioid toxicity; it is not indicated in this case.

99. D. Naloxone. The low Glasgow Coma Score (GCS), pinpoint pupils and respiratory rate point toward opioid toxicity. It would be appropriate to try a dose of naloxone and review response. The other most obvious culprit drug for causing low GCS is diazepam. However, the antidote for this drug, flumazenil, should only be given in circumstances where it is certain that pure benzodiazepine toxicity has occurred, such as iatrogenic overdose. This is because flumazenil has significant adverse effects, including lowering the seizure threshold. If the benzodiazepine was taken as part of a mixed overdose with pro-convulsive drugs, or if the patient has epilepsy, this may precipitate seizures. Activated charcoal is useful for acute oral overdoses, but not for toxicity caused by reduced drug elimination. It should also be avoided in patients unable to protect their own airway as a result of a reduced level of consciousness. There is no history of paracetamol overdose and it is not eliminated by the kidneys, so there is no immediate indication for acetylcysteine. Sodium bicarbonate is used in the treatment of tricyclic antidepressant toxicity (e.g. amitriptyline); his antidepressant, fluoxetine, is a selective serotonin reuptake inhibitor.

100. D. Temporarily stop acetylcysteine and give chlorphenamine. When administered intravenously at high doses (such as in paracetamol poisoning), acetylcysteine can cause an anaphylactoid reaction. Like anaphylaxis, anaphylactoid reactions are mediated by histamine and involve symptoms such as urticaria, angioedema and bronchospasm. However, in contrast to anaphylaxis, they do not involve IgE antibodies. This means that the reactions tend to build up more gradually, such that they can usually be identified and treated before they become too severe.

At this stage, the management would be to stop the acetylcysteine and administer an IV antihistamine (H₁-receptor antagonist), such as chlorphenamine. Once the reaction has subsided, it is usually safe to restart the infusion at a lower rate. Adrenaline, administered by IM injection, is the key treatment for anaphylaxis, but it is not required for anaphylactoid reactions unless they are very severe or the diagnosis is in doubt. Ranitidine is an H₂-receptor antagonist used to suppress gastric acid production. It has little, if any, role in the treatment of anaphylactic and anaphylactoid reactions.

Index

Page numbers followed by "*t*" indicate tables, and "*b*" indicate boxes.